Emergencies Around Childbirth

Supporting readers to perform effectively in urgent or emergency situations that can occur in a hospital, at a birth centre or at home, this fully updated fourth edition presents the necessary knowledge and skills for student and practising midwives.

With contributions from highly experienced midwives, this practical guidebook incorporates a new chapter on legal issues for safe practice, as well as additional content on professional issues. It also includes an essential new chapter on cardiac problems, recognising that midwives are often the lead professional caring for women with cardiac anomalies, as many are undiagnosed until the emergency. The book continues to provide key, up-to-date information on high-risk medical and obstetric situations, from serious infection to uterine complications to resuscitation.

Emergencies Around Childbirth is essential reading for practising and student midwives and those who teach them.

Maureen Boyle is Senior Lecturer in Midwifery at the University of West London, UK.

Emergencies Around Childbirth

A Handbook for Midwives

Fourth Edition

Edited by Maureen Boyle

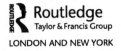

Routledge
Taylor & Francis Group

LONDON AND NEW YORK

Designed cover image: Blurred rainbow colored light flare background. (Getty Images. Credit: Lazy_Bear)

Fourth edition published 2025
by Routledge
4 Park Square, Milton Park, Abingdon, Oxon, OX14 4RN

and by Routledge
605 Third Avenue, New York, NY 10158

Routledge is an imprint of the Taylor & Francis Group, an informa business

First edition published by Radcliffe Publishing 2002
Third edition published by Taylor and Francis 2017

British Library Cataloguing-in-Publication Data
A catalogue record for this book is available from the British Library

ISBN: 978-1-032-46543-2 (hbk)
ISBN: 978-1-032-46542-5 (pbk)
ISBN: 978-1-003-38219-5 (ebk)

DOI: 10.4324/9781003382195

Typeset in Minion Pro
by Apex CoVantage, LLC

Contents

List of contributors   vii

List of abbreviations   ix

List of figures   xiii

List of tables   xv

List of boxes   xvii

1   An overview of the professional issues that support safe practice   1
Kate Nash and Julie Jones

2   Legal issues in emergency care   17
Anne O'Loghlen-Pinion and Kate Nash

3   Maternal and newborn resuscitation   33
Jenny Brewster

4   Antepartum Haemorrhage   56
Luisa Acosta

5   Cardiac conditions   76
Maureen Boyle

6   Thromboembolism in pregnancy   87
Judy Bothamley

7   Pre-eclampsia and associated conditions   103
Maureen Boyle

8   Malpresentations   124
Maureen Boyle

9   Cord prolapse   143
Clare Gordon

10   Shoulder dystocia   152
Debra Sloam

11   Uterine complications   165
Marie Hall

12   Primary postpartum haemorrhage   181
Jessica Scoble

13   Amniotic fluid embolism: (anaphylactoid syndrome of pregnancy)   194
Maureen Boyle

14   Serious infection   204
Judy Bothamley

15   Other causes of potential maternal collapse   222
      Andrea Aras-Payne
16   Birth trauma and post-traumatic stress disorder   234
      Reina Fisher-van Werkhoven
17   Postpartum psychosis   247
      Reina Fisher-van Werkhoven

Index   **259**

Contributors

Luisa Acosta
University of West London
United Kingdom

Andrea Aras-Payne
University of West London
United Kingdom

Judy Bothamley
University of West London
United Kingdom

Maureen Boyle
University of West London
United Kingdom

Jenny Brewster
University of West London
United Kingdom

Reina Fisher-van Werkhoven
University of West London
United Kingdom

Clare Gordon
University of West London
United Kingdom

Marie Hall
Imperial College Healthcare NHS Trust
United Kingdom

Julie Jones
University of West London
United Kingdom

Kate Nash
University of Winchester
United Kingdom

Anne O'Loghlen-Pinion
University of the West of England Bristol
United Kingdom

Jessica Scoble
University of West London
United Kingdom

Debra Sloam
University of West London
United Kingdom

Abbreviations

ABG	Arterial Blood Gas		Hb	Haemoglobin
ACS	Acute Coronary Syndrome		HbA1c	Glycated Haemoglobin (A1c)
AED	Automated External Defibrillator		hCG	Human Chorionic Gonadotrophin
AES	Anti-Embolic Stockings		HELLP	Haemolysis, Elevated Liver Enzymes and Low Platelet Count
AFLP	Acute Fatty Liver Disease of Pregnancy		HIE	Hypoxic-Ischemic Encephalopathy
AN	Antenatal		HQIP	Healthcare Quality Improvement Partnership
APH	Antepartum Haemorrhage			
ARM	Artificial Rupture of Membranes		HSE	Health Service Executive
BAPM	British Association of Perinatal Medicine		ICU	Intensive Care Unit (see ITU)
			ITU	Intensive Therapy Unit (see ICU)
BMI	Body Mass Index		IUD	Intrauterine Death
BNP	Brain Natriuretic Peptide		IUGR	Intrauterine Growth Restriction (see also FGR)
BP	Blood Pressure			
BPI	Brachial Plexus Injury		IV(I)	Intravenous (infusion)
CPR	Cardio-Pulmonary Resuscitation		IVF	In Vitro Fertilisation
CS	Caesarean Section		LFT	Liver Function Tests
CEMD	Confidential Enquiries into Maternal Deaths		LMWH	Low Molecular Weight Heparin
			MBRRACE-UK	Mothers and Babies: Reducing Risk through Audits and Confidential Enquiries across the UK
CMACE	Centre for Maternal and Child Enquiries (now MBRRACE-UK)			
COVID-19	Coronavirus Disease 2019		MC&S	Microscopy, Culture and Sensitivity
CT	Computerised Tomography		MEWS	Maternity Early Warning Score
CTG	Cardiotocograph		MEOWS	Maternity Early Obstetric Warning System
DIC	Disseminated Intravascular Coagulation			
			MOH	Major (or Massive) Obstetric Haemorrhage
DVT	Deep Vein Thrombosis			
ECG	Electrocardiogram		MRI	Magnetic Resonance Imaging
ECMO	Extracorporeal Membrane Oxygenation		NHS	National Health Service
			NICE	National Institute for Health and Care Excellence
ESC	European Society for Cardiology			
EWS	Early Warning Systems		NICU	Neonatal Intensive Care Unit
FBC	Full Blood Count		OASIS	Obstetric Anal Sphincter Injury
FH(R)	Fetal Heart (Tate)		ONS	Office for National Statistics
FGR	Fetal Growth Restriction (see IUGR)		OP	Occipito-Posterior
			PAS	Placenta Accreta Spectrum
GAS	Group A Streptococcus (infection)		PE	Pulmonary Embolism
GP	General Practitioner		PMH	Perinatal Mental Health

PPCM	Peripartum Cardiomyopathy	**SCAD**	Spontaneous Coronary Artery Dissection
PPH	Postpartum Haemorrhage		
PTS	Post-Thrombotic Syndrome	**SD**	Shoulder Dystocia
RCOG	Royal College of Obstetricians and Gynaecologists	**SOB**	Shortness of Breath
		SROM	Spontaneous Rupture of Membranes
RCP	Royal College of Physicians	**UKOSS UK**	Obstetric Surveillance System
ROM	Rupture of Membranes	**VBAC**	Vaginal Birth After Caesarean
RUQ	Right Upper Quadrant	**VBG**	Venous Blood Gas
SADS/MNH	Sudden Arrhythmic Death Syndrome with a Morphologically Normal Heart	**VE**	Vaginal Examination
		V/Q	Ventilation and Perfusion Scan
		VTE	Venous Thromboembolism
SARS-CoV-2	Severe Acute Respiratory Syndrome Coronavirus 2	**WHO**	World Health Organisation

Disclaimers

The words women and woman are used throughout this book; however, we acknowledge that for anyone who is receiving maternity care, this should be individualised and respectful, including the gender nouns and pronouns they prefer.

This book contains information obtained from authentic and highly-regarded sources. While all reasonable efforts have been made to publish reliable data and information, neither the authors nor the publisher can accept any legal responsibility or liability for any errors or omissions that may be made. The publishers wish to make clear that any views or opinions expressed in this book by individual authors are personal to them and do not necessarily reflect the views/opinions of the publishers. The information or guidance contained in this book is intended for use by medical, scientific or healthcare professionals and is provided strictly as a supplement to the medical or other professional's own judgement, their knowledge of the patient's medical history, relevant manufacturer's instructions and the appropriate best practice guidelines. Because of the rapid advances in medical science, any information or advice on dosages, procedures or diagnoses should be independently verified. The reader is strongly urged to consult the relevant national drug formulary and the drug companies' and device or material manufacturers' printed instructions and their websites before administering or utilising any of the drugs, devices or materials mentioned in this book. This book does not indicate whether a particular treatment is appropriate or suitable for a particular individual. Ultimately it is the sole responsibility of the medical professional to make his or her own professional judgements so as to advise and treat patients appropriately. The authors and publishers have also attempted to trace the copyright holders of all material reported in this publication and apologise to copyright holders if permission to publish in this form has not been obtained. If any copyright material has not been acknowledged, please write and let us know so that we may rectify it in any future reprint.

Figures

2.1 Spheres of accountability 22
2.2 Maternity statistics taken from the NHS Resolution annual report and account 2021/22: NHS Resolution Annual report and accounts 2021/22 23
3.1 Aortal and inferior vena caval compression in dorsal position 35
3.2 Adult in-hospital resuscitation algorithm 37
3.3 Hand position for chest compressions 38
3.4 Electrode pad placement for defibrillation 39
3.5 (a) Left uterine displacement from left side of patient; (b) Left uterine displacement from right side of patient 41
3.6 Obstetric Cardiac Arrest 42
3.7 Minimum equipment for newborn resuscitation and the support of transition of infants at birth in the pre-hospital setting 47
3.8 The 'C' grip for holding the mask 48
3.9 Newborn life support algorithm 49
3.10 Head position for optimum airway opening 50
3.11 Two-person jaw thrust 50
3.12 Finger positions for neonate chest compressions 51
4.1 Placental abruption (revealed, concealed and mixed) 59
4.2 Placenta praevia 63
5.1 Normal Sinus Rhythm 82

6.1 Triad of factors associated with venous thrombosis 88
6.2 Obstetric thromboprophylaxis risk assessment and management: antenatal 90
6.3 Obstetric thromboprophylaxis risk assessment and management: postnatal 91
8.1 Classifications of breech presentation (a) Extended breech, (b) Flexed breech (c) footling breech 125
8.2 Løvset's manoeuvre in maternal semi-recumbent/lithotomy position 131
8.3 Assisted birth of the head: Mauriceau-Smellie-Veit with maternal semi-recumbent/lithotomy position 132
8.4 Transverse and Oblique lie: (a) Transverse lie, (b) Oblique lie 134
9.1 Management of cord prolapse – at hospital and at home 146
9.2 Knee-chest position 147
9.3 Exaggerated Sims position 147
10.1 Shoulder dystocia 153
10.2 McRoberts position 156
10.3 Suprapubic pressure 157
10.4 Release of the posterior arm 158
12.1 Manual removal of placenta (a) stage 1: separation, (b) stage 2: removal 186
12.2 Rubbing up a contraction 187
12.3 Internal bimanual compression 189

Tables

1.1	A summary of the principles and values to be upheld within The Code – Professional standards of practice and behaviour for nurses and midwives	2
1.2	An overview of possible human factors that contribute to risk	4
1.3	Functions of record keeping	10
1.4	Critical points to include within record keeping	11
2.1	Applying the Human Rights Act to midwifery practice	20
2.2	Overview of the NMC Code and requirements for informed consent	24
2.3	Good practice guide – the principles of obtaining consent during labour	27
3.1	Normal blood gas levels	36
3.2	Drugs used during a cardiac arrest	40
3.3	Fetal adaptations in utero	45
3.4	Drugs used in newborn resuscitation	52
4.1	Causes of APH	57
4.2	Possible risk and predisposing factors for placenta abruption and placenta praevia	58
4.3	Signs and symptoms of placental abruption and placenta praevia	61
4.4	Placenta praevia classification	63
4.5	The Royal College of Obstetricians and Gynaecologists definitions used for assessing the severity of an APH	67
5.1	Cardiac/respiratory signs and symptoms	79
9.1	Associations with cord prolapse and cord presentation	144
9.2	Checklist to manage cord prolapse	148
12.1	Maternal symptoms of primary PPH by amount of blood loss	184
16.1	Pre-disposing and precipitating factors	237

Boxes

1.1 The five elements required to sustain a positive working culture 6
2.1 Definitions 17
2.2 Governing legislation of the Nursing and Midwifery Council, the regulatory body of midwives, nurses and nursing associates 18
2.3 St. George's Healthcare Trust, v S (1998) 19
2.4 Principles of valid consent, adapted from the RCOG 25
2.5 Overview of the Montgomery v Lanarkshire Health Board Case 25
2.6 Summary of the Bolam Test 25
2.7 Key outcomes of the Montgomery Case 25
2.8 Principles of the Mental Capacity Act 28
3.1 Definition 33
3.2 Newborn resuscitation 43
3.3 Risk/predisposing factors for neonatal resuscitation 44
3.4 Oxygen saturation levels in the newborn infant 48
4.1 Definitions 56
4.2 Placenta accreta spectrum (PAS) 64
4.3 Team members for managing a massive APH 68
4.4 Blood tests 69
5.1 Definition 76
5.2 Changes to the cardiovascular system in pregnancy 77
5.3 Pre-disposing/Risk Factors 78
5.4 Signs and Symptoms of cardiac disorders 78
5.5 Red flags in a pregnant woman presenting with chest pain 79
5.6 Initial care of a woman with suspected cardiac complications 80

5.7 Midwifery assessment and care of a woman with suspected cardiac issues 81
5.8 Blood tests 81
5.9 Cardiac Failure 83
5.10 Acute coronary syndrome/ischemic heart disease 83
5.11 Aortic Dissection (AD) 84
5.12 Cardiac Valve Compromise 84
6.1 Definitions 87
6.2 Thrombophilia conditions 89
6.3 Prophylactic measures that may be used to prevent thromboembolism 92
6.4 Guidance for correct use of compression stockings 93
6.5 Women who will be considered for antenatal prophylaxis with LMWH 94
6.6 Symptoms and Signs of DVT 94
6.7 Clinical manifestations of PE 95
6.8 Investigations for diagnosis of PE 96
6.9 Midwife's responsibilities in suspected pulmonary embolism emergency 96
6.10 Checklist for midwives regarding the use of LMWH around the time of birth 98
7.1 Definitions 103
7.2 Pre-disposing/risk factors 105
7.3 Signs and symptoms of pre-eclampsia 106
7.4 Women's self-assessment of pre-eclampsia symptoms 107
7.5 PET screening 108
7.6 Medications commonly used in pre-eclampsia 110
7.7 Summary of midwifery care in the antenatal period for the woman with pre-eclampsia 111

7.8	Summary of midwifery care in labour for the woman with pre-eclampsia	112
7.9	Potential maternal complications	112
7.10	Eclampsia	113
7.11	Immediate care of a seizure	114
7.12	Care for women receiving a magnesium sulphate (MgSO₄) infusion	114
7.13	HELLP	115
7.14	HELLP syndrome: signs, symptoms and possible laboratory findings	116
7.15	Optimal care for women with HELLP syndrome	116
7.16	Potential signs and symptoms for hepatic haematoma	117
7.17	Acute Fatty Liver of Pregnancy (AFLP)	117
7.18	Pre-disposing/risk factors for AFLP	117
7.19	Swansea Criteria for diagnosis of AFLP	118
7.20	Potential complications of AFLP	119
8.1	Malpresentation	124
8.2	Breech presentation	124
8.3	Predisposing and risk factors to a breech presentation	126
8.4	Possible contraindications for ECV	127
8.5	External Cephalic Version (ECV)	128
8.6	Vaginal Examination (VE)	129
8.7	Suggested contra-indications to planned vaginal breech birth	130
8.8	Løvset's manoeuvre in maternal semi-recumbent/lithotomy position	131
8.9	Vaginal breech birth checklist	133
8.10	Transverse Lie	133
8.11	Suggested causes and associations with transverse or oblique lie	134
8.12	Compound presentation	135
8.13	Causes, risks and associations with compound presentation	135
8.14	Brow presentation	136
8.15	Suggested risks and associations with brow presentation	136
8.16	Face presentation	137
8.17	Suggested risks and associations with face presentation	137
8.18	Mechanism of face presentation birth	138
8.19	Possible complications which are commonly associated with all malpresentations	139
9.1	Definitons	143
9.2	Filling the bladder following a cord prolapse	145
10.1	Shoulder Dystocia	152
10.2	Risk/Predisposing factors for shoulder dystocia	154
10.3	Signs of potential shoulder dystocia	155
10.4	Multidisciplinary team present at shoulder dystocia	155
10.5	Possible maternal complications following a shoulder dystocia	158
10.6	Possible infant complications following a shoulder dystocia	159
11.1	Uterine rupture	165
11.2	Risk/pre-disposing factors for uterine rupture	166
11.3	Potential signs and symptoms of uterine rupture	169
11.4	Uterine inversion	171
11.5	Risk/pre-disposing factors for uterine inversion	172
11.6	Signs and symptoms	173
12.1	Definition	181
12.2	Causes of PPH	182
12.3	The 4 T's	182
12.4	Risk factors for PPH	182
12.5	Manual removal of placenta	185
12.6	First line drugs	187
12.7	Second line drugs	188
12.8	Fluid overview	189
12.9	Bimanual compression	189
12.10	Risks for women who have had a massive obstetric haemorrhage	190
12.11	Disseminated Intravascular Coagulation (DIC)	191
13.1	Amniotic Fluid Embolism (AFE)	194
13.2	Possible risk/pre-disposing factors for AFE	196
13.3	UKOSS8 case definition for AFE	197
13.4	Potential investigations	199
14.1	Definitions	204
14.2	Risk factors for development of infection and sepsis	206
14.3	Signs and symptoms of sepsis	207
14.4	Assessment of skin changes in women with darker skin	207

14.5   Head-to-toe Assessment to
       identify features of infections that
       may lead to sepsis in pregnant
       and postpartum women   208
14.6   Investigations for sepsis   209
14.7   Sepsis Six   209
14.8   Definition   209
14.9   Risk factors for hospitalisation
       with Covid-19 in pregnancy   210
14.10 Features of deteriorating
       maternal illness from Covid-19
       infection   211
14.11 Members of MDT involved in the
       care of women admitted with
       Covid-19   211
14.12 Assessment of respiratory
       function by the midwife   211
14.13 Laboratory and other
       investigations for Covid-19   212
14.14 Medication which may be used in
       the care of women with Covid-19   213
14.15 Definition   213
14.16 Common symptoms of influenza   215

14.17 Investigations for respiratory
       illness/influenza   215
14.18 Summary of considerations for
       care when a woman is admitted
       with influenza   216
15.1   Emergency care   224
16.1   Post-traumatic stress
       disorder (PTSD)   234
16.2   Definitions of conditions
       associated with PTSD   236
16.3   Examples of intrusive symptoms
       and avoidance   238
17.1   Definitions   247
17.2   Possible risk/pre-disposing factors 249
17.3   Examples of psychotic phenomena   250
17.4   Questions to identify depression/
       anxiety   251
17.5   MBRRACE-UK red glags for
       severe maternal illness   253
17.6   MBRRACE-UK amber flags to
       prompt heightened awareness of
       change in mental state   253

An overview of the professional issues that support safe practice

KATE NASH AND JULIE JONES

Introduction   1
Accountability and duty of care   3
Risk assessment and management   3
Working together: teamwork, multi-professional
    training and creating a positive culture   6
Communication and record keeping   8
Conclusion   11
References   12

INTRODUCTION

You uphold the reputation of your profession at all times. You should display a personal commitment to the standards of practice and behaviour set out in the Code. You should be a model of integrity and leadership for others to aspire to. This should lead to trust and confidence in the profession from patients, people receiving care, other healthcare professionals and the public.[1]

The terms professional and professionalism are used widely within the midwifery literature and help shape the roles and responsibilities of midwives both within their work and personal lives. The National Health Service (NHS) Constitution[2] was developed to specify the rights that the public has when using the NHS and sets out a list of principles that guide the NHS and govern the way that it operates. A central tenet embedded within these principles is for the public to be treated with a professional standard of care by appropriately qualified and experienced professionals. It should also be noted that this professional standard of behaviour also applies to interactions between professionals.

The concept of professionalism is multifaceted[3] and can be partly explained as encompassing a specific set of skills, knowledge, attitudes and behaviours which carry certain responsibilities and duties. The Nursing Midwifery Council (NMC) is the professional regulator for nursing and midwifery in the United Kingdom and has created a structure and set of professional rules and standards for both professions (see Table 1.1). The criteria for the professional behaviours, attitudes, knowledge, skills and proficiencies of midwives are also set out by the NMC and are neither negotiable nor discretionary.[4] These rules and standards reinforce the professionalism of midwifery and must inform and underpin midwifery practice at all times.[1] Midwives commit to upholding these standards when they join the NMC register and subsequently renew their registration. They are an essential part of protecting the public and the delivery of a high standard of safe midwifery care.[1] They also provide a benchmark upon which midwifery practice can be scrutinised and for which midwives may be called to account

Table 1.1 A summary of the principles and values to be upheld within The Code – Professional standards of practice and behaviour for nurses and midwives[1]

Prioritise People

- Treat people as individuals and uphold their dignity
- Listen to people and respond to their preferences and concerns
- Make sure that people's physical, social and psychological needs are assessed and responded to
- Act in the best interests of people at all times and respect people's right to privacy and confidentiality

Practice Effectively

- Always practise in line with the best available evidence
- Communicate clearly and work cooperatively
- Share your skills, knowledge and experience for the benefit of people receiving care and your colleagues
- Keep clear and accurate records relevant to your practice
- Be accountable for your decisions to delegate tasks and duties to other people
- Have in place an indemnity arrangement which provides appropriate cover for any practice you take on as a nurse or midwife in the United Kingdom

Preserve Safety

- Recognise and work within the limits of your competence
- Be open and candid with all service users about all aspects of care and treatment, including when any mistakes or harm have taken place
- Always offer help if an emergency arises in your practice setting or anywhere else
- Act without delay if you believe that there is a risk to patient safety or public protection
- Raise concerns immediately if you believe a person is vulnerable or at risk and needs extra support and protection
- Advise on, prescribe, supply, dispense or administer medicines within the limits of your training and competence, the law, our guidance and other relevant policies, guidance and regulations
- Be aware of and reduce as far as possible any potential for harm associated with your practice

Promote Professionalism and Trust

- Uphold the reputation of your profession at all times
- Uphold your position as a registered nurse or midwife
- Fulfil all registration requirements
- Cooperate with all investigations and audits
- Respond to any complaints made against you professionally
- Provide leadership to make sure people's wellbeing is protected and to improve their experiences of the healthcare system

and ultimately removed from the register should they fail to uphold them.

This chapter aims to explore the various components that are essential for the professional practice of midwives. Whereas each component can be considered on an individual basis, it is important to be aware that they are mutually dependent and coexist together to support and inform the care that midwives must provide at all times. Issues such as communication, record keeping and teamwork might

seem an obvious consideration in the provision of safe and effective care; however, consecutive published reports into failing Trusts and maternal deaths have shown that these are areas which often fall short of the required standard.[5] Because of this, they urgently need to be improved to prevent unnecessary maternal and neonatal morbidity and mortality.

Responding to emergencies around childbirth can be both a stressful and potentially devastating time for all those involved. It is during such times that the provision of a high standard of professionalism by the practitioners involved is crucial in minimising the potential psychological and physiological sequelae for the mother and her family both during and following the event. It is hoped that through reading this chapter, the midwife will gain an understanding of what it means to be a professional and how accountability, effective leadership, a positive safety culture, multi-professional collaboration, communication and training are a vital part of achieving this.

ACCOUNTABILITY AND DUTY OF CARE

There are many definitions of accountability presented within the literature; however, it is best explained in terms of how it can be applied to midwifery. The roles and responsibilities of a midwife are set in statute and midwives are personally answerable for the actions and omissions that they make during their working lives, and have a duty of care to the women, babies and families that they care for. Midwives are accountable to both the criminal and civil courts to ensure that their activities conform to legal requirements, to their employer to follow their contract of duty and to the NMC to ensure that the rules and standards that govern midwifery practice are adhered to.[6] Midwives are also accountable to the women and babies to whom they have a duty of care and must be able to provide evidence that this duty has been met. Midwives can, therefore, be held to account by a range of higher authorities with whom they have a legal relationship in order to provide justification for their actions.[7] Failure to do this can result in disciplinary or legal action, the application of sanctions and possible removal from the register or recognised training programme (for student midwives).

It is important that midwives have the necessary knowledge, skills and proficiencies to enable them to fulfil their professional responsibilities. The NMC Standards of Proficiency for registered midwives sets out the standards that midwives must meet when they qualify and which they must maintain consistently throughout their careers in order to remain on their professional register.[8,4] Midwives must keep their knowledge and skills up to date and ensure that they have undertaken sufficient practice hours in order to maintain their skills and proficiency.

The International Confederation of Midwives (ICM) has considered the implications of midwives' accountability and emphasised the importance of midwives *not* undertaking any actions for which they have not received the appropriate training.[9] This is also supported by the NMC Code,[1] which stipulates that midwives must not provide any care or undertake any treatment that they have not been trained for and, in an emergency, they should only act within the limits of their knowledge and competence. It is important, however, that midwives, if necessary, should call for help from other health or social care professionals with the necessary skills and experience to provide assistance in the provision of care.[1]

The accountability of midwives also extends to any delegation of tasks they might make, and midwives must ensure that they only delegate those tasks and duties that are within the other person's scope of competence.[1] Whilst Health Care Support Workers can document unsupervised tasks within the maternity records on their own responsibility, it is the midwife who has delegated the task who is accountable and should ensure the counter-signing of these at the end of the shift.

RISK ASSESSMENT AND MANAGEMENT

Having the expert knowledge and skill to recognise, assess and manage risk, both at an individual level and within the wider realms of the maternity unit and healthcare organisation, is an integral part of ensuring that midwives maintain their accountability and uphold their duty of care. Risk assessment forms part of the broader clinical governance strategy within healthcare organisations, which is crucial to their ability to carry out their functions effectively and safeguard the provision of quality care. It is paramount that midwives are able to identify risk and initiate referral and the implementation of appropriate care and information. However, it is important that maternity units and Trusts have systems and processes in place to facilitate this and ensure that risk assessment and management are undertaken in a systematic and robust way.

The publication of An Organisation with a Memory[10] emphasised the need for healthcare organisations to learn from critical safety incidents to improve care and act to reduce risks and increase safety. A holistic systems approach to understanding failure in healthcare was advocated which emphasised the inherent presence of human factors within an organisation that may predispose individuals to make mistakes. The report stressed the importance of considering the broader environmental context to help minimise those circumstances and situations which may contribute to the occurrence of error. Far from being random, the report found that human errors tended to fall into recurrent patterns whereby the same set of circumstances may provoke individuals to make the same mistake. Risk management strategies should, therefore, focus on removing such situational 'error traps'[11]. This has become a predominant theme in more recent publications that have sought to expose the human factors that may lead to mistakes being made and consider ways that these can be minimised.[11,12] Table 1.2 provides an overview of human factors that are often identified as a contributing factor in patient safety incidents,[13] alongside some examples that are pertinent for the provision of optimum care during childbirth emergencies.

Following the publication of An Organisation with a Memory,[10] the National Patient Safety Association (NPSA) was developed in 2001 with the aim of identifying and reducing risks to patients receiving NHS care and assisting all those involved in healthcare to identify and learn when things go wrong. Historically, patient safety incidents were not always reported locally, often because of fears of disciplinary action, and it was recognised that there was a need to move from blaming individuals to understanding the underlying factors within the system that are more often responsible for incidents.[14]

The key functions developed by the NPSA were later transferred to the NHS Commissioning Board Special Health Authority in 2012.

The National Reporting and Learning System (NRLS) is a central database which was established in 2003 and receives confidential reports of patient safety incidents from healthcare staff across England and Wales. Clinicians and safety experts analyse these reports to identify common risks to patients and opportunities to improve patient safety. Resources of the NRLS include the publication and dissemination of Patient Safety Alerts through the Central Alerting System (CAS) and the provision of regular feedback from the data collected to identify themes and causes. All healthcare organisations within England and Wales reported any patient safety incidents to the NRLS whose data the NHS Commissioning Board Authority use to analyse risk, promote learning and tackle important patient safety issues at their root cause.[14] This has been replaced by the Patient Safety Incident Management System in 2021.

The National Health Service Litigation Authority (NHSLA) was established in 1995 as a Special Health Authority whose duties include the provision of legal and professional advice to the NHS and Department of Health (DH), assisting the NHS with risk management and managing claims made against the NHS. This is now replaced by NHS Resolution.[15] As part of its safety and learning service, the NHS Resolution publishes annual reports based on analysis drawn from its national database. The latest report includes maternity claims between

Table 1.2 An overview of possible human factors that contribute to risk

Human factors that may contribute to patient safety incidents[12]	Possible examples during childbirth emergencies
• Cognition and mental workload • Distractions • The physical environment • Physical demands • Service/product design • Teamwork • Process design	• Stress and fatigue • Several professionals in the room • Lack of communication or people talking at once if a clear leader is not identified • Peripheral noise • Poor lighting and clutter • Possible need to make complicated drug calculations/lack of prefilled syringes for high-risk drugs • Lack of equipment, for example, on Resuscitaire/PPH trolley • Seeing what you expect to see – remember to check labels/drugs

1 April 2022 and 31 March 2023.[15] During this time, 64% of clinical claims came from maternity care/obstetrics. This has informed the strategic priority three within this report which is to promote collaboration to improve maternity outcomes.

NHS Resolution is a partner in the Safer Births Initiative with The Kings Fund, Royal College of Obstetricians and Gynaecologists (RCOG), Royal College of Midwives (RCM), Centre for Maternal and Child Enquiries, Mothers and Babies: Reducing Risk through Audits and Confidential Enquiries across the UK (MBRRACE – UK) and the NRLS. There are many initiatives and strategies in place at a strategic level to assess and manage risk and which may feed into and inform the day-to-day practice of midwives on the front line. Lessons can be learnt from the analysis of safety incidents at both national and local levels. Many of the initiatives implemented within the workplace today have been done so in response to previous lessons learnt, and there are many tools available to promote effective risk management and safe working within maternity. Whilst it is important that safety incidents do not elicit a 'knee jerk' response, midwives have a responsibility to act immediately should they believe that there is a risk to the safety of women and babies.[1]

More recently, a number of high-profile cases and reports have been published that have reviewed the safety of the NHS and maternity services.[16,17,4] A key issue that lies at the heart of these is that of culture. The Health and Care Professions Council (HCPC) have emphasised the role that organisations themselves play in the development of professionalism[3] and how culture can exert a significant influence on the professional behaviour of practitioners and either help or hinder the extent to which they are able to carry out their professional duties.

Recently published reports following investigations into failing Trusts have revealed that poor organisational culture is synonymous with poor patient care and its associated impact on morbidity and mortality rates.[16,17,5] Various initiatives implemented over the past decade have also sought to address the culture within which midwives work. The challenge of historical interprofessional and departmental barriers, drive for increased transparency and a commitment to report, investigate and learn from incidents to improve patient safety all serve to improve the clinical environment and promote a culture of openness and safety. Despite this, the Confidential Enquiry into Maternal Deaths and Morbidity 2018–2020[18] has revealed that only 22% of the women who died were considered to have received good care, which could not have been improved. Improvements to care were required in the remaining 78% of maternal mortalities and such improvements were judged as having the potential to change the outcome in 38% of these cases.[18] A key concern for the enquiry assessors was a lack of multidisciplinary team working and integration of critical care, particularly recognising that critical care is a treatment, not a place.

The Nursing and Midwifery Order 2001 grants the NMC authority to regulate midwifery and nursing in the United Kingdom. The Order also contains an additional set of powers for the NMC to set rules related to midwifery.

In 2017, the Professional Midwifery Advocate (PMA) role was established with a focus on leadership, support, advocacy and quality improvement through the implementation of the A-Equip model.[19] This model, 'Advocating and Education for Quality Improvement' was developed in response to the cessation of the statutory role of Supervisors of Midwives. There is a requirement for those midwives who wish to become a PMA within NHS Trusts to complete post-graduate training, which is available through completing a post-graduate taught module.

The A-EQUIP model has four functions which the PMA will use to support and interact with midwives.

1. Education and Development (formative)
2. Personal action for quality improvement
3. Clinical supervision (restorative)
4. Monitoring, evaluation and quality control

Clinical supervision is supplied through the PMA by offering either one-to-one or group sessions of restorative clinical supervision (RCS). This is led by the midwife, who decides what she/he wishes to discuss, and the PMA facilitates discussion and reflection, enabling the midwife themselves to find solutions and take appropriate actions. This role has slowly become established in Trusts since 2017, and the value of supporting staff in this way has been recognised at a strategic level. There are more funds being made available from NHS England to train PMAs. They can also support the aim of creating a positive working culture where every member of staff feels valued, which will now be discussed in more depth.

WORKING TOGETHER: TEAMWORK, MULTI-PROFESSIONAL TRAINING AND CREATING A POSITIVE CULTURE

Creating a positive culture

Whereas a positive working culture can increase patient safety, a negative working culture, which encompasses the elements of poor engagement, a lack of teamwork and suboptimal communication, can expose women and babies to unnecessary harm and the devastating impact that this can have on people's lives.[20,21,22] It has been suggested that leadership is the most influential factor in shaping organisational culture,[23] and the need for Trusts to develop appropriate leadership strategies and behaviours to improve the delivery of care is well recognised.[22,23] Such strategies have the potential to make a significant difference to the outcomes and experiences for both women and their partners and midwives have a significant role to play in the delivery of such strategies.[24,25]

A substantial review of the published literature surrounding leadership and leadership development in healthcare was undertaken[25] and identified five key elements necessary for sustaining positive work cultures that ensure high-quality, compassionate care for patients. A summary of these five elements is shown in Box 1.1.

The importance of all staff having shared values and mutually agreed on objectives[26] has been emphasised as this enables practitioners to work together effectively to coordinate their efforts, knowledge and resources to deliver highly complex clinical care successfully.[24] This is particularly important when responding to emergencies within childbearing, where everyone is working together towards the common goal of optimising outcomes for the woman and baby using the best available methods. Effective leadership is important when coordinating the activities of team members in response to an emergency situation and leadership duties should include ensuring that the evolving plan of care is clear to all, information is shared, resources are procured and the environment is managed so that team members are able to complete their roles and responsibilities effectively where possible.[27]

There may be occasions where situational leadership is required, such as when the initial clinician responding to the emergency assumes leadership until more senior help is available.[28] A lack of leadership was a feature in three deaths from postpartum haemorrhage in a previous Confidential Enquiries report and the need for clinicians to step up to assume responsibility for the coordination of care was emphasised.[29] Perceived hierarchies within the team may deter junior clinicians from speaking up,[28] and a key recommendation from the Kings Fund Inquiry was the need to build upon multiprofessional relationships to support and enable team working so that clinicians are empowered to speak up, raise concerns and assume leadership responsibilities when needed.[27]

Investing in staff teambuilding on labour ward is a key element of improving the function and capability of the multiprofessional team, and both management and lead clinicians should strive to develop creative ways to engage staff and provide opportunities for team building.[22] Whilst resource issues often mean that staff are unable to leave the workplace to attend team building days, other ways of developing staff engagement and team working include regularly scheduled in-house forums and training opportunities. Labour ward forums, case reviews, CTG review meetings and perinatal mortality meetings provide an opportunity to enhance team working and communication and break down interprofessional barriers. Such meetings may also offer the potential for the debriefing of staff following an emergency and provide an opportunity for individual and team learning whilst events remain fresh.[27] However, it is important that these forums

---

BOX 1.1: The five elements required to sustain a positive working culture[25]

- Shared vision to improve care and optimise outcomes
- Clear, aligned objectives for all teams, departments and individual staff
- Supportive and enabling people management and high levels of staff engagement
- Learning, innovation and quality improvement embedded in the practice of all staff
- Effective team working

are managed in such a way that the focus remains on the problem or incident itself rather than the allocation of individual blame. In this way, individuals are able to give and receive both constructive and positive feedback in order to learn from incidents and help foster a culture of safety.

Teamwork and multiprofessional training

Midwives have a duty to maintain their knowledge and skills to ensure that they practice safely and effectively.[1] The deployment of a well-trained and skilled workforce is at the heart of safe maternity care[27] and important to ensure the prompt recognition of and response to emergency situations during childbirth. The failure of staff to recognise or respond appropriately to an acute situation is an ongoing theme within the Confidential Enquiries,[29,30] and there may be occasions when junior members of staff feel overwhelmed or lack the required skill and confidence to respond appropriately when faced with an emergency situation in the hospital or the community.[17]

The effectiveness of local interprofessional training is recognised within the obstetric literature, and 'it has long been recognised that professional groups who work together should also train together to promote understanding of each other's practice and foster good team working'.[20] Maternity units within the UK are required to implement local interprofessional training around childbirth emergencies in order to improve clinical skills whilst developing communication and team working.[31,32,33] This is particularly significant when responding to emergencies during childbirth, as optimal teamwork is essential in order to prevent avoidable morbidity and mortality for women and babies.[31,32,33]

Local interprofessional training is associated with significant improvements in clinical outcomes.[17] It helps reduce interprofessional stereotyping and flattens hierarchies whilst facilitating collaboration and a positive working environment.[21,34] It also provides clinicians with the opportunity to refine and develop existing leadership and clinical skills within a safe environment and develop the confidence to take charge of and refer appropriately within an escalating clinical situation.

The SaFE study group (Simulation and Fire-drill Evaluation) received a research grant from the Department of Health to conduct a regional randomised controlled trial with the aim of reviewing obstetric emergencies training and determine if including teamwork training in the obstetric emergencies courses improved the team's management even further. Eight hospitals across the South West of England took part in the SaFE study, and the trial demonstrated the importance of teamwork and clear communication and revealed improvements in knowledge, clinical skills and teamwork during simulated emergencies following training.[35,36,37]

More recently, studies have continued to demonstrate the value of interprofessional training using simulation. A large retrospective cohort study was undertaken in eight public hospitals in Southern Australia to assess the introduction of Practical Obstetric Multi-professional Training (PROMPT) into maternity units and evaluate the effects on organisational culture and perinatal outcomes in maternity units.[38] The results showed significant improvements in staff attitudes towards safety and teamwork in addition to improvements in neonatal outcomes. Other studies have also reported significant improvements in communication[39] and safety culture[40] as well as clinical outcomes.[36,41] The Royal College of Obstetricians and Gynaecologists (RCOG) caution, however, that not all studies have shown an improvement in outcomes following the introduction of training and recommend that hospitals monitor the neonatal injury rate after the introduction of training to ensure it is effective.[42]

It is imperative that emergency training prepares clinicians for all possible outcomes and to consider the wider clinical picture at all times during an emergency. This has been referred to as situational awareness,[28] whereby clinicians survey their environment and think ahead to ensure they remain aware of the various factors that may impact care, including the possibility of all eventualities within their planning.[26] The importance of keeping a 'critical mind, anticipating risk factors and explaining observations rather than accepting them'[29] forms a part of developing situational awareness and may help prevent delays in recognising and responding to emergencies within childbirth.

COMMUNICATION AND RECORD KEEPING

Communication

Whilst the most recent Confidential Enquiries into maternal deaths show a decrease in the overall rate of maternal death across the United Kingdom, a lack of optimal communication and teamwork remains a continuing theme from previous enquiries.[18,30,29,] Many factors contribute to suboptimal communication, and having an explicit strategy to facilitate communication within acute situations is important to ensure that individuals, teams and departments communicate effectively.[18] The use of the SBAR (situation, background, assessment, recommendation) tool can lead to improved communication between team members, and its use is recommended to improve communication during emergencies in childbirth.[27]

The multiprofessional development and use of evidence-based clinical guidelines and care pathways have been shown to facilitate the organisation of multiprofessional care, communication and teamwork.[43] There is some evidence that care pathways are effective interventions for improving teamwork, increasing the organisational level of care processes, and decreasing the risk of burnout for healthcare teams in an acute hospital setting.[44] The European Pathway Association (E-P-A) has defined a care pathway as 'a complex intervention for the mutual decision making and organisation of care processes for a well-defined group of patients during a well-defined period'.[45,46] Defining characteristics of care pathways include having clearly stated goals and objectives of care that are evidence-based and the coordination and sequencing of the care process and activities of the multiprofessional team.[46] In this way, they are a useful tool used to facilitate the coordination, communication and documentation of care by the multiprofessional team during an emergency. However, they should be communicated, reviewed and adapted to the requirements of the individual woman or baby.

The use of proformas and early warning systems are other tools that can be used to facilitate communication and have been shown to reduce mortality and improve care.[47,48] Care bundles such as the United Kingdom (UK) Sepsis Trust 'Sepsis Six Care Bundle'[49] should be used as a matter of urgency when dealing with a confirmed diagnosis of sepsis,[50,51,52] and the use of MEOWs charts can provide a framework to encourage the undertaking of observations and recognition and escalation of abnormalities.

It is vital that documented findings are escalated and acted upon appropriately, although published reports suggest that this is not always the case.[4,16,17] The findings of the report into the Morecambe Bay investigation and the Ockenden report have shown that there was evidence of a lack of situation awareness, with a deficiency in understanding of basic observations, their clinical significance and how they should be managed. There were many instances where symptoms and signs, observations, progress in labour and the concerns of patients, parents and families were recorded but were not underpinned by a clinical plan or escalation of clinical decision-making.[4,17] Clear communication and record keeping enable observations to be shared with others to help maintain an ongoing awareness of the clinical situation, and staff should have a low threshold for seeking assistance should they have any concerns or are unsure.[26] Effective interprofessional communication is essential to ensure that all those involved with the care are aware of significant risk factors or concerns.

Multiprofessional communication is a vital component of the overall safety culture of a maternity unit, and the importance of learning lessons from safety incidents has been discussed previously in this chapter. Members of the multidisciplinary team need to engage to provide mutual support and review the evidence when things go wrong. Through systematic multiprofessional scrutiny of cases, feedback can be provided and acted upon to ensure that any necessary improvements to the systems and processes in place are made. It also enables any local training or individual practitioner behavioural, knowledge and competency issues that may become apparent to be dealt with constructively. The use of cross monitoring has been advocated as a means of monitoring the actions of other team members to facilitate situation awareness and the self-correction of tasks in order to reduce errors in the provision of healthcare.[26,53] This enables the actions of the members of the team during an emergency to be monitored in a supportive way by colleagues with the purpose of sharing the workload, facilitating communication between teams and ensuring that a safe standard of care is provided.

When faced with immediate concerns regarding maternal and fetal well-being, most women would value safety and good communication with staff to make autonomous choices.[54] The Being Open Framework[55] emphasises the importance of effective communication with patients when things go wrong, and midwives have a duty of candour to the women that they provide care for.[1] Communication between staff and women has a significant influence on the maternal experience and women's perception of the care they have received.[32] Effective communication is of paramount importance when responding to childbirth emergencies. A phenomenological study undertaken to explore women's experiences of their birth emergencies[56] found that the quality of women's interactions with midwives and doctors was integral to how they felt about their experience. Non-verbal cues such as facial leakage, whereby the facial expressions of clinicians revealed their own anxiety, perpetuated the fear and distress that women felt both during and after the event. Women valued supportive interactions from clinicians, and issues with communication included poor communication, a lack of interaction and inadequate or inappropriate explanations.

Compassion in Practice, the national strategy for nurses, midwives and care staff, was launched in December 2012 and emphasises the government's commitment to the delivery of high-quality, compassionate care by nurses, midwives and care staff.[57] Part of this was ensuring that the six 'Cs' (care, compassion, competence, communication, courage and commitment) are embedded within clinical practice. The NMC Code is also clear about the need for nurses and midwives to communicate clearly and treat people as individuals with kindness, respect and compassion.[1] Whilst this may seem to be stating the obvious, recent surveys into women's experiences suggest that this is not always being achieved.[16,17] Whereas the findings from the most recent survey of women's experiences of maternity care[58] showed that improvements were made in some areas, a significant proportion of women expressed concerns about communication between maternity staff and themselves. Creating an open safety culture and having access to good quality multiprofessional simulation training ensures midwives have the necessary skills, knowledge and confidence to respond appropriately to emergencies during childbearing. It stands to reason that when clinicians feel supported and prepared, they will feel less anxious and be empowered to offer effective support and care to women.

Record keeping

Record keeping is an integral part of the professional practice of midwives, and midwifery records can serve to reflect the standards of midwifery practice provided.[1] Ultimately, midwives can be called to account through their records as to whether they have met their duty of care. This is because records provide the evidence that care has been provided as well as the justification for such care. Records completed to a high standard adhere to the principles of good record keeping and provide evidence that midwives are practicing in a safe and competent way. Such principles have been set out within the NMC guidance in the Code.[1]

The Data Protection Act section 68 (2) has defined health records as 'consisting of information relating to the physical or mental health or condition of an individual made by, or on behalf of, a health professional in connection with the care of that individual'.[59] This includes all records relevant to the midwives' scope of practice and the principles of good record keeping apply to all types of records and communication methods and are not just confined to the maternity notes.[1] Such records are legal documents that can be called as evidence within a court of law, coroner's inquests and fitness to practice panels. Within a court of law, it is generally viewed that if something is not recorded, then it has not been done,[6,60] and failure to maintain a good standard of record keeping is one of the main reasons that midwives and nurses appear at an NMC Fitness to Practice panel.[6]

Record keeping serves many vital functions, and an overview of these are included in Table 1.3, alongside a list of the various different formats that records might take.

The principles of good record keeping specify that records should be clearly written (in indelible ink if handwritten) and be factual, accurate, follow a logical sequence and use accepted professional terminology so that they can be understood by both colleagues and women.[1] Notes should be contemporaneous or when this is not possible be written as soon as is possible following the event, identifying the time when written.[1] Records should also identify any risks or problems that have arisen

Table 1.3 Functions of record keeping

The types of records used within midwifery practice	Various purposes of record keeping
• Handwritten/computer clinical notes • Emails and letters to and from other health professionals • Laboratory reports • X-rays • Printouts from monitoring equipment • Incident reports and statements • Photographs • Videos • Tape recordings of telephone conversations • Text messages	• Provides an accurate account of care planning, decision making, treatment and care given, as well as responses to care and further action taken • Promotes the ability to detect problems at an early stage, detailing the reasoning behind any action taken • Demonstrates continuity of care • Facilitates and supports inter-professional and client communication • Supports clinical audit/research, allocation of resources and service planning • Helps to address complaints and/or legal processes • Improves accountability

and show the actions taken to deal with them, including assessment details, reviews, actions and plans for future care.

Record keeping can be especially difficult during an emergency situation when a high level of stress may be present. The allocation of a scribe to contemporaneously record events as they unfold should be used where possible.[61] The Royal College of Obstetricians and Gynaecologists has recommended the use of proformas which can be adapted for local use, and provides guidance for critical points to include in record keeping during specific childbirth emergencies.[42,52] An adaption of these is presented as an example in Table 1.4.

Local training in record keeping has been recommended as part of multiprofessional childbirth emergency training ('skills drills') provided by maternity units to ensure that records include the required critical elements.[42,62] It should be assumed that all records will be scrutinised following a childbirth emergency in order to ensure that a safe standard of care was provided, learn lessons and provide answers for women and their families. It is important that documentation is accurate and reflects the reality of what occurred during the emergency. This was investigated as part of the previously mentioned SaFE trial (Simulation and Fire-drill Evaluation) by comparing a written record with a videotape of the simulation and an electronic record of the force applied to the baby during

the simulation of shoulder dystocia.[61] The authors also sought to compare the quality of record keeping with and without the use of a proforma. Both video and force recording for each simulation were obtained, which enabled the comparison of the written records with the actual events. The study findings suggested that record keeping during childbirth emergencies is a complex process fraught with many influencing factors. Although the use of a proforma demonstrated improved completeness of documentation, it may have reduced the accuracy of recording in some areas, and the immediate written recollection of events by clinicians may often be both inaccurate and incomplete.[61]

The authors concluded that there were different virtues associated with the use of a proforma and writing longhand and postulated that writing longhand may encourage more careful thought than simply ticking preformatted boxes. The use of a proforma, however, appeared to act as an aide-memoire for more comprehensive documentation, although it may encourage the practitioners to record things of which they have no true recollection and miss items that are not included within the proforma.[61] The use of a scribe within an emergency situation to record events contemporaneously may circumvent this by increasing the accuracy of recordings whilst having the benefit of helping to ensure all critical components of care are documented.[61]

Table 1.4 Critical points to include within record keeping (adapted from RCOG guidelines[42,52])

Childbirth Emergency	Critical points to include within record keeping
Shoulder Dystocia	• Time of delivery of the head and time of delivery of the body • Position of fetal head at delivery • Which shoulder was anterior at the time of the dystocia • Manoeuvres performed, their timing and sequence • Degree of axial traction applied • Maternal perineal and vaginal examination • Estimated blood loss • Assessment of the mother • Staff in attendance and the time they arrived • General condition of the baby (Apgar score) • Umbilical cord blood acid-base measurements • Neonatal assessment of the baby
Postpartum Haemorrhage	• The staff in attendance and the time they arrived • The sequence of events • The time of administration of different pharmacological agents given, their timing and sequence • The time of surgical intervention, where relevant • The condition and overall assessment of the mother throughout the different steps • Identification and timing of the fluid and blood products given

As well as the potential for maternal psychological sequelae to occur as a result of childbirth emergencies, there is evidence that those midwives directly involved with the emergency may also suffer a degree of traumatisation during and following the event.[63] It is important to bear in mind how individual perceptions of events may become distorted and, in turn, impact the quality and completeness of subsequent record keeping. A recent prospective observational study that assessed the quality of midwifery documentation by reviewing the intrapartum notes and partograms of 61 consecutive women found that fatigue may also play a role in suboptimal documentation towards the middle and end of the shift.[63] The provision of support from senior staff or a PMA through RCS may help improve the standard of record keeping following such events.

Social media

Within today's society, the use of social media is commonplace and firmly embedded within the working and personal lives of most practitioners via Facebook, X, and various other electronic vehicles. Midwives have a professional duty to maintain the confidentiality of those in their care, and this duty extends to both their online professional and personal lives.[64] The NMC has published guidance for Social Networking,[65] and midwives may put their registration at risk as well as jeopardise their professional integrity by behaving online in a way that may be deemed inappropriate or unprofessional.

CONCLUSION

The NHS Constitution has set out the standards that those accessing their services should expect.[2] Midwives are knowledgeable and skilled practitioners who must behave in a way that reflects high standards of personal integrity and justifies the trust placed in them by the women and families who access their care. This chapter has introduced the reader to an overview of the components that are essential to professional practice and which must entwine together to underpin midwifery care.

The adverse aspects of risk and patient safety have been emphasised within maternity services in recent years, and this has been a result of both individual tragedies and a wider concern that has been expressed about the infrastructure in place to support maternity services.[20] Whilst much of the language that centres on risk and patient safety is negative[20] it is important to remember that midwives hold a privileged position in society today and have the potential to shape the experiences and outcomes for women and their families during a momentous period in their lives. The provision of good quality, safe midwifery care is accomplished through the tireless commitment of individual clinicians and the robust processes and systems of care that are in place within maternity units and hospitals. It is vital that all midwives have an understanding of what professionalism means and how it must be promoted and enhanced to safeguard the future of midwifery and maternity care.

REFERENCES

1. NMC (Nursing and Midwifery Council). The code: professional standards of practice and behaviour for nurses and midwives. London: NMC; 2015a. [Accessed 29 July 2023]. Available from: www.nmc.org.uk/standards/code/

2. Department of Health (DH). The NHS constitution. London: Crown Copyright; 2015. [Accessed 3 August 2023]. Available: www.gov.uk/government/publications/the-nhs-constitution-for-england/the-nhs-constitution-for-england

3. Health and Care Professions Council (HCPC). Professionalism in healthcare professionals. London: Health and Care Professions Council; 2011. [Accessed 3 August 2023]. Available from: www.hcpc-uk.org/globalassets/resources/reports/professionalism-in-healthcare-professionals.pdf

4. Nursing Midwifery Council (NMC). Standards of competence for registered midwives. 2020. [Accessed 3 August 2023]. Available from: www.nmc.org.uk/globalassets/sitedocuments/standards/nmc-standards-for-competence-for-registered-midwives.pdf

5. Independent Maternity Review. Ockenden report – final: findings, conclusions, and essential actions from the independent review of maternity services at the Shrewsbury and Telford Hospital NHS Trust (HC 1219). Crown; 2022. [Accessed 20 July 2023]. https://assets.publishing.service.gov.uk/government/uploads/system/uploads/attachment_data/file/1064302/Final-Ockenden-Report-web-accessible.pdf

6. Dimond B. Legal aspects of midwifery. 4th ed. London: Quay Books Division, MA Healthcare Ltd.; 2005.

7. Griffith R, Tengnah C, Patel C. Law and professional issues in midwifery. Exeter: Learning Matters; 2010.

8. Nursing Midwifery Council (NMC). Standards framework for nursing and midwifery education: NMC. 2023a. [Accessed 3 August 2023]. Available from: www.nmc.org.uk/standards-for-education-and-training/standards-framework-for-nursing-and-midwifery-education/

9. International Confederation of Midwives (ICM). Position statement: professional accountability of the midwife. 2023. [Accessed 29 September 2023]. Available from: www.internationalmidwives.org/08h_en_professional-accountability-of-the-midwife.pdf

10. Department of Health. An organisation with a memory. London: Crown Copyright; 2000. [Accessed 29 September 2023]. Available from: www.elft.nhs.uk/r_02-an-organisation-with-a-memory-l-donaldson.pdf

11. Carthey J. Understanding safety in healthcare: the system evolution, erosion and enhancement model. J Public Health Res. 2013;2(3). Available from: <doi:10.4081/jphr.2013.e25>

12. National Health Service (NHS) England. Human factors in healthcare a concordat from the national quality board. 2013. [Accessed 23 September 2023]. Available from: www.england.nhs.uk/wp-content/uploads/2013/11/nqb-hum-fact-concord.pdf

13. Stephenson T. The national safety patient agency. Arch Dis Child. 2005;90:226–228. Available from: <doi:10.1136/adc.2004.065896>

14. National Patient Safety Agency. Transfer of patient safety function to the NHS commissioning board special health authority. 2012. [Accessed 3 August 2023]. Available from: www.npsa.nhs.uk/corporate/news/transfer-of-patient-safety-function/

15. NHS Resolution. Annual report and accounts. 2023. [Accessed 3 August 2023]. Available from: https://resolution.nhs.uk/

wp-content/uploads/2023/07/4405-NHSR-Annual-Report-and-Accounts_Rollout_A_Access2.pdf

16. Francis R. Report of the mid Staffordshire NHS foundation trust public inquiry. London: HMSO; 2013.

17. Kirkup B. The report of the Morecambe Bay investigation. London: The Stationary Office; 2014. [Accessed 26 August 2023]. Available from: www.gov.uk/government/uploads/system/uploads/attachment_data/file/408480/47487_MBI_Accessible_v0.1.pdf

18. Knight M, Kenyon S, Brocklehurst P, Neilson J, Shakespeare J, Kurinczuk JJ, On behalf of MBRRACE-UK, editors. Saving lives, improving mothers' care – lessons learned to inform future maternity care from the UK and Ireland confidential enquiries into maternal deaths and morbidity 2018–20. Oxford: National Perinatal Epidemiology Unit, University of Oxford; 2022. [Accessed 2 August 2023]. Available from: www.npeu.ox.ac.uk/assets/downloads/mbrrace-uk/reports/maternal-report-2022/MBRRACE-UK_Maternal_MAIN_Report_2022_UPDATE.pdf

19. NHS England. A-equip midwifery supervision model. n.d. [Accessed 2 August 2023]. Available from: www.england.nhs.uk/mat-transformation/implementing-better-births/a-equip/a-equip-midwifery-supervision-model/

20. Kings Fund. Safe births: everybody's business: an independent inquiry into the safety of maternity services in England. London: The Kings Fund; 2008. [Accessed 3 August 2023]. Available from: www.kingsfund.org.uk/sites/files/kf/field/field_publication_file/safe-births-everybodys-business-onora-oneill-february-2008.pdf

21. Cornthwaite K, Edwards S, Siassakos D. Reducing risk in maternity by optimising teamwork and leadership: an evidence-based approach to save mothers and babies. Best Pract Res Clin Obstet Gynaecol. 2013;4:571–581. [Epub 3 May 2013]. Available from: <doi:10.1016/j.bpobgyn.2013.04.004>

22. West MA, Lyubovnikova J. Illusions of team working in health care. J Health Organ Manag. 2013;27(1):134–142. Available from: <doi:10.1108/14777261311311843>

23. West M, Armit K, Loewenthal L, Eckert R, West T, Lee A. Leadership and leadership development in healthcare: the evidence base. London: Faculty of Medical Leadership and Management; 2015. [Accessed 20 September 2023]. Available from: www.kingsfund.org.uk/leadership-leadership-development-health-care-feb-2015.pdf

24. Department of Health. Delivering high quality midwifery care: the priorities opportunities and challenges for midwives. London: Crown Copyright; 2009. Available from: <doi:10.1016/j.midw.2009.11.006>

25. Midwifery 2020. Delivering expectations. 2010. [Accessed 3 August 2023]. Available from: https://assets.publishing.service.gov.uk/media/5a7c95cae5274a7b7e3216cd/dh_119470.pdf

26. Deering S, Johnstone LC, Colacchio K. Multidisciplinary teamwork and communication training. Semin Perinatol. 2011;35(2):89–96. Available from: <doi:10.1053/j.semperi.2011.01.009>

27. Thomas V, Dixon A. Improving safety in maternity services: a toolkit for teams. London: The Kings Fund; 2012. [Accessed 3 August 2023]. Available from: www.kingsfund.org.uk/publications/improving-safety-maternity-services

28. Leonard M, Graham S, Bonacum D. The human factor: the critical importance of effective teamwork and communication in providing safe care. Qual Safety Heal Care. 2004;13(Supp 1):i85–i90. Available from: <doi:10.1136/qhc.13.suppl_1.i85>

29. Paterson-Brown S, Bamber J, On behalf of the MBRRACE-UK. Haemorrhage chapter writing group: prevention and treatment of haemorrhage. In: Knight M, Kenyon S, Brocklehurst P, Neilson J, Shakespeare J, Kurinczuk JJ, On Behalf of MBRRACE-UK, editors. Saving lives, improving mothers' care – lessons learned to inform future maternity care from the UK and Ireland confidential enquiries into maternal deaths and morbidity 2009–12. Oxford: National Perinatal Epidemiology Unit, University of Oxford; 2014. p. 45–55.

30. Centre for Maternal and Child Enquiries (CMACE). Saving mothers' lives: reviewing maternal deaths to make motherhood safer: 2006–08. The Eighth Report on Confidential Enquiries into Maternal Deaths in the United Kingdom. BJOG. 2011;118(Suppl. 1):1–203.

31. Royal College of Obstetricians and Gynaecologists RCOG. Green-top guideline no. 50 umbilical cord prolapse. London: RCOG; 2014. [Accessed 3 August 2023]. Available from: www.rcog.org.uk/media/3wykswng/gtg-50-umbilicalcord prolapse-2014.pdf

32. Royal College of Obstetricians and Gynaecologists RCOG. Joint RCOG and RCM statement: Kirkup report into maternity services at Morecambe Bay NHS trust. 2015. [Accessed 3 August 2023]. Available from: www.rcog.org.uk/en/news/joint-rcog-and-rcm-statement-kirkup-report/

33. Royal College of Midwives RCM. Joint statement from the royal college of midwives and the royal college of obstetricians and gynaecologists on the Kirkup report into maternity services at Morecambe Bay. 2015. [Accessed 3 August 2023]. Available from: www.rcm.org.uk/news-views-and-analysis/news/joint-statement-from-the-royal-college-of-midwives-and-the-royal

34. Siassakos D, Fox R, Hunt, L, Farey J, Laxton C, Winter C, et al. Attitudes towards safety and teamwork in a maternity unit with embedded team training. Am J Med Qual. 2011;26:132–137. Available from: <doi:10.1177/1062860610373379>

35. Draycott TJ, Sibanda T, Owen L, Akande V, Winter C, Reading S, Whitelaw A. Does training in obstetric emergencies improve neonatal outcome? BJOG. 2006;113(2):177–182. Available from: <doi:10.1111/j.1471-0528.2006.00800.x>

36. Siassakos D, Crofts JF, Winter C, Weiner CP, Draycott TJ. The active components of effective training in obstetric emergencies. BJOG. 2009a;116(8):1028–1032. Available from: <doi:10.1111/j.1471-0528.2009.02178.x>

37. Siassakos D, Hasafa Z, Sibanda T, Fox R, Donald F, Winter C, et al. Retrospective cohort study of diagnosis-delivery interval with umbilical cord prolapse: the effect of team training. BJOG. 2009b;116:1089–1096. Available from: <doi:10.1111/j.1471-0528.2009.02179.x>

38. Shoushtarian M, Barnett M, McMahon M, Ferris J. Impact of introducing practical obstetric multi-professional training (PROMPT) into maternity units in Victoria, Australia. BJOG. 2014;121(13):1710–1718. Available from: <doi:10.1111/1471-0528.12767>

39. Noblot E, Raia-Barjat T, Lajeunesse C, Trombert B, Weiss S, Colombié M, et al. Training program for the management of two obstetric emergencies within a French perinatal care network. Eur J Obstet Gynecol Reprod Biol. 2015 June:101–105. Available from: <doi:10.1016/j.ejogrb.2015.03.019>

40. van der Nelson HA, Siassakos D, Bennett J, Godfrey M, Spray L, Draycott T, Donald F. Multiprofessional team simulation training, based on an obstetric model, can improve teamwork in other areas of health care. Am J Med Qual Official J Am Coll Med Qual. 2014;29(1):78–82. Available from: <doi:10.1177/1062860613485281>

41. Draycott TJ, Crofts JF, Ash JP, Wilson LV, Yard E, Sibanda T, et al. Improving neonatal outcome through practical shoulder dystocia training. Obstet Gynecol. 2008;112(1):14–20. Available from: <doi:10.1097/AOG.0b013e31817bbc61>

42. Royal College of Obstetricians and Gynaecologists RCOG. Green-top guideline no. 42 shoulder dystocia. 2nd ed. London: RCOG; 2012a. [Accessed 3 August 2023]. Available from: www.rcog.org.uk/media/ewgpnmio/gtg_42.pdf

43. Deneckere S, Euwema M, Van Herck P, Lodewijckx C, Panella M, Sermeus W, et al. Care pathways lead to better teamwork: results of a systematic review. Soc Sci Med. 2012;75(2):264–268. Available from: <doi:10.1016/j.socscimed.2012.02.060>

44. Deneckere S, Euwema M, Lodewijckx C, Panella M, Mutsvari T, Sermeus W, et al. Better interprofessional teamwork, higher level of organized care, and lower risk of burnout in acute healthcare teams using

care pathways: a cluster randomized controlled trial. Medical Care. 2013;51(1):99–107. Available from: <doi:10.1097/MLR.0b013e3182763312>

45. European Pathway Association. Clinical care pathways. n.d. [Accessed 3 August 2023]. Available from: www.e-p-a.org/clinical-care-pathways/index.html

46. Vanhaecht K, De Witte K, Sermeus W. The impact of clinical pathways on the organisation of care processes. PhD dissertation, Katholieke Universiteit Leuven; 2007.

47. Daniels R, Nutbeam T, McNamara G, Galvin C. The sepsis six and the severe sepsis resuscitation bundle: a prospective observational cohort study. Emergency Medicine Journal. 2011;28(6):459–460. Available from: <doi:10.1136/emj.2010.095067>

48. Miller RR, Dong L, Nelson NC, Brown SM, Kuttler KG, Probst DR, et al. Multicenter implementation of a severe sepsis and septic shock treatment bundle. American Journal of Respiratory and Critical Care Medicine. 2013;188(1):77–82 Available from: <doi:10.1164/rccm.201212-2199OC>

49. UK Sepsis Trust. Clinical tools. 2021. [Accessed 3 August 2023]. Available from: https://sepsistrust.org/professional-resources/clinical-tools/

50. Royal College of Obstetricians and Gynaecologists. Green-top guideline no. 64a: bacterial sepsis in pregnancy. 2012b. [Accessed 3 August 2023]. Available from: www.rcog.org.uk/media/ea1p1r4h/gtg_64a.pdf

51. Royal College of Obstetricians and Gynaecologists. Green-top guideline no. 64b: bacterial sepsis following pregnancy. 2012c. [Accessed 3 August 2023]. Available from: www.rcog.org.uk/media/bfnkzznd/gtg_64b.pdf

52. Churchill D, Rodger A, Clift J, Tuffnell D, On Behalf of the MBRRACE-UK Sepsis Chapter Writing Group. Think sepsis. In: Knight M, Kenyon S, Brocklehurst P, Neilson J, Shakespeare J, Kurinczuk JJ, On Behalf of MBRRACE-UK, editors. Saving lives, improving mothers' care – lessons learned to inform future maternity care from the UK and Ireland confidential enquiries into maternal deaths and morbidity 2009–12.

Oxford: National Perinatal Epidemiology Unit, University of Oxford, 2014. p. 27–43.

53. Agency for Healthcare Research and Quality. Labor and delivery: cross monitoring: team STEPPS training video. Rockville, MD; Oct 2014. [Accessed 3 August 2023]. Available from: www.ahrq.gov/professionals/education/curriculum-tools/teamstepps/instructor/videos/ts_ld crossmon/crossMonitorIntern.html

54. Kingdon C, Neilson J, Singleton V, Gyte G, Hart A, Gabbay M, Lavender T. Choice and birth method: mixed-method study of caesarean delivery for maternal request. BJOG. 2009;116(7):886–895 Available from: <doi:10.1111/j.1471-0528.2009.02119.x>

55. National Patient Safety Agency and National Reporting and Learning Service. Being open – communicating patient safety incidents with patients, their families and carers. London: NPSA/NRLS; 2009. [Accessed 3 August 2023]. Available from: www.nrls.npsa.nhs.uk/

56. Mapp T, Hudson K. Feelings and fears during obstetric emergencies – 1. British Journal of Midwifery. 2005;13(1):30–35. Available from: <doi:10.12968/bjom.2005.13.1.17319>

57. Department of Health/NHS Commissioning Board. Compassion in practice: nursing, midwifery and care staff: our vision and strategy. London: Crown Copyright; 2012. [Accessed 3 August 2023]. Available from: www.england.nhs.uk/wp-content/uploads/2012/12/compassion-in-practice.pdf

58. Care Quality Commission (CQC). National findings from the 2017 survey of women's experiences of maternity care. 2018. [Accessed 3 August 2023]. Available from: www.cqc.org.uk/news/stories/most-women-report-better-experiences-maternity-care

59. Data Protection Act. Meaning of 'accessible record'. 1998. [Accessed 24 September 2023]. Available from: www.legislation.gov.uk/ukpga/1998/29/section/68

60. Andrews A, O'Malley M. The ball's in your court. Midwives. 2009;12(5):24–25. PMID: 24902241.

61. Crofts JF, Bartlett C, Ellis D, Fox R, Draycott TJ. Documentation of simulated shoulder

dystocia: accurate and complete? BJOG. 2008;115(10):1303–3018. Available from: <doi:10.1111/j.1471-0528.2008.01801.x>

62. Deering S, Poggi S, Hodor J, Macedonia C, Satin AJ. Evaluation of residents' delivery notes after a simulated shoulder dystocia. Obstetrics & Gynecology. 2004;104:667–670. Available from: <doi:10.1097/01.AOG.0000137347.94987.01>

63. Sheen K, Slade P, Spiby H. An integrative review of the impact of indirect trauma exposure in health professionals and potential issues of salience for midwives. Journal of Advanced Nursing. 2014;70(4):729–743. Available from: <doi:10.1111/jan.12274>

64. National Health Service (NHS) England. Confidentiality policy. 2014. [Accessed 3 August 2023]. Available from: www.england.nhs.uk/wp-content/uploads/2013/06/conf-policy-1.pdf

65. Nursing Midwifery Council. Guidance on using social media responsibly. London: NMC; 2015b. [Accessed 3 August 2023]. Available from: www.nmc.org.uk/globalassets/sitedocuments/nmc-publications/social-media-guidance-30-march-2015-final.pdf

2

Legal issues in emergency care

ANNE O'LOGHLEN-PINION AND KATE NASH

Introduction	18	Intrapartum and emergency care	26
Protected title and function of the midwife	18	Capacity	27
Defining law	18	Rights of the fetus	28
Human rights and the Human Rights Act 1998	19	Conclusion	28
Accountability	21	Further reading and resources	29
Duty of care, negligence and liability	22	References	29
Informed consent	23		

BOX 2.1: Definitions

Informed consent "is the intentional communication process where benefits, risks and alternatives of a treatment or procedure are disclosed (a right to know) allowing independent acceptance or rejection by patients on the basis of their own preferences, personal values or goals".[1]

Autonomy can be defined as the right to 'self-determination' or the right to make one's own choices.[2] A woman has control over her own body and makes her own decisions about medical treatment.[3]

Paternalism is the opposite of autonomy; a medical practitioner advises or decides what is best without concern for the woman's wishes or feelings.[4]

Coercion is when one person communicates to another that there will be negative consequences if that second person pursues a particular course of action.[5]

Capacity- A person must be assumed to have capacity unless it is established that they lack capacity. A person lacks capacity if they are unable to make a decision for themselves in relation to the matter because of an impairment or a disturbance in the functioning of the mind or brain.[6]

Negligence is a legal mechanism when an action or failure of a health care professional to act causes harm to a person.[4] If a woman is not informed of the risks of complications and if one or more arises, a case of negligence can be brought.[7]

Trespass or battery is when a competent adult refuses treatment and is overridden[2] or when consent is coerced, presumed or provided without information, the consent is invalid and treatments/interventions should not take place. Trespass to a person can be termed a 'tort'.[4]

Clinical Governance- Healthcare is controlled and influenced by the government, and Parliament has direct control over NHS England.[8,4]

INTRODUCTION

Midwives must practice within an ethical and legal framework at all times and can be held to account for what they do and fail to do. This chapter will provide an overview of the general principles of the law relevant to healthcare before considering the associated legal issues that midwives must be cognisant of in relation to emergencies around childbirth.

As a registered midwife, you are legally and professionally accountable for your actions, irrespective of whether you are following the instruction of another or are using your own initiative. This is because midwives have a duty of care, meaning they have a legal obligation to provide and demonstrate a minimum standard of acceptable care and behaviours. They should also avoid acts or omissions that could foreseeably harm others in accordance with the law of negligence. Care and treatment must also be based on the law of consent; that is, consent to care should be informed and provided of the person's free will.

There are other legal requirements that midwives must adhere to around equality and human rights. These issues will be explored within this chapter as we consider the complexities that may exist when providing midwifery care during an emergency. A glossary of terms is provided at the start of this chapter, and an overview of resources is provided at the end. Examples and case studies, along with signposting to further reading, will be threaded in throughout the chapter.

PROTECTED TITLE AND FUNCTION OF THE MIDWIFE

The Nursing Midwifery Council (NMC) is the independent regulator for nurses, nursing associates and midwives in the United Kingdom (UK) and maintains the register of professionals eligible to practice. Following successful completion of midwifery training, students must apply to gain entry to the Midwifery Register held by the NMC before they can practice as a midwife. This is a legal requirement as midwives must be registered before they can legally practice as a midwife.

This is because Midwifery is a protected function in the UK, meaning it's a criminal offence for any person other than a registered midwife or a registered medical practitioner to provide care to people in childbirth, except in emergencies or when in training as a student midwife or medical student. It's also a criminal offence for someone to falsely represent themselves as being a registered midwife and use the protected title of 'Midwife', or falsely represent themselves as possessing midwifery qualifications.

As well as the title and function of the role of the midwife being protected by law, midwives themselves must provide assurance that they are of good character, and are required to notify the NMC of any convictions or cautions they receive. Student midwives are obliged to inform their Education Institute and also sign an annual declaration of good character as a student.[9] Further information is available in Box 2.2.

DEFINING LAW

Law can be defined as a system of rules of a particular country, group, or area of activity, usually made by the government, that are used to order the way in which a society behaves.[10] Underpinning this definition is the notion of a legal system that supports the creation and implementation of the law, alongside the implementation of compliance with the rules that are laid down by the law. Whilst ethical

---

BOX 2.2: Governing legislation of the Nursing and Midwifery Council, the regulatory body of midwives, nurses and nursing associates

As the independent regulator for nurses, midwives and nursing associates, the NMC has a set of governing legislation. The main legislation is the Nursing and Midwifery Order 2001 ('the Order'), a series of orders made by the Privy Council and Rules made by our Council sit underneath the Order.

Further information about the legislation that governs the NMC can be found on their website: Our legislation – The Nursing and Midwifery Council (nmc.org.uk)

Further information about declaring criminal convictions and cautions to the NMC can be found on their website Criminal convictions and cautions – The Nursing and Midwifery Council (nmc.org.uk).

principles and the law are often intertwined, they are inherently different as the law refers to rules of conduct which are prescribed by an authority such as a society or community, whereas ethics refer to moral principles or a set of values.

Types of law

Legislation is made up of Acts of Parliament (Statute law) and Case law, otherwise known as Common law. An Act of Parliament includes Acts such as the Equality Act (2010)[11] and the Health and Social Care Act[12] (2012). Statutory law results from a bill or proposal for a statute and usually starts with a dilemma or problem followed by consultation and debate. Once debated and approved by the House of Commons and House of Lords, it is ready to receive royal assent. This is when the King formally agrees to make the bill into an Act of Parliament, and it becomes law[4,13].

Case law or Common law refers to a law that is developed through decisions made by the court rather than by relying solely on statutes or regulations. Common or Case law is an important source of law influencing healthcare and has evolved from legal cases whose outcomes shape the course of subsequent decisions. An example of case law is presented in Box 2.3, which shows how the case should introduce a new principle or develop an existing statute to become case law.[4]

Human rights are also protected by common law and decisions that have been passed in the law courts in the United Kingdom (UK) throughout the years. This is particularly important in the areas of clinical negligence and consent. The right to autonomy and the requirement for health professionals to seek informed consent is a fundamental part of the law of negligence.[15] The UK has also signed up to the Convention on the Elimination of all Forms of Discrimination against Women.[16]

HUMAN RIGHTS AND THE HUMAN RIGHTS ACT 1998

The Human Rights Act[17] is the main law protecting human rights and freedoms in the UK and is derived from the European Convention on Human Rights (ECHR). The UK law has adopted 16 of the key rights (Articles) from the convention and made them enforceable by law.[18] The values of human rights are grounded in the idea that all humans are born free and are equally worthy of respect.[19,20] Autonomy, respect, dignity and equity are fundamental human rights principles[21] creating a legal foundation that forms the provision of individualised and high-quality care. These principles are central to midwifery practice and are enshrined within the Code[22] and NHS Constitution, forming the basis of personalised maternity care.[23] The Code[22] sets out the fundamental principles that must underpin everything a midwife does, providing the professional benchmark for midwifery practice alongside the NMC Standards of Proficiency for Midwives.[24]

The Human Rights Act places a legal duty on all public officials, including health services, to uphold standards by ensuring that human rights are respected in everything they do.[18] All legislation, including health and social care law, should be compatible with human rights or be 'human rights compliant', and services should be designed and applied in a way that respects, protects and fulfils human rights.[25]

BOX 2.3: St. George's Healthcare Trust, v S (1998)

A court of appeal reviewed the case of a woman with severe pre-eclampsia who had declined an Induction of Labour (IOL) at 36 weeks gestation. The IOL was considered lifesaving and the woman was unlawfully detained under the Mental Health Act 1983 because of her decision to decline an IOL and subsequent caesarean section. Whereas a previous court had authorised the Trust to perform a caesarean without the woman's consent, the appeal outcome emphasised that competent pregnant women have the right to decide whether they undertake medical treatment. This is evidenced in the citation which follows, and further detail can be found at www.global healthrights.org/wp-

A woman "is entitled not to be forced to submit to an invasion of her body against her will, whether her own life or that of her unborn child depends on it"[14] (Judge L.J.).

A human rights approach is built into the Care Quality Commission (CQC), whose core purpose is to respect diversity, promote equality and ensure everyone receives safe and good quality care.[26] This approach is supported by the Equality Act,[11] which seeks to eliminate discrimination and advance equality of opportunity. Although the Human Rights Act and CQC provide a solid legal and regulatory framework to work within, evidence of suboptimal care, including a reported lack of dignity and respect, still exists within maternity care.[20,27,28]

An overview of the key principles of the Human Rights Act and how they can be applied to midwifery practice is provided in Table 2.1. This has been adapted from the British Institute of Human Rights' *Midwifery and human rights: a practitioners guide*.[25,15]

Human Rights principles and legislation are entrenched within maternity care and midwifery practice. It is vital that midwives and maternity healthcare professionals appreciate how human rights legislation informs and influences their practise and the responsibilities it imposes on them whilst working in healthcare settings.

Table 2.1 Applying the Human Rights Act to midwifery practice (adapted from the British Institute of Human Rights' *Midwifery and human rights: a practitioners guide*)

Article 2 – Protects the right to life

- Good quality maternity care provision will anticipate and prevent risk to life.
- When women's choices are not accommodated, they may choose to have an unassisted birth which could pose a risk to life. Midwives and maternity professionals should support women in their decision making, including when choices are made outside of the guidelines.
- An unborn baby does not have the right to life. Women and birthing people are responsible for the choices and decisions made in childbirth.

Link to practice: all women have a right to access life-saving maternity services. Women should not be denied access to care based on their immigration status and should not be charged for their care at the point of access and especially in an emergency situation. Women should be informed that maternity care will not be withheld, regardless of their ability to pay. Confidential Enquiries remind us of the importance of equitable care.

Article 3 – Right to be free from inhuman and degrading treatment

- Gaining informed consent- and the right to physical autonomy and integrity. No medical treatment can be carried out without consent (also links to Article 8).
- Failing to give sufficient, objective and unbiased information for someone to make an informed choice, including not providing adequate interpreting services will also violate Article 8.

Link to practice: midwives must assess and respond to the need for timely pain relief during and after childbirth, including in an emergency situation, and to monitor the effects of pain relief when provided. This would include effectiveness and side effects.

Article 8 – Right to respect for private and family life, home and correspondence

- Supporting choice.
- Protecting privacy.
- Involving and supporting birth partners and family members.
- Ensuring women who do not speak English can understand and are able to participate in care.

Link to practice: women have the legal right to choose their place of birth. It is the professional duty of all midwives to attend a birth at home even if they don't agree with the decision. A full discussion of the risks and benefits (without coercion) should take place, formulating in a care plan.

(Continued)

Table 2.1 *(Continued)* Applying the Human Rights Act to midwifery practice (adapted from the British Institute of Human Rights' *Midwifery and human rights: a practitioners guide*)

Article 9 – The right to freedom of thought, conscience and religion

- Choices based on beliefs such as preferences about the birth partner, the birth environment and the gender of health professionals in attendance.

Link to practice: a woman may decline a blood transfusion in life-threatening circumstances due to a religious conviction -this may be the case of a Jehovah Witness.

Article 14 – Prohibits discrimination in the application of other human rights and entitles people to equal treatment in their maternity care

- Entitles people to equal treatment in their maternity care.
- It is unlawful to discriminate on the grounds of disability, race, religion, immigration status and national origin. In addition, the Equality Act,[11] protects people against discrimination and harassment.
- Midwives should consider their unconscious bias, avoid assumptions and use preferred pronouns.

Link to practice: a woman with a disability may require the opportunity to tour a birth environment and be given the opportunity to get in and out of a birth pool to see what extra support might be needed to ensure an optimum and non-discriminatory labour experience.

ACCOUNTABILITY

To be accountable is to be answerable for what you do and fail to do, which is the approach adopted by the Nursing Midwifery Council. As a midwife, you have a duty of care and legal liability to those in your care. When delegating an activity, for example, to a maternity support worker or student, you must ensure that it has been appropriately delegated.[22] Employers also have a duty to ensure their staff are trained and supervised properly until they are competent. Under contract law, employers must pay any damages for negligence liability through the principle of vicarious liability; that is, employers are liable for the negligent actions or omissions of their employees during the course of their employment.[29]

As a midwife, you are accountable to your profession and professional standards. The professional standards that nurses, midwives and nursing associates must uphold in order to be registered to practise in the UK are presented in The Code,[22] which also stipulates that you keep to the laws of the country in which you are practising.

Furthermore, the NMC specifies that you should:

- only delegate tasks and duties that are within the other person's competence
- make sure that everyone they delegate tasks to is adequately supervised and supported
- confirm that the outcome of any task they have delegated to someone else meets the required standard.[22]

As a midwife, you are accountable for your actions to a range of authorities that you have a legal relationship with and to whom you must justify your actions.

An overview of the four spheres of accountability in midwifery practice is presented in Figure 2.1:[30]

Difficulties may occur when there is a conflict of interest between these parties, putting the midwife in a precarious position. Under human rights law, all Trusts and their employees are obliged to respect women's decisions in childbirth and cannot compel a woman to receive care in a hospital. Challenges may occur, however, when midwives are not permitted to attend a homebirth due to staffing issues. Midwives may find themselves in a position where they either disobey their employer and put the woman first or obey their employer

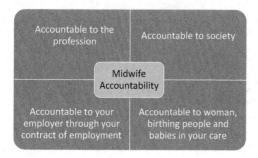

Figure 2.1 Spheres of accountability

and neglect their duty of care. If a midwife does not attend a woman, and the woman or her baby die or suffer harm as a consequence, there is a risk that the Trust could have breached Article 2 of the European Convention on Human Rights, the right to life.[15] In these situations, midwives must escalate their concerns, ensure this is documented and communicate with the woman and local ambulance services as per local guidance/policy.

DUTY OF CARE, NEGLIGENCE AND LIABILITY

Duty of care refers to the obligations placed on people to act towards others in a certain way, in accordance with certain standards. The law imposes a duty of care on healthcare practitioners in conditions where it is reasonably foreseeable that the practitioner might cause harm to patients through their actions or omissions.[29] These obligations prevail when the practitioner has assumed some sort of responsibility for the person's care, which can be basic personal care or a complex procedure.[29]

To execute their legal duty of care, healthcare practitioners must act in accordance with the relevant standard of care, usually deemed to be the standard expected of an ordinarily competent practitioner performing that particular role or task. Failure to implement the duty to the relevant standard may be regarded as negligence. When a person receiving care suffers harm, the law examines who has a duty of care to that person and whether there was negligence in order to attribute responsibility and liability for that harm.

Midwives and maternity healthcare professionals have a duty of care towards the woman and her baby. Actions to ensure safety and quality of care include information giving, shared decision making, gaining informed consent, keeping clear and accurate documentation, medicines management, carrying out midwifery procedures competently and appropriate delegation of tasks to other staff as well as applying the duty of candour principles.[31,32]

Obstetric-related incidents can be catastrophic and lifechanging, spanning the course of the lifespan of a newborn and causing lifelong trauma to those involved. The Clinical Negligence Scheme for Trusts (CNST) handles all clinical negligence claims against member National Health Service (NHS) bodies. Whilst membership in the scheme is voluntary, all Trusts in England belong to the scheme, which is under the auspices of NHS Resolution, formerly known as the NHS Litigation Authority. NHS Resolution provides expertise to the NHS on resolving concerns and disputes and providing compensation payments with the aim of sharing learning for improvement and preserving resources for patient care. A strategic priority of NHS Resolution is to collaborate with maternity services through schemes such as the early notification scheme (provides a faster and more caring response to families whose babies have suffered harm) and maternity incentive scheme (if Trusts meet ten safety actions, they recover an element of their contribution to the CNST).[33]

Obstetric-related claims represent the CNST's biggest area of spending. If a woman or baby is harmed during pregnancy or childbirth through clinical negligence, a claim for personal injury compensation may be made. Recent data from 2021–2022 reveals that obstetric claims represented 12% of total clinical claims in number; however, they accounted for 62% of the total value of all new claims at a cost of almost £6 billion (See Figure 2.2). Findings also suggest that whilst the number of claims has increased in recent years, 77% of these claims are resolved outside of court with less than 1% of claims resulting in a full court trial. Claims that result in court proceedings tend to result in a judgement in favour of the NHS. Often, litigants want an apology or an explanation rather than damages,[34] which is closely related to the duty of candour and dispute resolution strategies, such as mediation, that are now much more commonplace.[33] Compensation payments are made to meet the expenses that occurred as a result of injury, including loss of earnings, and in recognition of the pain and suffering experienced by an individual.[35]

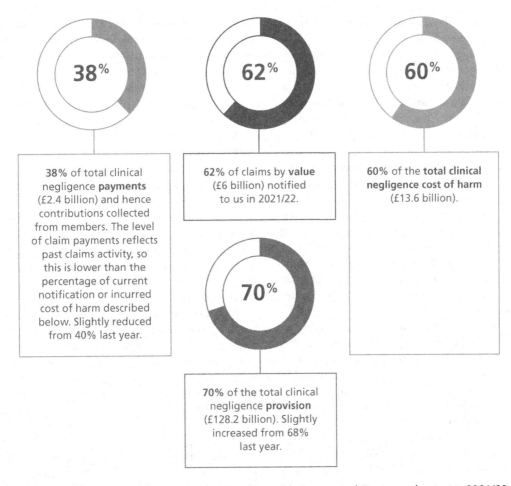

Figure 2.2 Maternity statistics taken from the NHS Resolution annual report and account 2021/22: NHS Resolution Annual report and accounts 2021/22

Findings from National Reviews have revealed that incivility and poor teamworking contribute to poor outcomes within maternity care, often through a range of factors that include a lack of teamworking and failure to recognise the need to escalate or to escalate appropriately when things go wrong.[27,36] Effective teamwork is vital for the provision of safe, effective and personalised care, particularly during an emergency where human factors such as lack of situational awareness, poor communication and inadequate leadership in a rapidly deteriorating clinical situation put women and babies at particular risk.

A consistent recommendation is that improvements in safety and quality of maternity care require more effective teamwork and the transformation of sometimes dysfunctional working cultures and wider infrastructure within organisations.[37] NHS Resolution, along with other key government reports, calls for ensuring a just and learning culture for all staff and patients following incidents within the NHS, which facilitates an open environment and learning from when things go wrong.[33,38]

INFORMED CONSENT

Informed consent is a legal requirement and ethical imperative in all circumstances, including during emergency care. This principle reflects the right for women to determine what happens to their own bodies and is a fundamental requirement of midwifery practice as set out within the NMC Code[22] as well as a legal requirement. A healthcare professional (or other healthcare staff) who does not respect this principle may be liable to legal action by the person who uses services and to action by their professional body.

While there is no English statute setting out the general principles of consent, consent is based on legal principles that are laid down in human rights legislation, case law and standards of professional conduct.[5] Case law has established that treating a patient without valid consent may constitute the civil or criminal offence of trespass or battery. Furthermore, if healthcare professionals (or other healthcare staff) fail to obtain appropriate consent and the person who uses services subsequently suffers harm as a result of treatment, this may be a factor in a claim of negligence against the healthcare professional/employer involved, constituting in a civil offence of assault or a criminal offence, and it is a breach of the duty of care and the professional code of conduct leading to professional malpractice.

Midwives are integral to the consent-giving process and will often be best placed to judge the extent to which the woman has understood, digested and deliberated upon the information provided.[39,40] Midwives have a legal duty to respect, protect and fulfil the legal right to make informed and autonomous decisions throughout the childbirth continuum, even if the decisions appear to be unwise to healthcare professionals (see Table 2.2).[35]

Consent may be considered invalid or fraudulent if there is evidence that manipulation, coercion or paternalism has been used by the midwife or healthcare professional to gain consent.[4] Women may perceive communication as threatening or unreasonable, particularly when decisions need to be made in a timely manner, such as within an emergency situation.[41] Any treatment, procedure or intervention should be *offered* to facilitate the option of voluntary acceptance or *the opportunity to decline* the offered intervention.[5]

The Royal College of Obstetricians and Gynaecologists (RCOG)[42] provides a useful summary of the key principles for obtaining valid informed consent, which is adapted and outlined within Box 2.4.

Montgomery v Lanarkshire Health Board 2015

Montgomery v Lanarkshire is a landmark case concerning informed consent which emphasises a woman's right to autonomy in decision-making during pregnancy and childbirth. See Box 2.5 for an overview of this case.

The Montgomery case shifts the law away from the conventional test for clinical negligence, known as the Bolam principle, based on the Bolam test, towards a more holistic, person-focused approach.[43,44,45] A summary of the Bolam Test is provided in Box 2.6. The Bolam test was established in 1957 after a judge ruled that the doctor was not negligent as they provided treatment in a manner considered appropriate by other doctors within the same medical field. The Bolam principle is used to establish whether a duty of care has been breached by demonstrating whether the care provided aligned with the opinion of experts within the field.

Whereas the Bolam Principles set out to establish via expert professional opinion whether negligence occurred due to a breach in duty of care, more recent cases such as the Montgomery v Lanarkshire

Table 2.2 Overview of the NMC Code and requirements for informed consent

NMC The Code[22]
Prioritise people
2   Listen to people and respond to their preferences and concerns. To achieve this, you must:
2.5 Respect, support and document a person's right to accept or refuse care and treatment.
4   Act in the best interests of people at all times. To achieve this, you must:
4.1 Balance the need to act in the best interests of people at all times with the requirement to respect a person's right to accept or refuse treatment.
4.2 Make sure that you get properly informed consent and document it before carrying out any action.
7   Communicate clearly. To achieve this, you must:
7.1 Use terms that people in your care, colleagues and the public can understand.

BOX 2.4: Principles of valid consent, adapted from the RCOG[42]

The person who uses services must have *capacity* to make an informed decision; that is, they must be:

- considered competent to give consent
- able to understand information provided
- can communicate their decision.

Consent must be provided *voluntarily:*

- in most cases, the decision to provide or withhold consent should be made by the people who use services themselves
- the person who uses services should not be coerced or influenced by carers, family or friends.

The person who uses services should be *fully informed* of the following by carers with enough time allowed to reflect and ask questions about the following:

- benefits and risks of the intended procedure
- alternative management strategies
- implications of not undergoing the proposed treatment.

BOX 2.5: Overview of the Montgomery v Lanarkshire Health Board Case

Montgomery was an insulin-dependent diabetic pregnant woman, predicted to give birth to a large baby (> 4kg). Montgomery's obstetrician chose not to disclose the increased risk (9–10%) of shoulder dystocia associated with diabetes, a large baby and a vaginal birth. There was no discussion around alternatives such as a caesarean birth despite Montgomery's expressed anxieties, asking if the baby's size would be a problem. There was a shoulder dystocia at birth, and consequently, the baby suffered cerebral palsy. The obstetrician reasoned that if every woman was told about shoulder dystocia, then every woman would want a caesarean, which isn't in the best interests of the woman.

BOX 2.6: Summary of the Bolam Test

The claimant was a voluntary patient at the defendant's mental health hospital who was injured during electro-convulsive therapy. He sued the defendant for negligence, arguing that the doctors had breached their duty of care by not giving him muscle relaxants or manually restraining him. Expert evidence showed that most doctors opposed the use of chemical relaxants. A small portion of competent doctors were also against the use of manual restraints as they thought it heightened the risk of injury.

Bolam v Friern Hospital – Case Summary – IPSA LOQUITUR

BOX 2.7: Key outcomes of the Montgomery Case

MONTGOMERY V LANARKSHIRE HEALTH BOARD 2015
Key outcomes

- The UK Supreme Court affirmed a woman's right to autonomy in childbirth.
- All risks and benefits of any medical procedure need to be explained, understood and consideration of what a reasonable person in that position would be likely to attach significance to the risk, underpinning the concept of shared decision-making.
- The law requires midwives and doctors to respect women's informed choices above what is believed to be best clinical practice.

case (Boxes 2.5 and 2.6) reflect an increasing legal endorsement of the importance of discourses that foster the *autonomy of the person who uses services*. This acts as an ethical counterbalance to what some might perceive to have been unhelpful paternalistic or autocratic professional practices,[46] and the outcomes of the Montgomery case have set the precedent for future cases.

Following the Montgomery ruling, there has been a rise in cases of obstetric negligence involving consent.[47] Specialist training around consent during childbirth and emergencies is especially important due to time constraints, the challenges of providing information in a labour environment and the sensitive nature of intimate examinations (see intrapartum and emergency care section). Practitioners must sensitively balance full disclosure of risks and benefits without overwhelming a woman whilst at the same time avoiding making assumptions or withholding valuable information, which constitutes coercion and/or manipulation. [45,46,48]

Data suggests a deterioration in care over the last five years, with a downward trend reported in those who use our services being treated with kindness, respect, dignity, understanding, information provision, and concerns being listened to during the intrapartum period.[49] Racial inequalities within maternity care have been highlighted recently,[50] and nearly half of women (n=1,340) surveyed in the Black Maternity Experience Survey[51] reported that they did not have pain relief options explained to them or receive the pain relief of their choice with no explanation of why. Women with multiple disadvantages have also reported less positive maternity experiences and outcomes than women without multiple disadvantages.[52,53]

Recent reports have shone a light on racism within maternity services and the association between safety and a culture of maternity care that listens to and respects the preferences and decisions made by women and families.[36,51] Midwives must be proactive in taking steps to identify personal unconscious and implicit bias, recognising that people may resort to prejudices and assumptions in acute or pressurised situations. It is vital that midwives are alert to this and challenge unacceptable behaviours and attitudes if encountered during their working lives. Relational-based models of care with a holistic and humanistic approach are strongly indicated to improve women's experiences, improve safety and are firmly in line with a midwife's legal and ethical duties of care provision.

INTRAPARTUM AND EMERGENCY CARE

The physiological process of labour and birth can present barriers to enabling informed consent. Factors such as time constraints, pain and influence of medication may present challenges to information-giving during childbirth.[54,55,46]

Changes can occur rapidly during labour, and time may be limited for detailed discussions and contemplating the alternatives in an emergency situation. Whilst the safety of the mother and baby is crucial, consideration needs to be given to the woman's preferences, consent and information giving. The request for consent is just one of the steps in a more complex path of the decision-making process, and the midwife has a pivotal role as an advocate with supporting the consent process. Ideally, this should be accompanied by a trustful relationship between professionals and women with transparent communication of the best available evidence and discussion of an individual's preferences.[1]

Intimate procedures such as vaginal examinations, often considered routine by practitioners,[40] require explicit consent as evidence suggests women have associated negative experiences and trauma from this procedure.[56,48] Negative perceptions of the consent process in labour and/or during an emergency may also significantly affect current and future childbirth experiences. [57,58]

Episiotomy remains a controversial intervention that is undertaken primarily to expedite birth. Recent findings suggest that often consent for episiotomy does *not* fulfil legal requirements as women report *not* being reliably informed about the procedure to enable consent,[8] with one study reporting a lack of consent in 42% of cases.[58] There was a reported lack of discussion around the risks of episiotomy or the opportunity to decline the procedure, and participants experienced unease, distress and disempowerment as a consequence.[59] The time-critical nature of birth was consistently reported as a barrier to informed consent, and, ideally, the potential for interventions during labour, such as episiotomy, vaginal examinations and interventions during an emergency, should be discussed antenatally as a first stage of consent and again at the point of intervention, providing the opportunity for the right to decline. Birth plans can provide opportunities to make explicit labour and birth preferences. It should be remembered, however, that they are not legal documents, nor do they provide written consent for certain treatments, but they offer an opportunity for information giving and planning. [4,45,58]

Themes of coercion and prioritising of the care provider's agenda not only contravene legal requirements but can also lead to birth trauma[60] and subsequent psychological sequelae. Van der

Table 2.3 Good practice guide – the principles of obtaining consent during labour

Principles of obtaining informed consent during labour
• Be culturally sensitive and approach every encounter with humility and understanding.
• Ask people what their needs are and have an open and non-judgemental attitude.
• Be aware of your unconscious biases and how they might interfere with interactions.[61]
• Ensure an adequate interpreter is present. Do not rely on a family member.[41]
• Remember, sub-optimal communication is high with vulnerable women.[62]
• Choose respectful, professional and neutral language: avoid overly emotive language based on personal preferences or what you believe a woman should do.
• Be aware of power imbalances and discuss risks and benefits without coercion (RCM i-learn; Human rights in maternity care: advocating for women).
• Aim to tailor information depending on the situation and individual instead of providing high quantities of information.[62,63]
• Consider appropriate timing of discussions: in-between contractions and not during procedures.[42]
• Give some time for deliberation where possible.
• Consent may be withheld and/or withdrawn at any time.[64]
• Be an advocate for women and families. Support the woman as she makes her decision, including if you are not acting as the lead caregiver.[65]
• Document the information you have given, the discussion you have had and the care you have provided, and share what is written with the woman.[65]
• Keep the principle of autonomy as a central focus of care and ensure women can decline, consent to care or withdraw consent at any time.[35,41,65]

Pijl et al.[58] argue that whilst consent for procedures in labour is *always* necessary, this consent does not always have to be fully informed but should be explicit at the point of intervening.

In particular, during obstetric emergencies, it may not be possible to disclose all potential risks and complications of those procedures without bias, otherwise known as the "framing effect".[1] This is when clinicians intentionally frame information provided toward the outcome preferred by them. Further research should explore the effectiveness of alternative ways to provide informed consent for emergency procedures that may include timely consultation and better patient information during antenatal care courses.[1]

During an emergency where there is loss of consciousness and no consent can be obtained, treatment should be provided on the basis of necessity; however, exactly what this constitutes is a matter of degree.[7,55] Whilst such 'emergencies' are likely to be exempt from the Montgomery ruling, depending on their nature and timing, complications of labour such as fetal compromise are not.[45] In an emergency, women may be unfamiliar with caregivers, moved to a different environment and may feel coerced to consent to invasive procedures.

A lack of consent in these instances may contribute to associated trauma post-birth.[4]

An overview of the principles of obtaining informed consent during labour and birth is presented in Table 2.3:

CAPACITY

The Mental Health Capacity Act 2005 provides a statutory framework for decision-making concerning adults lacking mental capacity. The act sets out a series of principles that underpin decision-making where a person lacks capacity, and treatment may be given where it is considered in their best interests to do so. It is important to see the person behind the decision to be made and to consider their previous requests, past and present wishes, feelings, beliefs and values that would have been taken into account if they had capacity.[7,66] Key principles of the Mental Capacity Act are outlined in Box 2.8:

A person is assumed to have capacity unless it is established that they lack it. Situations where women decline treatment or refuse to consent to procedures can be emotive for those healthcare professionals involved, particularly if it is

BOX 2.8: Principles of the Mental Capacity Act[6]

- A person must be assumed to have capacity unless it is established that he lacks capacity.
- A person is not to be treated as unable to make a decision unless all practicable steps to help him to do so have been taken without success.
- A person is not to be treated as unable to make a decision merely because he makes an unwise decision.
- An act done or decision made under this Act for or on behalf of a person who lacks capacity must be done or made in his best interests.
- Before the act is done or the decision is made, regard must be had to whether the purpose for which it is needed can be as effectively achieved in a way that is less restrictive of the person's rights and freedom of action.

considered that the wellbeing of the woman, birthing person or fetus is at risk and the principles of autonomy should be kept in mind at all times.[35]

The Mental Capacity Act covers how people who know they may lose their capacity can plan ahead and seek legal representation to make an advance decision. This covers refusals of treatment only and is legally binding. An advance statement can also be made. Advance statements cover a wider range of issues and are not legally binding; however, they can be consulted once the person has lost capacity.[67]

A person's ability to recall information given to them during the consenting process is indicative (although not conclusive) of their capacity at the time that information was given. Prospective studies based on recall of risks of epidural analgesia disclosed during the active labour process and when obtaining informed consent found no significant difference in recall between patients with mild or moderate pain and those with severe pain,[68] and that consent was obtained with a high degree of reliability.[69]

In England and Wales, no other person has the right to consent on behalf of an adult (although it

is good practice to discuss treatment with the family). Therefore, consent or refusal of consent cannot be delegated to the next of kin or other family members.[3,35]

RIGHTS OF THE FETUS

In UK law, the fetus does not have a legally enforceable right to life until it is born.[25] Decisions made in labour are entirely those of the woman and cannot be overridden by health professionals unless the woman is assessed as lacking mental capacity. The majority of women will act in accordance with the desire to protect their unborn child;[18] however, they are free to make choices against medical advice and cannot be forced to accept treatment whether or not it is said to be in their unborn child's interest. This is in accordance with Article 2 of Human Rights Act.[15] It is important that women have access to information to inform their decision, recognising the burden this may also place on them, particularly at times when they are likely to be scared, vulnerable, in pain or simply limited in capacity to absorb information.[48]

CONCLUSION

This chapter has introduced the reader to some of the key principles of the law and considered these in relation to midwifery practice and the management of emergency situations. Midwives are legally and professionally accountable for their actions and their omissions, irrespective of whether they are following the instruction of another or using their own initiative, and have a legal duty of care to those women and babies they provide care for. Informed consent is a legal requirement and ethical imperative in all circumstances, including during emergency care, and case law has established that treating a person without valid consent may constitute the civil or criminal offence of trespass or battery. Midwives have a legal duty to respect, protect and fulfil the right to make informed and autonomous decisions throughout the childbirth continuum, even if the decisions appear to be unwise to healthcare professionals. Often best placed to judge the extent to which the woman has understood, digested and deliberated upon information provided, midwives are integral to the consent-giving process. The time-critical nature of birth has consistently been reported as a barrier to informed consent, and midwives must be proactive in taking steps to identify personal implicit bias, recognising that people may resort to prejudices and assumptions in acute or pressurised situations. Relational-based models of care with a holistic and humanistic approach are strongly indicated to improve women's experiences and improve safety and are firmly in line with a midwife's legal and ethical duties of care provision.

FURTHER READING AND RESOURCES

Further resources for eLearning and relevant websites are provided in what follows:

eLearning

- Human rights in maternity care: advocating for women RCM i-learn module introducing human rights and how it affects maternity care.
- Maternity insights: closing the loop, learning from harm NHS Resolution eLearning module to support clinicians working in maternity services to learn from harm and raise awareness of the early notification scheme.

Websites

- The British Institute of Human Rights BIHR Midwifery and Human Rights: A practitioner's guide.
- Birthrights, a registered charity protecting human rights in childbirth.
- NHS Resolution
- Montgomery v Lanarkshire Health Board
- RCM Informed decision making

REFERENCES

1. Valente EP, Mariani I, Covi B, Lazzerini M. Quality of informed consent practices around the time of childbirth: a cross-sectional study in Italy. Int J Environ Res Public Health. 2022;19:7166. Available from: <doi:10.3390/ijerph19127166>
2. Avery G. Law and ethics in nursing and healthcare: an introduction. 2nd ed. Los Angeles: Sage; 2017. ISBN:978-1-4129-6173-8.
3. Brooks H, Sullivan WJ. The importance of patient autonomy. International Journal of Obstetric Aesthesia. 2002;11:196–203. Available from: <doi:10.1054/ijoa.2002.0958>
4. Clarke E. Law and ethics for midwifery. London: Routledge; 2015. ISBN:9781315691053.
5. McKenzie G. Understanding consent in maternity care: offers, threats, manipulation and force. Practising Midwife. 2021;24(6). Available from: <doi:10.55975/CPPU8540>
6. Mental Capacity Act. 2005. [Accessed 1 July 2023]. www.legislation.gov.uk/ukpga/2005/9/contents
7. McHale J. Consent and the capable adult patient. In: Tingle J, Cribb A, editors. Nursing law and ethics. 4th ed. Chapter 7. Chichester: Wiley Blackwell; 2014.
8. Hodgson J. The legal dimension: legal system and method. In: Tingle J, Cribb A, editors. Nursing law and ethics. 4th ed. Chapter 1. Chichester: Wiley Blackwell; 2014.
9. Nursing and Midwifery Council. Standards for pre-registration midwifery programmes. 2023. [Accessed 7 July 2023]. Available from: www.nmc.org.uk/Standardsforpre-registrationmidwiferyprogrammes-thenursingandmidwiferycouncil
10. Cambridge Dictionary. Dictionaries. Cambridge University Press; 2023. [Accessed 7 July 2023].
11. Government Equalities Office and Equality and Human Rights Commission. Equality act (2010): guidance. 2013. [Accessed 8 September 23]. Available from: www.gov.uk/guidance/equality-act-2010-guidance
12. Health and Social Care Act. 2012. [Accessed 8 September 2023]. Available from: www.legislation.gov.uk/HealthandSocialCareAct2012
13. UK Parliament. What is an act of parliament? 2023. [Accessed 7 September 2023].
14. Global Health & Human Rights Database. St. George's healthcare NHS trust v. S | Global health & human rights database. 2024. [Accessed 14 March 2024]. Available from: globalhealthrights.org
15. Birthrights. Human rights in maternity care: the key facts. Human rights

in maternity care: the key facts. 2017. [Accessed 1 June 2023]. Available from: www.birthrights.org.uk/factsheets/human-rights-in-maternity-care/

16. Birthrights. Human rights in maternity care: the key facts. 2023. [Accessed 1 June 2023]. Available from: https://birthrights.org.uk/factsheets/human-rights-in-maternity-care/

17. UK Public General Acts. Human Rights Act. 1998. [Accessed 17 July 2023]. www.legislation.gov.uk/ukpga/1998/42/contents

18. Schiller R. Why human rights in childbirth matter. London: Pinter & Martin; 2018.

19. Prochaska E. Human rights in maternity care. Midwifery. 2015;31(11):1015–1016. [Accessed 1 July 2023]. Available from: https://doi-org.ezproxy.uwe.ac.uk/10.1016/j.midw.2015.09.006

20. Ham L. Human rights in childbearing 1: basic human rights and their application in childbearing. Practising Midwife. 2022;25(8):14–17. Available from: <doi:10.55975/EKQN7825>

21. Philbin N, Schiller R. Progressive understanding of human rights in maternity care: from individual rights to systemic issues. In: Downe S, Byrom, S, editors. Squaring the circle. Chapter 7. London: Pinter & Martin; 2021.

22. Nursing and Midwifery Council. The code: professional standards of practice and behaviour for nurses, midwives and nursing associates. 2018. [Accessed 9 July 2023]. Available from: https://www.nmc.org.uk/standards/code/

23. NHS England. Three year delivery plan for maternity and neonatal services. 2023. [Accessed 9 July 2023]. Available from: https://www.england.nhs.uk/wp-content/uploads/2023/03/B1915-three-year-delivery-plan-for-maternity-and-neonatal-services-march-2023.pdf

24. Nursing and Midwifery Council. Standards of proficiency for midwives. 2019. [Accessed 7 July 2023]. Available from: https://www.nmc.org.uk/globalassets/sitedocuments/standards/standards-of-proficiency-for-midwives.pdf

25. British Institute of Human Rights. Midwifery and human rights: a practitioner's guide. 2016. [Accessed 1 June 2023]. Available

from: www.bihr.org.uk/media/14cgvytg/guide_midwifery-human-rights-practitioners-guide.pdf

26. Care Quality Commission, CQC. Our human rights approach for how we regulate health and social care services. 2019. [Accessed 17 July 2023]. Available from: https://www.cqc.org.uk/about-us/our-updated-human-rights-approach

27. Ockenden D. Ockenden report final. 2022. [Accessed 1 July 2023]. Available from: https://assets.publishing.service.gov.uk/government/uploads/system/uploads/attachment_data/file/1064302/Final-Ockenden-Report-web-accessible.pdf

28. Kirkup B. Reading the signals maternity and neonatal services in East Kent – the report of the independent investigation. 2022. [Accessed 17 July 2023] Available from: https://assets.publishing.service.gov.uk/government/uploads/system/uploads/attachment_data/file/1111992/reading-the-signals-maternity-and-neonatal-services-in-east-kent_the-report-of-the-independent-investigation_print-ready.pdf

29. Royal College of Nursing. Accountability and delegation. 2023. [Accessed 7 July 2023]. Available from: https://www.rcn.org.uk/Professional-Development/Accountability-and-delegation

30. Griffith R, Tengnah C, Patel C. Law and professional issues in midwifery (transforming midwifery practice series). Los Angeles: Sage Publications; 2013.

31. Dimond B. Legal aspects of midwifery. 4th ed. London: Quay Books; 2013.

32. Nursing and Midwifery Council. The professional duty of candour. 2022. [Accessed 1 July 2023]. Available from: https://www.gmc-uk.org/professional-standards/professional-standards-for-doctors/candour-openness-and-honesty-when-things-go-wrong/the-professional-duty-of-candour#:~:text=Every%20health%20and%20care%20professional,to%20cause%2C%20harm%20or%20distress

33. NHS Resolution. Being fair Supporting a just and learning culture for staff and patients following incidents in the NHS. 2022. Available from: https://resolution.nhs.uk/resources/being-fair-report/

34. Foster C. The legal perspective. In: Tingle J, Cribb A, editors. Nursing law and ethics. 4th ed. Chapter 6. Negligence. Chichester: Wiley Blackwell; 2014.

35. Gillman L, Petrocnik P. Legal issues relating to midwifery education and practice. In: Marshall J, editor. Myles professional studies for Midwifery education and practice: concepts and challenges. Chapter 7. London: Elsevier; 2019.

36. Ockenden D. Emerging findings and recommendations from the independent review of maternity services at the Shrewsbury and Telford hospital NHS trust. 2020. [Accessed 1 July 2023]. Available from: https://www.donnaockenden.com/downloads/news/2020/12/ockenden-report.pdf

37. Harris J, Beck S, Ayers N, Bick D, Lamb B, Aref-Adib MT, et al. Improving teamwork in maternity services: a rapid review of interventions. Midwifery. 2022;108. ISSN:0266-6138. Available from: <doi:10.1016/j.midw.2022.103285>

38. Williams N. Gross negligence manslaughter in healthcare: the report of a rapid policy review. 2018. [Accessed 1 July 2023]. Available from: https://assets.publishing.service.gov.uk/government/uploads/system/uploads/attachment_data/file/717946/Williams_Report.pdf

39. Farsides B. An ethical perspective-consent and patient autonomy. In: Tingle J, Cribb A, editors. Nursing law and ethics. 4th Ed. Chapter 7B. Chichester: Wiley Blackwell; 2014.

40. Lee N, Kearney L, Shipton E, Hawley G, Winters-Chang P, Kilgour C, et al. Consent during labour and birth as observed by midwifery students: a mixed methods study. Women Birth. 2023;36(6):e574–e581. Available from: <doi:10.1016/j.wombi.2023.02.005>

41. Golden P. Coercion or consent? British Journal of Midwifery. 2018;26(7):482–483. Available from: https://doi-org.ezproxy.uwe.ac.uk/10.12968/bjom.2018.26.7.482

42. Royal College of Obstetricians and Gynaecologists. Obtaining valid consent. 2015, [Accessed 1 July 2023]. Available from: https://rcog.org.uk/guidance/browse-all-guidance/clinical-governance-advice/obtaining-valid-consent-clinical-governance-advice-no-6/

43. Bolton H. The Montgomery ruling extends patient autonomy. BJOG. 2014:1273.

44. Farrell AM, Brazier M. Not so new directions in the law of consent? Examining Montgomery v Lanarkshire health board. Journal of Medical Ethics. [online]. 2016;42(2):85–88. Available from: <doi:10.1136/medethics-2015-102861>

45. Chan SW, Tulloch E, Cooper ES, Smith A, Wojcik W, Norman JE. Montgomery and informed consent: where are we now? BMJ. [Online]. 2017;357:j2224. [Accessed 7 July 2023]. Available from: https://doi.org.ezproxy.uwe.ac.uk/10.1136/bmj.j2224

46. Nicholls J, David AL, Iskaros J, Lanceley A. Patient-centred consent in women's health: does it really work in antenatal and intrapartum care? BMC Pregnancy Childbirth. 2022;22:156. Available from: <doi:10.1186/s12884-022-04493-6>

47. Wald DS, Bestwick JP, Kelly P. The effect of the montgomery judgement on settled claims against the national health service due to failure to inform before giving consent to treatment. Int J Med. 2020;113(10):721–725. Available from: https://doi-org.ezproxy.uwe.ac.uk/10.1093/qjmed/hcaa082

48. Kingma E. Harming one to benefit another: the paradox of autonomy and consent in maternity care. Bioethics. 2021;35:456–464. Available from: <doi:10.1111/bioe.12852>

49. CQC. Maternity survey 2022. 2023a. [Accessed 17 July 2023]. Available from: www.cqc.org.uk/publication/surveys/maternity-survey-2022

50. Knight M, Bunch K, Patel R, Shakespeare J, Kotnis R, Kenyon S, Kurinczuk JJ, On behalf of MBRRACE-UK, editors. Saving lives, improving mothers' care core report – lessons learned to inform maternity care from the UK and Ireland Confidential Enquiries into Maternal Deaths and Morbidity 2018–20. Oxford: National Perinatal Epidemiology Unit, University of Oxford; 2022.

51. Peter M, Wheeler R. The Black maternity experiences survey a nationwide study of Black women's experiences of maternity services in the United Kingdom. 2022.

[Accessed 9 July 2023]. Available from: www.squarespace.com/The+Black+Maternity+Experience+Report.pdf

52. Rayment-Jones H, Harris J, Harden A, Khan Z, Sandall J. How do women with social risk factors experience United Kingdom maternity care? A realist synthesis. Birth. 2019. Available from: https://doi-org.ezproxy.uwe.ac.uk/10.1111/birt.12446

53. McLeish J, Redshaw M. Maternity experiences of mothers with multiple disadvantages in England: a qualitative study. Women and Birth. 2019;32(2):178–184.

54. Grady C. Enduring and emerging challenges of informed consent. The New England Journal of Medicine. [online]. 2015;372(9): 855–862. Available from: <doi:10.1056/NEJMra1411250>

55. Stohl H. Childbirth is not a medical emergency: maternal right to informed consent throughout labour and delivery. Journal of Legal Medicine. 2018;38:329–353. Available from: <doi:10.1080/01947648.2018.1482243>

56. Klerk H, Boere E, van Lunsen RH, Bakker JJ. Women's experiences with vaginal examinations during labour in the Netherlands. Journal of Psychosomatic Obstetrics and Gynaecology. 2018;39(2):90–95. Available from: <doi:10.1080/01674 82X.2017.1291623>

57. Hayes-Klein. Informed consent in childbirth: making rights into reality. 2013. [Accessed 17 July 2023]. Available from: www.birthrights.org.uk/2013/07/10/informed-consent-in-childbirth-making-rights-into-reality/

58. van der Pijl M, Essink MK, van der Linden T, Verweij R, Kingma E, Hollander MH, et al. Consent and refusal of procedures during labour and birth a survey among 11,418 women in the Netherlands. BMJ. 2022:015538. Available from: <doi:10.1136/bmjqs-2022-015538>

59. Djanogly T, Nicholls J, Whitten M, Lanceley A. Choice in episiotomy-fact or fantasy: a qualitative study of women's experiences of the consent process. BMC Pregnancy and Childbirth. 2022;22:139. Available from: <doi:10.1186/s12884-022-04475-8>

60. Reed R, Sharman R, Inglis C. Women's descriptions of childbirth trauma relating to care provider actions and interactions. BMC Pregnancy Childbirth. 2017 Jan 10;17(1):21. Available from: <doi:10.1186/s12884-016-1197-0> PMID: 28068932; PMCID: PMC5223347.

61. Esegbona-Adeigbe S. Transcultural midwifery practice: concepts, care and challenges. London: Elsevier; 2022. ISBN:978-0-3238-7230-0.

62. Cook A. Midwifery perspectives: the consent process in the context of patient safety and medico-legal issues. Clinical Risk. 2016;22(1–2):25–29. [Accessed 7 July 2023]. Available from: https://doi-org.ezproxy.uwe.ac.uk/10.1177/1356262216672614

63. Kennedy S, Lanceley A, Whitten M, Kelly C, Nicholls J. Consent on the labour ward: a qualitative study of the views and experiences of healthcare professionals. European Journal of Obstetrics and Gynecology and Reproductive Biology. 2021;264:150–154. Available from: <doi:10.1016/j.ejogrb.2021.07.003>

64. CQC. Regulation 11: need for consent. 2023b. [Accessed 17 July 2023]. Available from: www.cqc.org.uk/guidance-providers/regulations-enforcement/regulation-11-need-consent

65. Royal College of Midwives. Informed decision making. 2022. Available from: www.rcm.org.uk/media/6007/informed-decision-making_0604.pdf

66. Hamilton SJ. A short guide to effective mental capacity assessment for midwives. The Practising Midwife. 2021;24(9). Available from: <doi:10.55975/GLLB6244>

67. Mind. Mental capacity act 2005. 2023. [Accessed 9 July 2023]. Available from: https://www.mind.org.uk/information-support/legal-rights/mental-capacity-act-2005/overview/

68. Affleck PJ, Waisel DB, Cusick JM, Van Decar T. Recall of risks following labor epidural analgesia. J Clin Anesth. 1998;10: 141–144.

69. Gerancher JC, Grice SC, Dewan DM, Eisenach J. An evaluation of informed consent prior to epidural analgesia for labour and delivery. International Journal of Obstetric Anesthesia. 2000;9:168–173.

3

Maternal and newborn resuscitation

JENNY BREWSTER

Maternal resuscitation   33
Physiological changes in pregnancy
    affecting resuscitation   34
Physiological changes when body systems
    are not maintained   35
Recognition of maternal collapse   36
Basic life support   36
Advanced life support   39
Modifications to resuscitation for pregnant
    women   41

Newborn resuscitation   43
Fetal physiology   44
Support during transition from in-utero to
    ex-utero life   46
Care following resuscitation   52
Summary of midwifery responsibilities   52
Further reading and resources   53
References   53

MATERNAL RESUSCITATION

BOX 3.1: Definition

The Royal College of Obstetricians and Gynaecologists (RCOG)[1] defines maternal collapse as 'an acute event involving the cardiorespiratory systems and/or central nervous systems, resulting in a reduced or absent conscious level (and potentially cardiac arrest and death) at any stage in pregnancy and up to six weeks after birth' (p. e20).

Cardiac arrest during pregnancy, intrapartum and the postnatal period is a rare event and probably will never be witnessed by the majority of midwives or those involved in maternity and obstetric care. However, if it does occur, it requires specific knowledge and skills due to the physiological changes that occur during pregnancy. According to the MBRRACE report published in 2022,[2] there were 229 maternal deaths during pregnancy and up to six weeks following birth in 2018–2020, with 86% of these occurring in the postnatal period. Midwives and all those working in this area should always be prepared for both this eventuality and the possibility that they may, either in the working or social environment, witness and assist in the resuscitation of a member of the public. A statement within The Code: Professional Standards of Practice and Behaviour for Nurses, Midwives and Nursing Associates[3] requires all registered personnel to assist in an emergency, be it whilst on or off duty. In all situations, the principles of basic life support should be initiated and employed until help and support arrive.

A study was carried out with data being collected between July 2011 and June 2014 to look at the incidence and management of cardiac arrests during pregnancy in the United Kingdom.[4] This study found that the incidence of cardiac arrest in pregnancy was 1:36,000 maternities, with a survival rate of 58%. There was a clear indication that

DOI: 10.4324/9781003382195-3

for those who survived, resuscitation was initiated promptly, including the use of perimortem caesarean section. A total of 25% of the cardiac arrests in this study were linked to anaesthesia, and several were identified as having co-morbidities which may have contributed to the cardiac arrest.

Maternal cardiac arrest is not only rare but can frequently be unexpected. Therefore, all those involved in maternity care should ensure that they remain proficient and up to date in their basic life support skills by attending regular multidisciplinary training and updating in resuscitation and maternal collapse,[1] including perimortem caesarean section. Everyone should also be familiar with the resuscitation equipment, which may vary slightly from hospital to hospital. A list of suggested contents may be found on the Resuscitation Council website.[5] The Resuscitation Council UK recommends that this equipment is checked regularly, with the frequency of these checks being agreed locally.[5] In any area where a maternal cardiac arrest may occur, including accident and emergency departments, it is recommended that this should also include the basic equipment of a pre-mounted scalpel blade, gloves and cord clamps in case a perimortem caesarean section is required.[1]

The RCOG highlights that any maternal collapse where the cause is not identified and treated appropriately can result in cardiac arrest. Therefore, when caring for all women, vigilance and accuracy in carrying out observations of vital signs are essential so that early signs of deterioration in condition can be recognised and managed. These should be clearly documented using an obstetric modified early warning score chart,[1] with MBRRACE recommending that the development of a national early warning score system should be made a priority.[6]

In the recognition and initial treatment of maternal collapse, it is important that the cause is identified using the ABCDE approach and appropriate management commenced.[1] The causes of cardiac arrest have been identified by the Resuscitation Council (UK)[7] as belonging to one of 8 categories, which are known by the 4 H's and the 4 T's. A modified version of these related to pregnancy is detailed in Figure 3.6. During the period 2018–2020, the most common causes of maternal death directly related to pregnancy were thrombosis and thromboembolism, while cardiac disease was the most common indirect cause of maternal death.[8]

The main focus of care for all women should be to be aware of any known risk factors and to

work continually to recognise these and any deterioration in condition to prevent maternal collapse where possible. However, when collapse does occur, the aim is to identify the cause as soon as possible and work to correct this whilst continually assessing the bodily functions and commencing general resuscitation.

PHYSIOLOGICAL CHANGES IN PREGNANCY AFFECTING RESUSCITATION

During pregnancy, there are many changes in the maternal body systems to support the growth and development of both the fetus and the uterus. Some of these changes will lead to cases of maternal collapse to a rapid onset of hypoxia and acidosis due to reduced oxygen-carrying capabilities. There may also be difficulties in ventilation and with performing effective chest compressions.

From around 20 weeks gestation, the weight of the gravid uterus may compress the inferior vena cava, reducing venous return by 10–30% when the woman is lying supine and cardiac output by up to 40%.[1,9] There are adaptations made by the body, such as the increase in systemic vascular pressure and an increase in heart rate, which provide some compensation.[10] However, the inferior vena cava may be completely compressed when the woman lies supine at term. This leads to supine hypotension, which alone may lead to maternal collapse and certainly hinders effective resuscitation. Supine hypotension may be relieved by turning the woman onto the left lateral position, where a tilt of 30% is recommended[9] (see Figure 3.1), or by manually displacing the uterus to the left. This will be discussed in modifications to resuscitation for pregnant women later in the chapter.

During pregnancy, there is an increase in the circulating blood volume of 30–50%, which leads to physiological anaemia caused by haemodilution and, thus, a reduction in the oxygen-carrying capacity of the blood.[1,11] The increased blood volume leads to an increase in the cardiac output as well as the maternal pulse rate, which in turn will affect cardiopulmonary resuscitation (CPR) attempts.[1] The amount of blood circulating to the uterus increases dramatically throughout the pregnancy in order to supply the fetus through the placenta with the oxygen and nutrients required for its growth and development. By term, 450–700mls

(a)

(b)

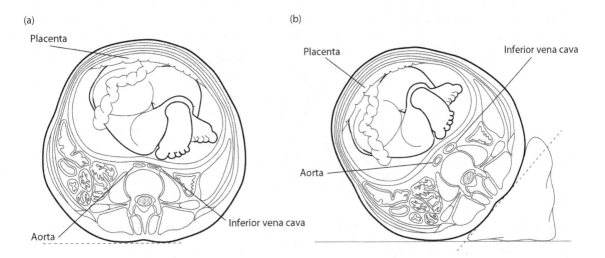

Figure 3.1 Aortal and inferior vena caval compression in dorsal position. (a) Showing compression of vessels by gravid uterus with the woman lying supine and (b) showing how compression is relieved by tilting the woman to the left

of blood per minute are flowing through the placental site, giving the potential for a massive haemorrhage.[12] This, however, may not be immediately apparent as the extra circulating volume masks the symptoms of haemorrhage, and up to 35% of the circulating blood volume may be lost before the woman becomes symptomatic.[1]

The respiratory system in pregnancy is subject to change and adaptation mediated by hormonal influences to support the increased metabolic requirements of the woman, her increased oxygen needs and the requirements of the feto-placental unit, and these changes will impact any resuscitation attempts. The growth of the uterus affects the functional capacity of the lungs, reducing the reserve capacity by up to 25%.[1,13] During pregnancy, the respiration rate increases slightly in rate, but also in depth to support the increase in oxygen requirements of up to 20%. These factors lead to the rapid onset of hypoxia when there is a lack of ventilation to the lungs.[1]

The anatomical changes to the respiratory system also mean that intubation can be more difficult during pregnancy due to weight gain, as well as the possibility of laryngeal oedema, which can reduce access and view.[14] A further risk of intubation is that of aspiration pneumonia, or Mendelson's syndrome. The action of progesterone relaxes the oesophageal sphincter and slows the emptying of the stomach. This increases the risk of acid reflux, which, if inhaled, can lead to adult respiratory distress syndrome.[1,14]

PHYSIOLOGICAL CHANGES WHEN BODY SYSTEMS ARE NOT MAINTAINED

For the body to survive cardiopulmonary collapse, blood circulation and respiration must be maintained with an adequate circulating volume. Once the heart stops beating, blood stops circulating around the body, the cells become hypoxic and the metabolism within the cells alters, leading to an acidotic state. The normal level of blood pH is between 7.35 and 7.45 (see Table 3.1).

Cells require oxygen to produce adenosine triphosphate (ATP), the energy source that is needed to power the cell's functions. As a by-product of this, carbon dioxide (CO_2) and water are produced. Carbon dioxide, which under normal circumstances is a stimulator of respirations, when combined with water, produces bicarbonate and hydrogen ions. Generally, the bicarbonate ions neutralise the hydrogen ions, but if levels of CO_2 build up in the body, this can alter the pH of the blood, making it acidic, which will cause damage to cells. The brain detects increases in hydrogen ions and will increase the respiratory rate to help remove this from the body.[16]

When oxygen is not supplied to the cells in sufficient amounts, the metabolism within the cells changes to be anaerobic, where lactic acid is the by-product. A build of this in the body also leads to an acidosis. The respiratory system fails, meaning that not only is the blood not supplied with oxygen, but

Table 3.1 Normal blood gas levels[15]

	Normal ranges in arterial blood	Significance
pH	7.35–7.45[2]	Acid-base balance is the maintenance of hydrogen ion balance that maintains normal cell function.
pCO_2	4.6–6.4 kPa	The partial pressure of carbon dioxide (CO_2) dissolved in arterial blood. CO_2 is a waste product of cell metabolism. Increasing the respiratory rate helps the body clear CO_2.
pO_2	11.0–14.4 kPa	The partial pressure of oxygen (PO_2) dissolved in arterial blood. This indicates the amount of oxygen available for the cells.
Lactate	0.5–2.2 mmol/L	Lactic acid is a by-product of anaerobic metabolism and is an indicator of hypoxia.
Base excess	−2 to +2	Base is another word for alkali. Measurement of the surplus amount of base within the blood.

carbon dioxide is no longer being excreted, leading to an increase in the levels in the capillaries. The kidneys are unable to excrete harmful substances as they are not supplied with filtrate or oxygen to assist with the breakdown of substances within the blood. Without oxygen, the brain cannot function, and this leads to a rapid death of the cells.

The arterial base deficit of blood measures the amount of buffering solutions that are available to physiologically correct the acid-base balance, the normal range being between -2 to +2 mmol/L. Serum lactate levels also look at the levels of acidosis and should be <2.5mmol/L, although they can be altered by liver damage or sepsis, so they may not always be an accurate indicator of acidosis. (Normal blood levels are given in Table 3.1).

RECOGNITION OF MATERNAL COLLAPSE

Many cases of maternal collapse are instantaneous, with no prior warning. In other cases, there may be signs of a deterioration in the woman's condition or signs of shock. Due to the increase in oxygen requirements and the need to excrete excess carbon dioxide, an increase in the respiration rate should be noted and acted on, as should other signs such as a weak, thready pulse and low blood pressure. Other signs of hypoxia that may be seen are disorientation, a fall in the level of consciousness, cold extremities, feeling clammy to the touch and/or showing signs of pallor or cyanosis. Once the heart stops beating, this will lead to irreversible brain and organ damage unless resuscitation is commenced immediately with the aim of maintaining blood circulation around the body to

supply oxygen to the tissues by artificially pumping the heart and ensuring oxygen enters the lungs.

BASIC LIFE SUPPORT

It is important to remember that the initial approaches to a maternal collapse are the same as those for any person found collapsed, whether this is in the hospital or community setting. The first person to recognise the collapse, whether this is in the health care or community setting, must put out a call for help and commence basic resuscitation. To improve the chances of survival, compressions should be started early and continued with little interruption. The use of a defibrillator at the earliest opportunity is also a priority in the resuscitation process. According to the Resuscitation Council (UK),[17] where a cardiac arrest occurs in the community setting, the return to spontaneous circulation is achieved in 30% of resuscitation attempts. However, only 9% will survive to hospital discharge. In the hospital setting, return to spontaneous circulation occurs in 53% of attempted resuscitations, with 23.6% surviving to leave hospital.

Annual updates in resuscitation training should be attended by all those working in health services. For those working in maternity, these sessions should include the modifications that are required for pregnant women.

Clear guidance on the sequence of events in the case of any collapse is provided by the Resuscitation Council (UK),[18] as well as guidance on the modifications that are recommended for pregnant women suffering a cardiac arrest after 20 weeks gestation.[19] These will be discussed in the next section. The algorithm for suspected cardiac arrests in hospital is shown in Figure 3.2.

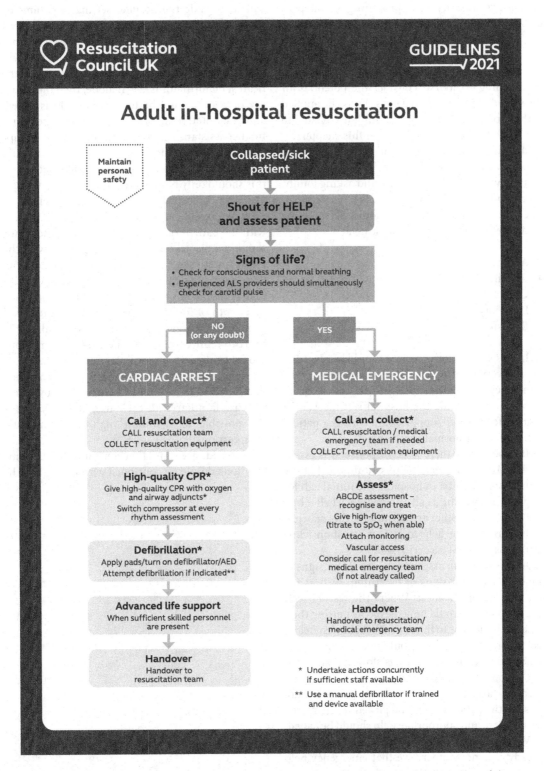

Figure 3.2 Adult in-hospital resuscitation algorithm (reproduced with the kind permission of the Resuscitation Council (UK))

The first priority in approaching a collapsed person, either in hospital, the home or in the street, is to ensure the personal safety of the rescuer. Therefore, it is essential to check floor areas for wires, spillages and other potential hazards before approaching, as well as consider the potential for the spread of infection, so gloves should be applied at the earliest opportunity. The guidance related to Covid-19 will be discussed later in this chapter.

An initial assessment should be made to see if they are able to respond or if they are unconscious by simply tapping the shoulders and asking loudly, 'Can you hear me?' Where there is a response, an assessment of the condition should be made by using the ABCDE approach, looking at

- Airway
- Breathing
- Circulation
- Disability
- Exposure

In this situation, the patient should be placed in the recovery position and, where appropriate, the emergency medical team should be called, or an ambulance if outside the hospital setting. Whilst waiting for further support, stay with the patient and observe for normal breathing.

In cases where there is no response, it is essential that the appropriate help is summoned at the earliest opportunity. In hospital, the initial call for help will be by using a call or emergency bell if by a bed space, but in other areas, initially, this may just be by shouting for help to attract attention while further assessment is carried out.[20]

At this point, an assessment is made for signs of life by looking for signs of breathing, such as the rise and fall of the chest. Where the rescuer feels safe to do so, this could be achieved by putting their ear and cheek close to the patient's face to listen and feel for breathing.[20] This should take no more than ten seconds. If the breathing is slow and laboured (agonal breathing), this should be treated as a sign of cardiac arrest.[18] As previously, if signs of life are present, the patient should be placed in the recovery position, and appropriate help should be called.

Where there is no sign of life, if not carried out already, it is now imperative that emergency help is called. In hospital, this would be the cardiac arrest team (using the emergency 2222 number in the UK), and, in cases of pregnancy, ensuring the obstetric team and obstetric anaesthetist are also

called. Outside the hospital setting, a paramedic ambulance should be called (in the UK by dialing 999). When using the 999 number, if possible, put the phone onto speaker, and the call handler will talk through what to do as well as advise where the nearest defibrillator is.[18,20] If alone, then the recovery position should be used while help is called, and resuscitation attempts only commenced once further assistance has been summoned.[18] If no support is available, then chest compressions should take precedence over getting the defibrillator, and this should only be collected once help arrives.

Chest compressions should be commenced as soon as possible at a rate of 100–120 per minute with the patient on a hard, flat surface. The hands should be placed one on top of the other with the fingers interlinked on the lower half of the sternum, the center of the chest[18,20] (see Figure 3.3). With each compression, the chest should be compressed to a depth of 5–6cms allowing the chest to recoil completely between each compression to allow the heart to refill with blood. The chest compressions should continue with minimal interruption.

Some Trusts have mechanical chest compression devices. These should only be used by teams who are familiar with their use, and only if it is not possible to maintain high-quality manual compressions.[21]

The guidance states that continuous chest compressions should be continued with rescue breaths

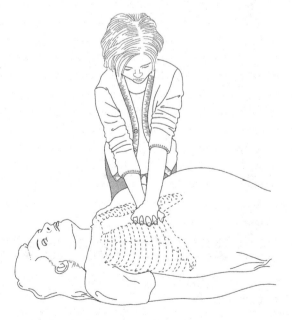

Figure 3.3 Hand position for chest compressions

only being given by a person who is trained and is willing to do so.[18] Where the cardiac arrest is a sudden event, the blood should be well-oxygenated and provide sufficient oxygen for a few minutes until further support or a defibrillator arrives. Within the hospital setting, adjuncts to help prevent the spread of infection whilst delivering breaths, such as a bag, valve and mask should be readily available on the crash trolley in each area. Once available, ventilation breaths should be delivered at a ratio of 30 compressions to two breaths.[18] Where qualified help is available, a Laryngeal mask airway may also be inserted by those trained to do so, or tracheal intubation may be attempted. If no airway device is available, direct mouth-to-mouth breaths may be given, or if there are concerns regarding hygiene or infection risks, compressions should be continued until further help arrives. Chest compressions should be continued until the rescuer is exhausted, someone can take over, a defibrillator advises that compressions are not required or, in the community setting, the call handler advises that the compressions should be stopped. Chest compressions are tiring, so it is ideal to have at least two people, and rotate between compressions and breaths every two or three cycles. In hospital, when the cardiac arrest team arrives, one person will coordinate a regular change around to ensure that no one becomes exhausted, generally with each rhythm check on the defibrillator.

ADVANCED LIFE SUPPORT

As soon as is possible, a defibrillator should be brought to the scene and the self-adhesive electrodes applied so that the cardiac rhythm can be analysed. Automated External Defibrillators (AEDs) are now available both in hospital and in many community settings. AEDs give clear directions as to how to use them, and the pads clearly show where they are to be placed (Figure 3.4). Compressions should continue if there is more than one rescuer present until the pads have been applied.[18] Once the pads are in place, the AED will advise to 'stand clear' while the cardiac rhythm is analysed and will then instruct as to whether cardio-pulmonary resuscitation (CPR) should continue or a shock be delivered.

The cardiac rhythms that may be reversed through a shock are ventricular fibrillation (VF) and pulseless ventricular tachycardia (VT). When the heart is in VT, cardiac output is massively reduced, and this can quickly deteriorate into VF.

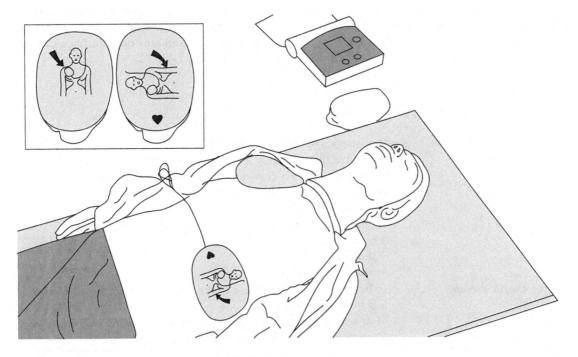

Figure 3.4 Electrode pad placement for defibrillation

The AED will instruct that the charge button be pressed. Before delivering the shock, the lead person must ensure that everyone is standing clear of the patient and, if in use, nasal cannula or an oxygen mask should be removed.[18] The shock works by depolarising the mass of the myocardium, allowing the pace-making tissue of the heart to resume control. Where there is a shockable rhythm, the chances of survival are greater than for a non-shockable rhythm unless the cause of the arrest can be identified and treated.[22] It is imperative that an AED is used at the earliest opportunity as, for each minute following collapse, the chance of survival reduces by 7–10%.[22] Once the shock has been delivered, CPR should be recommenced. The AED will automatically ask for compressions to be paused every two minutes to reassess the cardiac rhythm and advise either a further shock or the continuation of compressions.

The other rhythms which may be seen in cases of cardiac arrest are asystole and pulseless electrical activity (PEA). In PEA, the electrical activity of the heart continues, but there is no pulse detectable, often due to massive blood loss, such as with a postpartum haemorrhage (PPH).[22] In these cases, CPR should be continued whilst attempts to treat the underlying condition are put in place.

Fluid replacement

As soon as there are any concerns about the condition of the women, intravenous (IV) access, if not already in place, should be obtained using a wide bore, 16-gauge cannula and intravenous fluid replacement commenced as prescribed in an effort to help stabilise the woman by maintaining her blood pressure and the chemical components of the body. IV access can be gained during an arrest situation on the arrival of additional help and support.

The type of fluids and drugs that are needed will depend on the cause of the arrest. The Resuscitation Council advises that IV fluids should only be used if hypovolaemia is thought to be the cause of the cardiac arrest.[7] However, if fluids are administered, caution is needed as, if they are cold, they could disturb the thermal balance of the body and lead to further difficulties with resuscitation. Care in maintaining accurate records of the fluids that are administered is also required, with consideration being given to the possibility of fluid overload, especially in situations complicated by pre-eclampsia (see Chapter 7) and sepsis (see Chapter 14).

Drugs

The drugs used during resuscitation will be administered by the resuscitation team, although the midwife should have a working knowledge of those frequently used so that she can anticipate and prepare the drugs in advance. Following intravenous administration of each individual medication, a flush of 20mls of normal saline should be given. The drugs most commonly used during a cardiac arrest are listed in Table 3.2

Table 3.2 Drugs used during a cardiac arrest

Adrenaline (epinephrine)	Non-shockable rhythm – give 1mg IV once access is available
	Shockable rhythm – give 1mg IV following the third shock.
	Repeat 1mg every 3–5 minutes whilst resuscitation continues.
	Works by increasing the heart rate and contractility of the cardiac muscle.[23]
Amiodarone	300mg given IV where VF or VT persists after three shocks.
	A further dose of 150mg IV is given where VT/VF persists after five shocks.
	Antiarrhythmic drug
Thrombolytic therapy	To be considered if the cause of the cardiac arrest is thought to be pulmonary embolus.
	After administration, CPR should be continued for 60–90 minutes.
Calcium Chloride	10mg IV to be given where magnesium toxicity is suspected.[22]

MODIFICATIONS TO RESUSCITATION FOR PREGNANT WOMEN

For pregnant women who suffer a cardiac arrest, the principles of resuscitation remain the same; however, some modifications are required due to the physiological changes that occur in pregnancy, which were discussed earlier in this chapter.

As soon as it is recognised that the woman has collapsed, specialist help should be summoned, with the obstetrician, obstetric anaesthetist and neonatologist (if the woman is still pregnant) being required in addition to the cardiac arrest team. CPR should be commenced for any person in cardiac arrest, ensuring that the chest compressions are of good quality and that these are disrupted as little as possible.[19]

Due to the weight of the pregnant uterus compressing the inferior vena cava and aorta, venous return and cardiac output can be affected, as discussed earlier in this chapter (See Figure 3.1). In order to achieve effective compressions, the woman must be lying flat on a hard surface. Current guidelines[1,19] recommend that from 20 weeks gestation, when the uterus is palpable above the umbilicus, the uterus should be manually displaced to the maternal left side to relieve this compression. This can be carried out from the left side using two hands (see Figure 3.5a) or from the right side with one hand (see Figure 3.5b), depending on how the resuscitation team is positioned.

If the woman is on a theatre table when the cardiac arrest occurs, then the theatre table can be tilted to an angle of 15 to 30°. Soft surfaces, such as a bed, pillows or soft wedges, do not allow chest compressions to be effective.[1]

To aid oxygen delivery and ventilation, and because of the increased risk of regurgitation in a pregnant woman, early intubation of the trachea by a skilled anaesthetist should be carried out.[1,19] However, intubation in a pregnant woman can be more difficult due to pregnancy-related oedema of the airways and difficulty in gaining clear vision.

In cases of maternal cardiac arrest, the best chance of survival for the woman is to deliver the fetus as soon as possible. Hypoxia will develop in the pregnant woman far more rapidly than in the non-pregnant person, and they are at risk of brain damage within 4–6 minutes of cardiac arrest.[1]

Therefore, preparation for a peri-mortem caesarean section (emergency hysterotomy) should be undertaken once the diagnosis of cardiac arrest has been made, with the aim of commencing the procedure within four minutes of the arrest if there is no return to spontaneous circulation by this time, with the fetus being delivered by five minutes from the arrest.[1,19] By delivering the fetus, the maternal oxygen consumption will be reduced, venous return and cardiac output will improve and the empty uterus will allow for easier and more effective chest compressions and ventilation.[1] All resuscitation trolleys within a maternity unit and other areas where maternal cardiac arrest may occur, such as Accident and Emergency areas, should be prepared for this eventuality, with a

(a)

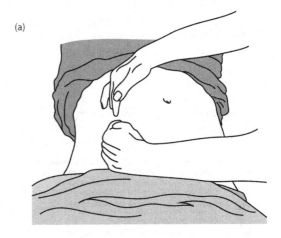

Figure 3.5a Left uterine displacement from left side of patient

(b)

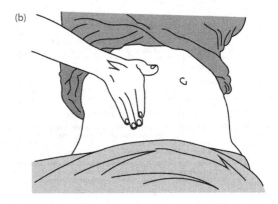

Figure 3.5b Left uterine displacement from right side of patient

pre-mounted scalpel handle and blade cord clamps and sterile gloves being an addition to the required equipment.[1,1]. Preparation should also be made for the potential resuscitation of a viable newborn, with appropriate equipment and the neonatologist present.

A peri-mortem caesarean section should be carried out by an experienced obstetrician where the resuscitation is taking place and should not be delayed by moving the woman to theatre. As there is no established circulation, no anesthetic is required, and there will be minimal blood loss. Where resuscitation is successful, there should be prompt transfer to theatre to complete the operation.[1] As a peri-mortem caesarean section is seen as being for the 'best interests of the patient,' this is performed without consent.[1]

An overview of the sequence of events for an obstetric cardiac arrest, including the 4T's and 4H's, plus a list of the drugs that may be used, can be seen in Figure 3.6.

According to the CAPS Study[4] in the United Kingdom (UK), during the study period of 2011 to 2014, there were 66 cardiac arrests occurring during pregnancy, with 28 of the women dying. Peri-mortem caesarian section was performed on 49 of these women, with 11 being in Accident and Emergency departments, and the earlier this was performed, the more likely a chance of survival. A total of 58 babies were born by peri-mortem caesarean section, with 46 being born alive, 32 of these to women who survived, with increased survival of the infant also being linked to an early delivery following the collapse of the woman.[4]

Whilst dealing with the arrest situation and the potential for a peri-mortem caesarean section, midwives will not only have to consider the needs of family members who may witness the arrest and subsequent interventions but also potentially will need to give support and consideration to other women and possibly their families if this occurs within a ward setting. In some cases, it may be

Obstetric Cardiac Arrest

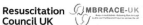

Alterations in maternal physiology and exacerbations of pregnancy related pathologies must be considered. Priorities include calling the appropriate team members, relieving aortocaval compression, effective cardiopulmonary resuscitation (CPR), consideration of causes and performing a timely emergency hysterotomy (perimortem caesarean section) when ≥ 20 weeks.

START

1 Confirm cardiac arrest and call for help. Declare 'Obstetric cardiac arrest'
- Team for mother and team for neonate if > 20 weeks

2 Lie flat, apply manual uterine displacement to the left
- Or left lateral tilt (from head to toe at an angle of 15–30° on a firm surface)

3 Commence CPR and request cardiac arrest trolley
- Standard CPR ratios and hand position apply
- Evaluate potential causes (Box A)

4 Identify team leader, allocate roles including scribe
- Note time

5 Apply defibrillation pads and check cardiac rhythm (defibrillation is safe in pregnancy and no changes to standard shock energies are required))
- if VF / pulseless VT ➔ defibrillation and first adrenaline and amiodarone after 3rd shock
- If PEA / asystole ➔ resume CPR and give first adrenaline immediately
- Check rhythm and pulse every 2 minutes
- Repeat adrenaline every 3-5 minutes

6 Maintain airway and ventilation
- Give 100% oxygen using bag-valve-mask device
- Insert supraglottic airway with drain port –or– tracheal tube if trained to do so (intubation may be difficult, and airway pressures may be higher)
- Apply waveform capnography monitoring to airway
- If expired CO₂ is absent, presume oesophageal intubation until absolutely excluded

7 Circulation
- I.V. access above the diaphragm, if fails or impossible use upper limb intraosseous (IO)
- See Box B for reminders about drugs
- Consider extracorporeal CPR (ECPR) if available

8 Emergency hysterotomy (perimortem caesarean section)
- Perform if ≥ 20 weeks gestation, to improve maternal outcome
- Perform immediately if maternal fatal injuries or prolonged pre-hospital arrest
- Perform by 5 minutes if no return of spontaneous circulation

9 Post resuscitation from haemorrhage - activate Massive Haemorrhage Protocol
Consider uterotonic drugs, fibrinogen and tranexamic acid
Uterine tamponage / sutures, aortic compression, hysterectomy

Version 1.1

Box A: POTENTIAL CAUSES 4H's and 4T's (specific to obstetrics)	
Hypoxia	Respiratory – Pulmonary embolus (PE), Failed intubation, aspiration
	Heart failure
	Anaphylaxis
	Eclampsia / PET – pulmonary oedema, seizure
Hypovolaemia	Haemorrhage – obstetric (remember concealed), abnormal placentation, uterine rupture, atony, splenic artery/hepatic rupture, aneurysm rupture
	Cardiac – arrhythmia, myocardial infarction (MI)
	Distributive – sepsis, high regional block, anaphylaxis
Hypo/hyperkalaemia	Also consider blood sugar, sodium, calcium and magnesium levels
Hypothermia	
Tamponade	Aortic dissection, peripartum cardiomyopathy, trauma
Thrombosis	Amniotic fluid embolus, PE, MI, air embolism
Toxins	Local anaesthetic, magnesium, illicit drugs
Tension pneumothorax	Entonox in pre-existing pneumothorax, trauma

Box B: IV DRUGS FOR USE DURING CARDIAC ARREST	
Fluids	500 mL IV crystalloid bolus
Adrenaline	1 mg IV every 3-5 minutes in non-shockable or after 3rd shock
Amiodarone	300 mg IV after 3rd shock
Atropine	0.5-1 mg IV up to 3 mg if vagal tone likely cause
Calcium chloride	10% 10 mL IV for Mg overdose, low calcium or hyperkalaemia
Magnesium	2 g IV for polymorphic VT / hypomagnesaemia, 4 g IV for eclampsia
Thrombolysis/PCI	For suspected massive pulmonary embolus / MI
Tranexamic acid	1 g if haemorrhage
Intralipid	1.5 mL kg⁻¹ IV bolus and 15 mL kg⁻¹ hr⁻¹ IV infusion

Obstetric Anaesthetists' Association   GUIDELINES
Promoting the highest standards of anaesthetic practice in the care of mother and baby   2021

Figure 3.6 Obstetric Cardiac Arrest (reproduced with the kind permission of the Resuscitation Council (UK))

appropriate for the family members to be brought in to observe the resuscitation so that they are aware that everything possible is being done.[24] However, this will require careful preparation by the professionals involved, with clear information given to the relatives at all times. If possible, it would be ideal for a midwife not directly involved in the hands-on resuscitation to stay with relatives to support them.

Following the resuscitation of a woman during pregnancy or the postpartum period, the family may have to face a number of outcomes and will need support and guidance during this difficult time. In the best situation, the resuscitation will have been successful, resulting in a healthy mother and baby. In others, the outcome may not be so good, with families having to face either the loss of the woman, the loss of the baby and, in some cases, the loss of both. In any situation, the family, and the mother if she survives, may need information and ongoing support to help them cope with what has happened.

Following any arrest situation, the personnel involved will also need support, guidance on where to gain further help if needed and clear debriefing. Where the resuscitation was unsuccessful, the information regarding the case should be reported to MBRRACE by the Trust.[25]

Resuscitation and Covid-19

Although the end of the Covid-19 pandemic was declared on 5 May 2023 by the World Health Organisation[26] and the risk of infection has been reduced by the uptake of immunisation, healthcare workers and those providing emergency care still need to take this into consideration for those they are caring for and themselves.[27] It is known that Covid-19 is transmitted through aerosol spray, but further research is required to see if chest compressions generate aerosol. The Basic Life Support guidelines,[18] along with the supporting video 'CPR Right Now,'[20] suggest that the rescuer looks for signs of breathing but may put their ear close to the patient's nose and mouth only if they feel safe to do so. When performing chest compressions, the face could be covered with a cloth, and breaths, even by a trained provider, should only be carried out if the rescuer is happy to do so.

Where there is a suspected or known case of Covid-19 within a healthcare setting, then FFP3 masks and eye protection should be worn before starting compressions. Each Trust will have specific guidance for these circumstances.

NEWBORN RESUSCITATION

BOX 3.2: Newborn resuscitation

Newborn resuscitation can be defined as the set of interventions immediately following birth to support the establishment of breathing and circulation when this does not happen spontaneously.

At any birth, all those present wait for the expected cry of the newborn infant, the parents to know that all is well, the midwives present observing that the first breath has been taken, replacing the fluid present in the lungs during the fetal period with air and making the transition from in-utero to ex-utero life. Gradually, as the oxygen starts to circulate through the body, an assessment of perfusion can be made by observing the baby's skin and/or mucous membranes change colour from blue to pink as normal respiration is established. In the vast majority of births, this is what happens immediately or following stimulation and opening of the airway. However, there are times when there is silence in the room.

The Resuscitation Council[28] 'Newborn Resuscitation and Support of Transition of Infants at Birth Guidelines' recognise that many newborn infants, rather than requiring resuscitation, need help and support with this transition from in-utero to ex-utero life. Most infants, about 85%, will breathe spontaneously, and a further 10% will establish respirations after drying, stimulation and ensuring that the airway is open. This means that intervention is only required for a small number of infants, with around 5% needing positive pressure ventilation, and chest compressions only being used in less than 0.3%.[28] In many circumstances, the potential for newborn resuscitation can be predicted,[29] with a list of conditions that may predispose to this being found in Box 3.3. Occasionally, the need for resuscitation is totally unexpected,

---

BOX 3.3: Risk/predisposing factors for neonatal resuscitation

Antenatal

Maternal medical conditions such as diabetes, heart disease

Pre-eclampsia

Anaemia

Haemorrhage

Maternal infection

Multiple pregnancy

Maternal substance abuse

Fetal Growth Restriction (FGR)

Serious congenital abnormality

Intrapartum

Placental abruption or placenta praevia

Prolapsed cord

Preterm labour

Precipitious labour

Prolonged rupture of membranes > 18 hours

Abnormal presentation or malposition of the fetus

Meconium stained liquor

Abnormal heart rate patterns on cardiotocograph (CTG)

Forceps or ventouse extraction

Caesarean section before 29 weeks gestation

Emergency caesarean section and/or general anaesthesia

This list is not extensive, and there may be other risk factors which predispose to the need for neonatal resuscitation; therefore, each case should be evaluated individually.

---

and this is the situation that every midwife must be prepared for, be it in the hospital or home birth situation. Therefore, for every birth, there should be professionals available who are trained and competent in newborn resuscitation. For home-birth situations, there should be two trained professionals present, with at least one being trained in ventilation and chest compressions for the newborn infant.[28]

Similarly to maternal collapse, it is essential that the midwife maintains skills and knowledge in newborn resuscitation, as, being the lead carer in 70% of normal births, the midwife may be the first and potentially the only professional present at the time of birth. In these situations, the midwife will need to be able to recognise the need for resuscitation and initiate and carry out the procedures needed for the transition to extra-uterine life to be completed. The midwife should also ensure that whenever taking over the care of any woman, the newborn resuscitation equipment (including drugs) has been checked and is working.

FETAL PHYSIOLOGY

As the fetus receives all its oxygen and nutritional requirements via the placenta in utero, adaptations are in place to ensure that the highest concentration of oxygen goes to the vital organs, such as the brain and myocardium, and to essentially bypass the lungs, which are redundant in terms of oxygen transfer until birth (see Table 3.3). The excretion of waste products also occurs via the placenta to the maternal circulation. As the carbon dioxide enters the maternal system, the pH is altered for a very short period of time, which again allows for greater levels of oxygen transfer from the maternal to the fetal system (the Bohr effect).[30]

During labour, the oxygen supply to the fetus may be affected by compression of the cord and/or the action of the uterine contractions on the placenta, restricting oxygen transfer. The fetus in good condition will be able to cope well with these transient falls in the oxygen levels by altering the heart rate and redistributing the blood flow so that the heart and brain, in preference to other internal organs and the peripheries, receive oxygenated blood. This is mediated by baroreceptors in the aortic arch and carotid sinuses, which react to the changes in the partial pressure of oxygen within the fetal blood and chemoreceptors in the brain, which are sensitive to the pH levels.

If hypoxia develops, the fetal heart rate is affected, with the cardiac muscle being maintained by anaerobic rather than aerobic metabolism. This is less efficient and leads to the buildup of lactic

Table 3.3 Fetal adaptations in utero

Ductus Venosus	Highly oxygenated blood from the umbilical vein bypasses the liver via the ductus venosus to join the inferior vena cava.
Foramen Ovale	Highly oxygenated blood entering the right atrium is diverted through to the left atrium and thus to the general circulation to ensure that the heart and brain receive the oxygen required.
Ductus Arteriosus	The fluid-filled lungs have high pulmonary arterial resistance. Blood from the pulmonary trunk diverts through the ductus arteriosus to the aorta, bypassing the lungs which are not used for oxygen transfer in utero.
Hypogastric arteries	Become the umbilical arteries, carrying deoxygenated blood away from the fetus to the placenta.
Higher Haemoglobin levels	To support the high oxygen requirements of the fetus, the haemoglobin levels are higher and also have a different structure, allowing a higher binding capacity.

acid, which causes acidosis in the blood, affecting the function of the cells.[31] Carbon dioxide levels also rise during a developing hypoxia, meaning there is an increase in hydrogen ions in the fetus, leading to respiratory acidosis.[32] These changes are reflected in the fetal cardiotocograph, tracing where initially there may be a rise in the baseline, followed by decelerations and the loss of variability and eventually bradycardia, as the hypoxia continues.[33]

As the baby is born, adaptations to the circulatory and respiratory systems should take place so that the neonate's oxygen supply comes from the lungs rather than the placenta. These changes are initiated by the first breaths that are taken, which push the fluid from the lungs into the interstitial spaces, filling the lungs with air and changing the pressure ratio so that the blood supply to the lungs increases. The foramen ovale closes, helping to establish pulmonary circulation, and the ductus venosus and arteriosus close anatomically over a period of time. Where this does not occur spontaneously, support and resuscitation may be needed.

Thermoregulation

It is of vital importance that the newborn is kept warm in the immediate period following birth, whether support with transition or resuscitation is required or not.[28] The room should be warm and free of draughts, with a recommended room of temperature of 23–25°C, this being increased to above 25°C for babies under 28 weeks gestation. Babies who get cold will be more difficult to resuscitate as they will be using their glucose stores to produce heat, thus increasing their oxygen requirements for normal cell metabolism.[30] The production of surfactant is also reduced in babies who are cold.

Babies under 32 weeks gestation should be placed in a polythene bag without pre-drying, leaving the face exposed, and placed under a radiant heater,[28,29] with a hat to cover the head. This allows easy access to those caring for the baby whilst the radiant heat circulates the evaporated fluid from the baby's skin, thus keeping the baby warm.

When to clamp and cut the cord

It is recommended[28,29] that, following discussing the options with the parents, the cord is not cut before one minute of age and ideally is left until after the first breath has been taken to allow for fetal blood in the placenta and cord to transfer to the newborn. However, where the infant requires resuscitation, the cord should be clamped and cut earlier to allow the baby to be moved to a suitable area unless a resuscitation platform which slides over the bed is available. A resuscitation platform allows for the cord to remain unclamped and the fetal/placental unit to provide oxygen to the newborn while resuscitation commences. The optimum time for delaying cord clamping has not been identified, only that it should be for at least one minute.

Where delayed cord clamping is used, decelerations in the heart rate following birth are less likely. This may be due to the increased circulatory support as the blood supply increases to the lungs for the first time. There is also an increase in the baby's haemoglobin levels initially and improved iron stores for the first 4–6 months of age.[29,34]

Equipment

The equipment for neonatal resuscitation varies according to the place of birth, so the midwife must ensure that she is familiar with what is available. The basic equipment needed for neonatal resuscitation are towels, a stethoscope, means of delivering breaths, heat and light. In maternity units, Resuscitaires are generally available, giving a flat working surface with heat, light, a pressurised gas device with a 'T' piece for delivering breaths to the newborn, suction and storage for any other equipment, such as laryngoscopes, laryngeal masks, a saturation monitor and endotracheal tubes.

The pressurised gas device should initially be powered by air, with oxygen being introduced later in the resuscitation if this is indicated by the O_2 saturation readings on the baby (see later in this chapter). The pressures for a term baby should be set at 30 cm water (H_2O) pressure and 25 cm H_2O pressure for a premature baby.[33] The latest guidelines[28,29] recommend the use of a 'T' piece with a positive end-expiratory pressure (peep) device, which is set at 5 cm H_2O pressure, to help maintain the inflation in the lungs for babies of all gestation.

Whilst the pressurised devices deliver constant pressure, midwives should also be familiar with and be able to use a bag/valve mask. At a home birth, this may be the only piece of equipment available or will be needed if the main system in hospital fails. Figure 3.7 indicates a suggested list of equipment that should be available at a home birth.

With both pieces of airway equipment, an appropriate-sized mask is required, which should fit over the nose and mouth without occluding the orbital ridges. For a good seal to be obtained, the mask should be rolled on from the cleft of the chin to the bridge of the nose. When holding the mask in place, the thumb and forefinger should hold the center stem of the mask in a 'C' hold, applying gentle downward pressure to obtain the seal. The remaining three fingers should form an 'E' on the jawline (see Figure 3.8), with the ring finger on the angle of the jaw. This should be used to lift the jaw into the mask, applying a single-handed jaw thrust.

For more advanced resuscitation, a laryngoscope with appropriately sized blade, laryngeal masks or 'Igel,' and a selection of endotracheal tubes with intubation stylets are required.

Air or Oxygen?

The aim of newborn resuscitation is to achieve ventilation of the lungs, removing the fluid present in-utero, replacing it with air and thus changing the resistance within the lungs so that blood previously diverted from the pulmonary artery to the aorta through the ductus arteriosus flows into the pulmonary circulation allowing gaseous exchange to take place. A systematic review by Davis et al.[33] found that, although little research exists into the subject due to the ethics of studying newborns, the findings suggested that using 100% oxygen in a newborn resuscitation as has traditionally happened, in fact, reduces the supply of cerebral oxygen and can delay the onset of spontaneous respirations. Babies resuscitated in air alone have been resuscitated as effectively, if not more so than those receiving 100% oxygen, and the guidelines[28,29] recommend that the resuscitation of babies over 32 weeks gestation commences in air. For babies from 28 to 32 weeks, 21–30% oxygen should be used initially, and 30% oxygen for babies under 28 weeks. An oxygen saturation monitor should be applied, usually to the right hand, in the early stages of resuscitation, with oxygen being titrated to achieve saturation levels, as shown in Box 3.4.

SUPPORT DURING TRANSITION FROM IN-UTERO TO EX-UTERO LIFE

The Resuscitation Council has clear guidelines for the systematic approach to aid the transition of babies at birth and for newborn resuscitation, outlined in Figure 3.10.

As the baby is born, the time of birth should be noted, and/or a timer started, so that clear timings of events can be observed. It is essential that the baby is then dried thoroughly and wrapped in a clean, warm, dry towel to minimise heat loss. Drying the baby will also act as stimulation, which, along with the stress of the birth and change in temperature, may be all that is needed to establish respirations.

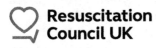

Resuscitation Council UK

Minimum equipment for newborn resuscitation and the support of transition of infants at birth in the pre-hospital setting

Introduction

This equipment list, developed for Resuscitation Council UK Newborn Life Support Subcommittee by the Pre-Hospital Newborn Life Support working group, represents a minimum recommended standard for those delivering care for planned or emergency births in the out-of-hospital setting.

All items should be latex free.

Thermal care
- Towels x 4
- Hat (small and large) x 2
- TransWarmer © (or similar)
- Clear plastic bag.

Airway management
- Portable suction equipment – battery operated with adjustable pressure (manual acceptable)
- Paediatric Yankeur catheter x 2
- i-gel/LMA size 1
- Laryngoscope with size 1 blade
- Sachet of lubricant gel
- 5 mL syringe (if inflatable cuffed LMA carried).

Breathing support
- Self-inflating paediatric resuscitation bag (approximately 500 mL volume)
- Face masks for positive pressure ventilation – appropriate to all gestations (e.g. Size 00, 0 and 1)
- Paediatric nasal cannula.

Additional items
- Cord clamps x 3
- Sharp scissors/umbilical cord scissors
- Gauze
- Clinical waste bag x 2
- Stethoscope
- Gloves
- Patient ID bracelet x 2
- Axilla thermometer
- Copy of the NLS algorithm
- Oxygen cylinder and saturation monitor with an appropriate probe.

Newborn Life Support Subcommittee | Minimum equipment for newborn resuscitation and the support of transition of infants at birth in the pre-hospital setting| Jan/2023 | Version 1

Figure 3.7 Minimum equipment for newborn resuscitation and the support of transition of infants at birth in the pre-hospital setting (reproduced with the kind permission of the Resuscitation Council (UK))

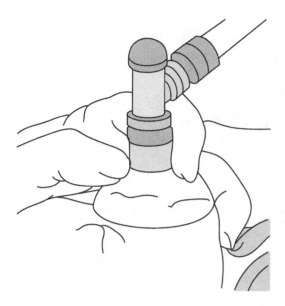

Figure 3.8 The 'C' grip for holding the mask

Time from birth	Acceptable (25th centile) right hand saturation (%)
2 minutes	65
5 minutes	85
10 minutes	90

While drying the baby, an assessment of the condition can be made. Although part of the assessment, the colour of the baby at birth is no longer considered to be a reliable assessment of the condition at birth with regards to oxygenation or of any improvement during a resuscitation process. However, babies who are acidotic at birth will look pale, almost white, thus indicating that intervention may be required.[28,31] Tone is an aid to assessing rapidly those babies where intervention may be needed. At birth, babies generally have a good tone and appear well-flexed. Those who are hypoxic will appear floppy. Also, the breathing activity should be observed. Normally, babies will breathe spontaneously soon after birth. Those in difficulty may demonstrate deep, intermittent gasping or not be breathing at all. Where the baby is not breathing effectively, action needs to be taken to inflate the lungs, remove the lung fluid and establish respirations.

In assessing the heart rate, a stethoscope should be used to ascertain the rate[28]:

- Normal (rate over 100 beats per minute)
- Slow (between 60–100 beats per minute)
- Very slow (less than 60 beats per minute)
- Absent

Assessing the heart rate initially gives a baseline and can also be used to demonstrate inflation of the lungs, with an increase in heart rate being one of the first signs of successful inflation.[31]

Following the initial assessment, where the baby has been found to have good tone, is breathing regularly and has a normal heart rate, delayed cord clamping should be continued for at least a minute, and the baby should be kept warm, ideally by skin-to-skin with the mother if she is happy with this.

Where there is poor tone, inadequate or no breathing and a slow or very slow heart rate, it should be immediately recognised that support with the transition from in-utero to ex-utero life is needed, and help should be summoned. At home, a paramedic ambulance should be alerted (by dialing 999 in the UK) and called to the house. In hospital in the UK, the call for help will be via the 2222 phone number, calling for the neonatal resuscitation team. Additional help from midwives or neonatal unit nurses may also be needed, with one being allocated to keep a note of the timing of the events to aid documentation at the end of the emergency. This may be in the form of a Trust specific proforma.

At this point, unless it is possible to perform the support required effectively, the cord should be clamped and cut and the baby should be moved to an appropriate area, such as the Resuscitaire. Where the baby has not taken the initial breath, the lungs will still be full of fluid, so oxygen transfer cannot take place without the placental support. Therefore, the priority in the resuscitation of the newborn is to establish and maintain an airway. Initially, the baby's head should be moved into the 'neutral' position[28] to open the airway (see Figure 3.10), accompanied by support of the lower jaw. This is where the face is parallel with the surface the baby is lying on. Airway obstruction in the newborn is usually due to lack of tone, causing

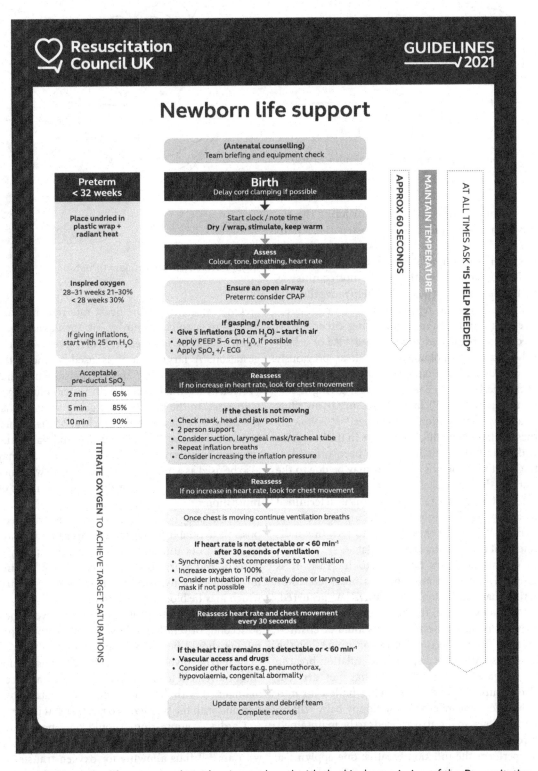

Figure 3.9 Newborn life support algorithm (reproduced with the kind permission of the Resuscitation Council (UK)

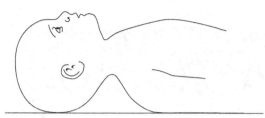

The neutral position is the correct head position for optimal airway opening

Figure 3.10 Head position for optimum airway opening

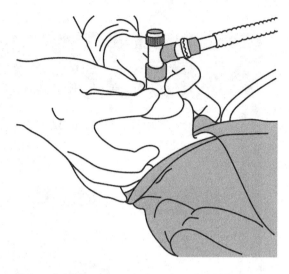

Figure 3.11 Two-person jaw thrust

the tongue to fall backwards, obstructing the airway rather than a mechanical obstruction. Many babies will respond and start spontaneous breathing purely with stimulation and an open airway.[31]

If spontaneous breathing does not commence, then assistance must be given to help move the fluid from the lungs and replace this with air for effective lung ventilation to begin. Using either the 'T' piece and pressurised ventilation device or a bag/valve mask and holding the mask as previously described, five inflation breaths should be delivered over a period of 2–3 seconds each, giving a sustained pressure of 30cm H_2O pressure in an effort to achieve the inflation of the lungs.[28,31] Following these inflation breaths, an increase in the heart rate will indicate that the lungs have been inflated. If the heart rate remains slow, this may be due to the fact that the lungs have not yet been inflated or that the heart is not able to respond. This is determined by observing chest movement during the inflation breaths. Where the chest is seen to rise, this indicates that the lungs have been inflated.

Where the heart rate fails to increase, it is essential that chest movement is observed, indicating that ventilation of the lungs has occurred, before moving on to further intervention. If chest movement has not been seen, it should be ensured that the head is in the neutral position, that the mask fits without leaks, and the inflation breaths are repeated. Where the help has not arrived, also ensure that the jaw is being pulled up into the mask. Remember that the floppy baby will be unconscious, so the airway needs to be maintained throughout. However, it is easier to have two people perform the inflation breaths, one applying a two-handed jaw thrust (see Figure 3.11) whilst the other gives the breaths, again observing for chest movement.

On reassessing, if the heart rate remains slow and there is no chest movement, then a laryngeal mask should be inserted in babies over 34 weeks gestation. A laryngoscope is used to move the tongue out of the way, and the mask, which has previously been lubricated with water-soluble gel, is inserted in the position it is going to sit so that the mask area lies over the trachea.[31] This is then connected to the 'T' piece or bag and valve and inflation breaths repeated. The laryngeal mask may also be used as a means to maintain an airway once established as an alternative to using the mask or intubation.

Suction may be considered when it has not been possible to establish the airway. This should always be carried out under direct vision using a laryngoscope and a large bore suction catheter, looking for particles of meconium, blood clots or vernix, which may be blocking the airways.[31]

Once chest movement has been observed, then 30 seconds of ventilation breaths at a rate of 30 per minute should be given in an attempt to provide oxygen to the myocardium. At all times, observe for chest movement to ensure that the airway has been maintained, with the head being in the neutral position and with the two-handed jaw thrust if used.

Cardiac compressions should only be considered once the fluid from the lungs has been replaced with air,[28,31] thus allowing for oxygen transfer to occur. If the heart rate remains below 60 beats per minute following the ventilation breaths, chest compressions should be commenced at a ratio of three compressions to one ventilation breath. The rate should be at a speed so that 90 compressions and 30 breaths are achieved in one minute. The aim is for 15 cycles to be performed in 30 seconds. The oxygen should be increased to 100% when compressions are performed.[28]

When performing cardiac compressions on a newborn, the hands should be placed around the chest to form a firm platform, and the thumbs should be placed together on the sternum, just below the nipple line (see Figure 3.13), with the chest being compressed by a third. It is also possible to perform compressions with two fingers placed centrally just below the nipple line, but this method is less effective and more tiring. However, where medical teams are working on the baby, this may be the only way in which the person performing compressions can reach the chest (see Figure 3.12). Reassessment of the heart rate should be carried out every 30 seconds, with compressions being continued if the heart rate remains below 60 beats per minute. In most cases, the heart rate will respond quickly once oxygenated blood starts circulating through the heart to the aorta and then to the coronary arteries.[28] The main reason for the heart not responding to chest compressions is that the lungs are not being ventilated, and the positioning of the airway should be checked once again.

Once the heart rate increases, chest compressions can stop, but ventilation of the lungs should be maintained until spontaneous breathing commences by giving breaths at a rate of 30 per minute, reassessing the heart rate every 30 seconds, and ensuring that the lungs are being ventilated by observing for chest movement.

As discussed earlier in this section, the application of a pre-ductal saturation probe should be made early in the resuscitation attempt, and the oxygen levels should be titrated accordingly.

Drugs

Drugs are seldom required in a neonatal resuscitation, and their use usually indicates that the myocardium is unable to function properly due to lactic acidosis. However, the effectiveness of drugs in the newborn resuscitation scenario is unknown, with some babies responding whilst others do not.[31] Where drugs are required, the quickest access route is via the umbilical vein, and an umbilical venous catheter (UVC) should be inserted under

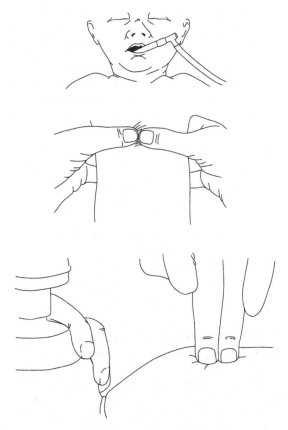

Figure 3.12 Finger positions for neonate chest compressions

aseptic conditions. A saline flush should be given between each drug. The drugs commonly used are outlined in Table 3.4.

Meconium

Any baby born in the presence of meconium (be it thin or significant) who cries at birth should be dried and handed to the mother for skin-to-skin contact. For babies who are not breathing at birth, the normal NLS algorithm should be followed. However, if it is not possible to achieve lung inflation after two rounds of inflation breaths, then a laryngoscope should be used to inspect the oropharynx and apply direct suction with a large bore suction catheter.[28,31] Where meconium or other particulate material such as blood or vernix is inhaled, it may indicate that the fetus in-utero has been hypoxic to the extent that the primitive breathing centers have been triggered, causing the fetus to take deep gasping breaths,[31] and this may

Table 3.4 Drugs used in newborn resuscitation

Drug	Dose	Effect
Adrenaline	20 micrograms/kg IV 100 micrograms/kg via ET tube if no access is available	Increases coronary artery perfusion pressure
Glucose	250mg/kg	Reduces incidence of hypoglycaemia in prolonged resuscitation attempts
Sodium Bicarbonate	1–2 mmol/kg slow IV	Reverses acidosis in prolonged resuscitation
Volume replacement	10ml/kg O negative blood or 0.9% sodium chloride	Considered if there is suspected blood loss

obstruct the airways. It is unlikely that normal breathing patterns will lead to this obstruction. The emphasis is to establish an airway and inflate the lungs, only reverting to suction if the inflation breaths are not successful in achieving this.

If the baby does not respond to the resuscitation attempt

Where it is difficult to inflate the lungs and/or increase the heart rate, the first consideration should be to check the neutral position, the application of the mask and the effectiveness of the jaw thrust. If airway adjuncts have been used, have these been inserted correctly? Once these facts have been checked, then other options must be considered, such as a blocked trachea, a pneumothorax, blood loss or an undiagnosed congenital abnormality.[31] If there is no heart rate at birth, and this is not established by ten minutes of age, the prognosis is poor even if spontaneous circulation is established. Generally, resuscitation would continue for 20 minutes before a discussion involving medical colleagues about discontinuing the attempt is made.

CARE FOLLOWING RESUSCITATION

Throughout any resuscitation attempt, the parents should be kept fully informed of the condition of their baby and what is happening. They will continue to need support and explanations following the resuscitation, but more especially so when the baby is not able to be resuscitated. Many maternity units have specialist midwives who offer support to parents following a birth where they need to explore the events further, as well as bereavement midwives who may become involved in their care at this point to give the appropriate information, support and guidance, although continued contact with the midwife present for the birth is often appreciated by the woman and the family.

Following successful resuscitation, the baby will need to be closely observed to ensure that there is no deterioration in the condition. The condition of the baby will determine if transfer to the neonatal unit is required, again with the parents in this situation needing guidance and support as well as the opportunity to visit the baby as soon as is possible. All babies who have been resuscitated should have skin-to-skin contact at the earliest opportunity and an early breastfeed, as their energy stores will have been depleted through the resuscitation. A blood glucose level test may be indicated to ensure the baby is not hypoglycaemic. As babies can lose heat rapidly, temperatures should be monitored, and the baby should be kept covered whilst with the mother. Heart rate and respirations according to the neonate's condition should also be monitored and documented,

As with all care, detailed records of the resuscitation should be made, including the time of birth, times for the varying interventions and the time that respirations were established. Where possible, one person scribing the events as they occur aids with the accurate documentation of the resuscitation.

SUMMARY OF MIDWIFERY RESPONSIBILITIES

- Ensure up-to-date knowledge of the theory and practice of both maternal and neonatal resuscitation. In most areas of work, this will involve a formal annual update. For those who may be working in areas, such as the community, where there is less support and backup, attendance at a recognised course may be beneficial.

- A good working knowledge of the equipment and drugs used for maternal and neonatal resuscitation within each area of work should be maintained. Remember that the equipment may vary from place to place.
- Ensure that equipment for both adult and newborn resuscitation is checked on a daily basis and again on taking over care. This includes levels of oxygen and air in cylinders on Resuscitaires.
- Observations of vital signs, in addition to a general assessment of health, should be carried out as frequently as appropriate for the woman and fetus/baby, ensuring that any deviations from what is expected are noted and escalated to the relevant practitioner. Maternal, fetal and neonatal conditions can deteriorate rapidly, so early identification is important to obtain a good outcome.
- Where possible, identify one person from the team to support the family/parents during any resuscitation situation. This enables explanations to occur at the time and may help the family to understand what is happening.
- Clear, contemporaneous and complete records must be kept, whether of routine assessments or in an emergency.

FURTHER READING AND RESOURCES

Chu J, Johnston TA, Geoghegan J, On Behalf of the Royal College of Obstetricians and Gynaecologists. Maternal collapse in pregnancy and the puerperium. BJOG. 2020;127:e14–e52.

The RCOG produces 'Green Top guidelines' on areas related to obstetrics and gynaecology. This guidance is specifically related to Maternal Collapse and includes guidance for resuscitation of the pregnant woman and perimortem caesarean section.

The Resuscitation Council, UK, produces a number of guidelines related to resuscitation. These can be found at 2021 Resuscitation Guidelines | Resuscitation Council UK and include the following:

- Perkins GD, Colquhoun M, Deakin CD, Smith C, Smyth M, Barraclough N, et al. Adult basic life support guidelines. 2021. [Accessed 13 April 2023]. Available from: www.resus.org.uk
- Soar J, Dealin CD, Nolan JP, Perkins GD, Yeung J, Couper K, et al. Adult advanced life support guidelines. 2021. [Accessed 12 April 2023]. Available from: www.resus.org.uk
- Wylie J, Madar J, Ainsworth S, Tinnion R, Chittick R, Wenlock N, et al. Newborn resuscitation and support of transition of infants at birth guidelines. 2021. [Accessed 7 June 2023]. Available from: Newborn resuscitation and support of transition of infants at birth Guidelines | Resuscitation Council UK

Resuscitation Council (UK). CPR right now. 2021. [Accessed 13 April 2023]. Available from: www.resus.org.uk/watch

A video representation of the basic life support guidance.

The Resuscitation Council (UK) has produced a number of interactive videos to help learn resuscitation skills. These can be found at: e-Lifesaver | Resuscitation Council UK.

Resuscitation Council (UK) NLS Subcommittee. Newborn life support. 5th ed. London: Resuscitation Council UK; 2021.

The Resuscitation Council (UK) runs newborn life support courses. This is the textbook related to this course, detailing the physiology and skills relating to the NLS guidance in detail.

Deakin CD, Soar J, Davies R, Patterson T, Lyon R, Nolan JP, et al. Special circumstances guidelines. 2021. [Accessed 13 April 2023]. Available from: www.resus.org.uk

The guidance for cardiac arrest in pregnancy can be found in the 'Specific health conditions' section of this publication.

REFERENCES

1. Chu J, Johnston TA, Geoghegan J. On behalf of the royal college of obstetricians and gynaecologists: maternal collapse in pregnancy and the puerperium. BJOG. 2020;127:e14–e52.
2. Knight M, Bunch K, Patel R, Shakespeare J, Kotnis R, Kenyon S, Kurinczuk JJ, On Behalf of MBRRACE-UK, editors. Saving lives,

improving mothers' care core report – lessons learned to inform maternity care from the UK and Ireland confidential enquiries into maternal deaths and morbidity 2018–20. Oxford: National Perinatal Epidemiology Unit, University of Oxford; 2022.

3. Nursing and Midwifery Council (NMC). The code: professional standards of practice and behavior for nurses and midwives. 2015, updated 2018. Available from: www.nmc-uk.org

4. Beckett VA, Knight M, Sharpe P. The CAPS study: incidence, management and outcomes of cardiac arrest in pregnancy in the UK: a prospective, descriptive study. BJOC. 2017;124:1374–1381.

5. Resuscitation Council UK. Quality standards: acute care equipment and drug list. 2013, updated 2020. [Accessed 11 April 2023]. Available from: https://www.resus.org.uk/library/quality-standards-cpr/acute-care-equipment-and-drug-lists

6. Gauntlett R, Knight M, On Behalf of the MBRRACE Critical Care Chapter Writing Group. Messages for critical care. In: Knight M, Bunch K, Tuffnell D, Shakespeare J, Kotnis R, Kenyon S, Kurinczuk JJ, On Behalf of MBRRACE-UK, editors. Saving lives, improving mothers' care core report – lessons learned to inform maternity care from the UK and Ireland confidential enquiries into maternal deaths and morbidity 2015–17. Oxford: National Perinatal Epidemiology Unit, University of Oxford; 2019.

7. Soar J, Dealin CD, Nolan JP, Perkins GD, Yeung J, Couper K, et al. Adult advanced life support guidelines. 2021. [Accessed 12 April 2023]. Available from: www.resus.org.uk

8. Bunch K, Knight M. Maternal mortality in the UK 2018–20: surveillance and epidemiology. In: Knight M, Bunch K, Patel R, Shakespeare J, Kotnis R, Kenyon S, Kurinczuk JJ, On Behalf of MBRRACE-UK, editors. Saving lives, improving mothers' care core report – lessons learned to inform maternity care from the UK and Ireland confidential enquiries into marternal deaths and morbidity 2018–20. Oxford: National Perinatal Epidemiology Unit, University of Oxford; 2022.

9. Lee AJ, Landau R. Aotocaval compression syndrome: time to revisit certain dogmas. Anesthesia & Analgesia. 2017 Dec;125(6):1975–1985. Available from: <doi:10.1213/ANE.0000000000002313>

10. Murray I, Hendley J. Change and adaptation in pregnancy. In: Marshall J, Raynor M, editors. Myles textbook for midwives. Edinburgh: Elsevier; 2020.

11. Rankin J. The haematological system – physiology of the blood. In: Rankin J, editor. Physiology in childbearing with anatomy and related biosciences. Edinburgh: Elsevier; 2017.

12. Howie J, Watson J, Marshall H. Postpartum haemorrhage and other third-stage problems. In: Rankin J, editor. Physiology in childbearing with anatomy and related biosciences. Edinburgh: Elsevier; 2017.

13. Rankin J. Respiration. In: Rankin J, editor. Physiology in childbearing with anatomy and related biosciences. Edinburgh: Elsevier; 2017.

14. Hayman R, Raynor M. Operative births. In: Marshall J, Raynor M, editors. Myles textbook for midwives. Edinburgh: Elsevier; 2020.

15. Bothamley J, Boyle M. Medical conditions affecting pregnancy and childbirth. 2nd ed. Abingdon: Routledge; 2021.

16. Waugh A, Grant A. Ross and Wilson anatomy and physiology in health and illness. 14th ed. Edinburgh: Elsevier; 2023.

17. Wyllie J, Lockey A, Hampshire S Executive summary of the main changes since the 2015 guidelines. 2021. [Accessed 10 April 2023]. Available from: www.resus.org.uk

18. Perkins GD, Colquhoun M, Deakin CD, Smith C, Smyth M, Barraclough N, et al. Adult basic life support guidelines. 2021. [Accessed 13 April 2023]. Available from: www.resus.org.uk

19. Deakin CD, Soar J, Davies R, Patterson T, Lyon R, Nolan JP, et al. Special circumstances guidelines. 2021. [Accessed 13 April 2023]. Available from: www.resus.org.uk

20. Resuscitation Council (UK). CPR right now. 2021. [Accessed 13 April 2023]. Available from: www.resus.org.uk/watch

21. Resuscitation Council (UK). Cardiopulmonary resuscitation, automated

defibrillators. 2018. Available from: https://www.resus.org.uk/sites/default/files/2020-05/CPR%20AEDs%20and%20the%20law%20%285%29.pdf

22. The PROMPT Editorial Team, editors. PROMPT course manual. 3rd ed. Cambridge: Cambridge University Press; 2017.

23. National Institute for Health and Care Excellence. British national formulary. 2023. [Accessed 13 April 2023]. Available from: www.bnf.nice.org.uk

24. Considine J, Eastwood K, Webster H, Smyth M, Nation K, Grief R, et al. Family presence during adult resuscitation from cardiac arrest: a systematic review in Resuscitation Col. 2022;180:11–23. [Accessed 5 June 2023]. Available from: <doi:10.1016/j.resuscitation.2022.08.021>

25. MBRRACE. Maternal deaths. 2023. [Accessed 6 June 2023]. Available from: www.npeu.ox.ac.uk

26. United Nations. WHO chief declares end to COVID-19 as a global health emergency. UN News. 2023. [Accessed 6 June 2023]. Available from: https://news.un.org/en/story/2023/05/1136367

27. Resuscitation Council (UK). Guidance: Covid-19: update to resuscitaiton council (UK) guidance for practice. 2022. [Accessed 6 June 2023]. Available from: https://www.resus.org.uk/library/additional-guidance/guidance-covid-19

28. Wylie J, Madar J, Ainsworth S, Tinnion R, Chittick R, Wenlock N, et al. Newborn resuscitation and support of transition of infants at birth guidelines. 2021. [Accessed 7 June 2023]. Available from: https://www.resus.org.uk/library/2021-resuscitation-guidelines/newborn-resuscitation-and-support-transition-infants-birth

29. Madar J, Roehr CC, Ainsworth S, Ersdal H, Morley C, Rudiger M, et al. European resuscitation council guidelines 2021: newborn resuscitation and support of transition of infants at birth. Resuscitation. 2021;161:291–326. Available from: <doi:10.1016/j.resuscitation.2021.02.014>

30. Blackburn S. Maternal, fetal and neonatal physiology: a clinical perspective. 5th ed. Missouri: Elsevier; 2017.

31. Resuscitation Council (UK) NLS Subcommittee. Newborn life support, 5th ed. London: Resuscitation Council UK; 2021.

32. Jackson K, Anderson M, Marshall JE. Physiology and care during the first stage of labour. In Marshall J, Raynor M, editors. Myles textbook for midwives. Edinburgh: Elsevier; 2020.

33. Davis PG, Tan A, O'Donnell CPF, Schulz A. Resuscitation of newborn infants with 100% oxygen or air: a systematic review and meta-analysis. The Lancet. 2004;364:1329–1333. [Accessed 9 June 2023]. Available from: https://pubmed.ncbi.nlm.nih.gov/15474135/

34. Gomersall J, Berber S, Middleton P, McDonald SJ, Niermeyer S, El-Naggar W, et al. On behalf of the international Liason committee on resuscitation neonatal life support task force: umbilical cord management at term and late preterm birth: a meta-analysis. Pediatrics. 2021;147(3):e2020015404.

4

Antepartum Haemorrhage

LUISA ACOSTA

Introduction 57
Risk/predisposing factors for APH 57
Placental abruption 59
Pathophysiology of placental
abruption 59
Clinical features of placental abruption 59
Specific care for women with placental
abruption 62
Placenta praevia 62
Pathophysiology of low-lying placenta and
placenta praevia 63
Clinical features of low-lying placenta and
placenta praevia 65
Specific care for women with low-lying
placenta and placenta praevia 66
Care for all women with APH (placental
abruption and placenta praevia) 66
Potential outcomes of APH 69
Follow-up/long-term issues 70
Summary of midwifery responsibilities 71
Further reading and resources 71
References 71

BOX 4.1: Definitions

Antepartum Haemorrhage (APH): bleeding from or into the genital tract after 24* weeks' gestation and before the birth of the baby.[1] (*The basis of this definition is in keeping with the national legal age of viability of the fetus in the UK.)

Intrapartum Haemorrhage: when antepartum bleeding occurs in the first or second stage of labour.

Obstetric Haemorrhage: encompasses antenatal, intrapartum and postpartum bleeding.

Placental Abruption: partial or complete separation of a normally situated placenta before the birth of the baby.

Placenta Praevia: when the placenta is attached to the lower uterine segment and completely or partially covers the internal uterine os.

Low-lying placenta: when the placenta is implanted within 20mm of the internal os but is not covering any part of the os.

Uterine rupture: when there is a complete (myometrial and peritoneal) or incomplete (myometrial only) tear of the uterine wall. See Chapter 11 for further details.

Vasa praevia: when fetal blood vessels travel through the placental membranes over or near the cervical os.

DOI: 10.4324/9781003382195-4

INTRODUCTION

Antepartum haemorrhage (APH) is known to occur in approximately 3–5% of all pregnancies and is considered a major cause of perinatal morbidity and mortality worldwide.[1] In the UK, the MBRRACE-UK report[2] identified six maternal deaths from APH between 2016 and 2018; three were due to placental abruption and three from placenta praevia/accreta. There are, however, no comprehensive statistics on the number of women who have suffered life-changing consequences from an APH.

Any amount of bleeding in the antenatal period is considered abnormal and could be serious, potentially resulting in rapid deterioration in the condition of the woman and baby. The visible blood loss may vary from spotting to major haemorrhage. However, the bleeding may also be concealed, and, therefore, assessment for signs of clinical shock is as important as estimating the amount of visible blood loss. Management of an APH requires prompt escalation and a multidisciplinary approach.

Causes of APH

Approximately half of women who present with a major or massive APH are found to have *placental abruption (PA)* or *placenta praevia (PP)*. Uterine rupture, although rare, may also lead to significant intrapartum and postpartum haemorrhage (see Chapter 11). The majority of minor antepartum bleeding can be attributed to 'unexplained'[1] APH causes, also described as 'unclassified'[3] causes or 'antepartum bleeding of unknown origin (ABUO)[4] and includes marginal placental bleeds and a 'show' at the start of labour. Sometimes, the cause may be identified later, for example, on inspection of the

placenta after the birth of the baby, but usually the origin of the bleed remains unexplained. Bleeding of unknown origin is associated with an increased risk of induction of labour and preterm birth.[4]

APH from *local causes* may be due to vaginal varicosities, a 'show', polyps, benign tumours, infections such as cervicitis/vaginitis and, more rarely, cervical cancer. Trauma to the genital tract can also cause bleeding, and midwives must be aware that APH is a known consequence of partner violence.

Ruptured *vasa praevia*, the only fetal cause of APH, occurs when there is a velamentous insertion of the umbilical cord (type 1) or there are blood vessels leading from the placenta to a succenturiate lobe (type 2).[5] The blood vessels are not protected by the placenta or the Wharton's jelly of the umbilical cord and run through the membranes across the lower segment of the uterus near or over the presenting part. Bleeding will occur if the blood vessels are severed when the membranes rupture. The blood lost is fetal blood and will be associated with acute fetal compromise.[6]

RISK/PREDISPOSING FACTORS FOR APH

APH cannot be predicted, and the risk factors are not always apparent. Although there are some overlapping risk factors for the different causes of APH (see Table 4.2), the underlying aetiology is often different. Yang et al.[7] noted that PA is more likely to occur due to conditions arising during pregnancy, whereas PP is more likely to occur due to conditions existing prior to pregnancy. However, PA is also considered to be the result of chronic processes that may be present before conception and during early pregnancy.[8]

Table 4.1 Causes of APH

Placental causes	Genital tract causes	Unclassified causes	Fetal causes
Placenta praevia	Uterine rupture	Marginal bleeds	Vasa praevia
Placental abruption	Genital tract trauma	'Show'	
	Varicosities		
	Polyps		
	Cervical ectropion		
	Cervical cancer		
	Infectionscervicitis/vaginitis		

Table 4.2 Possible risk and predisposing factors for placenta abruption and placenta praevia

Placental Abruption[3,9,10,11,12,13,14,15]	Placenta Praevia[3,16,17,18,19,20]
Socio-demographic and lifestyle risk factors	
• Maternal age > 35 and < 20 years • Multiparity >3 • Smoking • Cocaine use • Alcohol abuse • Socio-economic disadvantage • Low BMI, dietary and folic acid deficiency • Stress and depression	• Advanced maternal age • Multiparity • Smoking • Cocaine and other drug abuse
Pre-pregnancy risk factors	
• Chronic hypertension • Asthma • Thrombophilia • Anaemia • Diabetes • Uterine anomalies • Endometriosis • Subfertility and assisted conception • Raised BMI • Migraine • Previous C/S • Previous miscarriage • Previous ischaemic placental disease • Previous stillbirth • Previous placental abruption	• Uterine scarring • Previous CS (the risk rises in association with the increase in number of previous CS) • Endometriosis • Assisted reproductive technologies • Previous induced abortion • Previous miscarriage • Fibroids • Previous manual removal of the placenta • Previous placenta praevia
Current pregnancy risk factors	
Acute factors:	
• Sudden decompression: Rupture of membranes in polyhydramnios or multiple pregnancy • Abdominal trauma • External cephalic version (ECV) • Acute vascular changes (e.g., cocaine use)	• Multiple pregnancy • Male infant • Early pregnancy bleeding • Anaemia
Chronic factors:	

• Inflammatory conditions: Chorioamnionitis/premature rupture of membranes (PROM)
• Ischaemic placental disease:
  Pregnancy-induced hypertension
  Pre-eclampsia
  Small for gestational age fetus
• Oligohydramnios
• Premature rupture of membranes
• Anaemia
• Placenta praevia – which can lead to abruption
• Placental abnormalities (e.g., circumvallate placenta)
• Multiple pregnancy
• Early pregnancy bleeding	

PLACENTAL ABRUPTION

Placental abruption (PA) is the premature separation of a normally implanted placenta prior to the birth of the baby. It is associated with abdominal pain, vaginal bleeding and fetal compromise.[11] PA is reported to occur in approximately 0.3–1.6% of pregnancies.[21,22] However, the incidence is difficult to estimate as the condition varies in severity and is often only confirmed after the birth of the baby by evidence of retroplacental bleeding or clot, suggesting that the incidence is higher than estimated.

PA is associated with significant maternal and neonatal complications. There is a strong association with fetal growth restriction,[10] preterm birth, birth-related asphyxia and significant perinatal mortality rates,[22] with more than half the perinatal losses to fetal death occurring before the woman arrives in hospital.

PATHOPHYSIOLOGY OF PLACENTAL ABRUPTION

The immediate cause of placental separation is when maternal blood supply to the decidua basalis is disrupted. The severed blood vessels bleed into the space between the decidua and the placental wall, where the accumulated blood forms a haematoma. The pressure exerted by this forces the placenta to separate from the uterus, causing the fetus to become deprived of oxygen and nutrients. The

condition of the fetus will depend on the remaining placental area, fetal reserves and the rapidity of recognition and treatment.

With a **revealed** haemorrhage, bleeding may track down between the membranes and uterus and appear externally. This occurs in approximately 80% of cases. In 20% of cases, the bleeding is more centrally located and may be retained behind the placenta. Here, the blood does not escape, and it is said to be a **concealed** haemorrhage. In severe cases, there is a build-up of pressure, and the blood infiltrates the myometrium, causing pain, uterine tenderness and irritability, as well as the diagnostic 'board-like' uterus. This is known as a Couvelaire uterus or uteroplacental apoplexy.

A **mixed** haemorrhage may have some revealed and some concealed bleeding.

The classification of haemorrhage from PA can be seen in Figure 4.1.

CLINICAL FEATURES OF PLACENTAL ABRUPTION

The aetiology of PA is mainly unclear, with many cases occurring in women with no identifiable risks.[23] PA has been referred to as 'accidental' haemorrhage, suggesting that the cause is traumatic and sudden. However, it is now understood that only a small proportion of cases occur spontaneously and involve trauma. PA is more likely to occur as the end result of underlying chronic processes starting

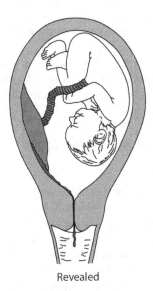
Revealed

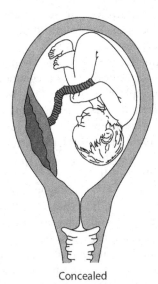
Concealed

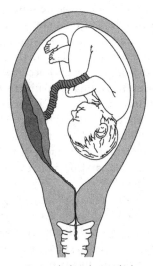
Concealed and revealed

Figure 4.1 Placental abruption (revealed, concealed and mixed)

weeks or months before the actual event,[24] despite its rapid clinical onset. Therefore, PA appears to be the result of a combination of both acute and chronic processes.[11]

Of the many associated risk factors (see Table 4.2), Brandt and Ananth found that the most common are previous PA, chronic hypertension, pre-eclampsia, cocaine and drug abuse and intimate partner violence.[11]

Acute Processes: Acute processes resulting in PA may be mechanical or 'shearing' in nature or may involve sudden decompression of an overdistended uterus.[11,13] Direct trauma to the abdomen and sudden decompression of the uterine cavity will cause the uterus to contract or expand and change shape, resulting in the inelastic placenta being forced to tear away from the uterine wall.[25]

Sudden decompression may occur with spontaneous rupture of membranes where there is polyhydramnios or in multiple pregnancies and after the birth of the first twin. Direct trauma to the abdomen has been associated with a six-fold increased risk of an abruption.[26] Examples of direct trauma include falls, road traffic accidents and intimate partner violence.[27] With road traffic accidents, it is proposed that sudden deceleration will cause high pressures within the uterus as well as a change in uterine shape, leading to the forced separation of the placenta.[13] Although rare, the external cephalic version may also result in an abruption due to mechanical forces changing the shape of the uterus.[28]

Acute vascular changes in pregnancy, which are associated with acute-onset abruption, involve vasoconstriction and sudden rise in blood pressure. Examples of this are fulminating pre-eclampsia or cocaine use (particularly in the 3rd trimester).[13,29]

Abruption may also occur as the end result of an acute inflammatory pathway. For example, chorioamnionitis from an ascending infection, particularly following preterm premature rupture of membranes, will result in bacterial colonisation, inflammation, subsequent cell destruction within the decidua, and possible early separation of the placenta.[9,30,31]

Other risk factors that have been more recently associated with acute PA are exposure to air and water pollution,[32] climate change and stressful life events,[33] although the underpinning mechanisms are not clearly understood.

Chronic Processes: Chronic processes that may lead to an abruption are secondary to inadequate placental implantation, involving defective spiral artery remodelling and shallow trophoblast invasion.[9,11] This is associated with poor placental perfusion, inflammation and thrombosis.[11] The outcome of these chronic processes can result in fetal growth restriction, pre-eclampsia and PA. These three conditions share similar underlying aetiology, which is based on ischaemic placental disease.[13,34]

Furthermore, women with a history of fetal growth restriction, preterm birth and pre-eclampsia in a previous pregnancy are also at an increased risk of abruption in a subsequent pregnancy[15] and have twice the risk of cardiovascular disease and stroke later in life,[35,36] suggesting that the chronic processes leading to placental ischaemia and abruption have a similar aetiology to those underpinning cardiovascular disease and stroke. Women who have experienced PA and who later develop cardiovascular disorders may also share similar lifestyle habits (for example, smoking) and underlying metabolic, inflammatory and genetic conditions,[36] placing them at higher risk.

Older maternal age is associated with PA due to decreased vascularisation of the uterus, predisposing to placental insufficiency.[14] This may also be compounded by lifestyle factors and underlying conditions, as mentioned previously.

When placental implantation occurs over uterine malformations or scarring (for example, fibroids, bicornuate uterus, previous caesarean section) and in the case of a circumvallate placenta, there is a greater risk due to the instability of the site and decreased vascularisation of the placental area.[37]

The more complications that occur in a previous pregnancy, the more the risk is for PA subsequently.[15] However, the greatest risk factor for PA is a previous abruption.[11,15]

Signs and symptoms of placental abruption

Diagnosis of an abruption is made by assessing the clinical features, as seen in Table 4.3. Ultrasound may assist in making a diagnosis but is not always reliable as the blood clots may look similar to the placental tissue.[38] Therefore, an abruption will be suspected if there is any bleeding, uterine pain or irritability and fetal compromise. Any pregnant woman involved in a road traffic accident or

Table 4.3 Signs and symptoms of placental abruption and placenta praevia

	Placental abruption (PA)[11]	Placenta praevia (PP)[3,38]
Bleeding	The amount of visible blood, whether acute or chronic, cannot be associated with the severity of the abruption. Blood may be red if it is fresh loss, but there may be brown blood or clots if it has been retained behind the placenta for any length of time. When there is no visible blood loss, retroplacental clots will be evident on inspection of the placenta after the birth of the baby. With an abruption resulting from acute processes, bleeding may be characterised by sudden onset. Bleeding from chronic processes may be characterised by more minor bleeds occurring intermittently throughout the pregnancy, often in the presence of oligohydramnios, fetal growth restriction and pre-eclampsia.	Bleeding is never concealed (as in a PA) and blood loss is fresh and red.
Shock	When haemorrhage occurs, regardless of whether it is revealed or concealed, signs of shock will occur when the woman is no longer able to compensate for the amount of blood lost. The heart rate and respiratory rate increase, and the BP will start to decrease. Peripheral circulation also decreases with skin becoming paler, cool and clammy, along with poor capillary refill and a weak pulse.	The level of hypovolaemic shock will correspond with the amount of blood loss. Due to increased blood volume, most healthy pregnant women with a normal BMI can tolerate up to 35% blood loss (or 1200–1500mls) before showing signs of shock.
Pain	Abdominal pain, which can be moderate or severe, is intermittent or continuous and the onset may be sudden or gradual. Backache may be present if the placenta is posterior.	Pain is not usually a feature because the placenta that is over the os will allow the blood to escape, thus avoiding the formation of a retroplacental clot. A small number of women may also present with uterine irritability alongside bleeding. This is similar to the presentation of PA and, indeed, coexisting abruption may be present.
Abdominal examination	In a concealed haemorrhage, there may be an increase in abdominal girth and the uterus may be firm or 'board-like' (Couvelaire) on palpation. The abdomen may be tender to touch, and the uterus will be generally irritable.	The uterus is usually soft and non-tender. There is often malpresentation and/or an unstable lie because the placenta occupies the space in the pelvis where the fetal head usually lies. Breech presentation is particularly common. With any presentation, the presenting part will remain high.
Fetal compromise	The woman may report a history of reduced or excessive fetal movements. Fetal heart sounds may be muffled or absent. On CTG, the fetal heart rate will show signs of hypoxia.	The fetal heart rate is usually normal, although fetal tachycardia, reflecting maternal tachycardia, may be present. When haemorrhage is severe, signs of fetal hypoxia will be present.
Altered mental status	Any deviation from the norm in the progression of pregnancy can cause anxiety. However, as hypovolaemic shock progresses, anxiety will increase, and the woman may become irritable, confused or lethargic and eventually may lose consciousness.[39]	

admitted with a history of partner violence should be deemed at high risk of an abruption regardless of their presentation.[13]

Symptoms may depend on the amount of blood loss and the extent of the detachment. Although these two factors do not always correlate with the degree of maternal/fetal compromise.[40] PA may be classified as mild, moderate or severe based on the following clinical features.

A **mild PA** involves minimal bleeding, which may be revealed or concealed. The detachment may have occurred at the edge of a normally located placenta.[23] There may or may not be slight uterine tenderness.[40,41] The condition of the woman and fetus are not compromised.[41] A mild abruption is not easy to diagnose, and treatment will be conservative.

A **moderate PA** is associated with significant haemorrhage where a large portion of the placenta has separated. The blood loss may be partially concealed and partially revealed – a mixed haemorrhage. The woman will show signs of shock and experience abdominal pain, uterine irritability or contractions.[41] Back pain may also be experienced.[25] The fetal condition will be compromised, and close monitoring is needed. The condition of both the woman and fetus may deteriorate rapidly.

A **severe PA** is associated with massive haemorrhage, and most or all of the placenta will have separated. The fetus will be severely compromised and may die. Rapid vaginal birth may occur due to hypertonic contractions.[25] The bleeding can be revealed or concealed. The woman will be shocked and in extreme pain when a large quantity of the blood loss is concealed behind the placenta. The board-like, 'Couvaliere' uterus will be evident. Coagulopathy is likely to occur as the damaged placenta will release thromboplastins into the circulation. See postnatal care in what follows for further detail.[23,41]

SPECIFIC CARE FOR WOMEN WITH PLACENTAL ABRUPTION

If a **mild PA** is suspected and if there are no further episodes of bleeding or other concerns, the pregnancy can continue, which will hopefully improve the outcome for the baby.[3] Careful monitoring throughout the pregnancy will be needed due to the increased chance of further bleeding and poor fetal growth.[3] Whilst in hospital, intravenous

access is needed, and blood is taken. This will include blood group and serum saved in case further haemorrhage occurs and cross-matching is necessary. If the gestation of the baby is between 24 and 34 + 6 weeks, antenatal corticosteroids can be administered to accelerate fetal lung maturity if an imminent birth is anticipated.[42] Anaemia must be corrected, and if the woman is rhesus negative, an intramuscular injection of anti-D immunoglobulin is needed. A Kleihauer test will be done to determine the dose required based on the presence of fetal blood in maternal circulation. The placental site will be determined by an ultrasound scan to exclude PP. After a period of observation, the woman may return home if no further bleeding has occurred in the preceding 24 hours and fetal monitoring is normal. It must be recognised that a mild PA can proceed to severe rapidly within this time.[13] Repeated episodes of bleeding will lead to a decision being made to expedite the birth of the baby.[23]

Where an abruption is **moderate or severe,** immediate birth may be necessary. Close monitoring and vigilant care are essential as both the woman and the fetus may deteriorate rapidly. See what follows for further discussion about the care of a woman experiencing a massive APH.

PLACENTA PRAEVIA

The term placenta praevia (PP) is used when the placenta partially or completely covers the internal cervical os. If the placenta is implanted within 20mm of the internal os but does not cover any part of the os, it is termed a low-lying placenta[19,43] (see Table 4.4). PP occurs in approximately one in 200 pregnancies at term and is associated with adverse maternal and neonatal outcomes and preterm birth.[19] The incidence is expected to rise due to the rising caesarean section rates, the increase in women of advanced maternal age and assisted birth technologies.[19,44]

PP is the most common cause of APH[45] and typically presents as painless bleeding in the third trimester. The unpredictability and possible severity of bleeding and frequent and prolonged hospital admissions pose significant challenges to the woman and the maternity team. Vaginal birth is not considered safe, and birth by caesarean section is therefore necessary.

There is a strong association of a low-lying placenta or PP with the placenta accreta spectrum (see Box 4.2), where the placenta is abnormally adherent or deeply invades the structures beyond the decidua basalis (for example, the myometrium and, more rarely, the surrounding visceral tissues) leading to massive haemorrhage when separation occurs, and sometimes the need for a hysterectomy. In 90% of the cases of placenta accreta spectrum, where the placenta is adherent, the women will have had a previous caesarean section alongside a PP in the current pregnancy.[46]

The risk factors for low-lying and PP can be seen in Table 4.4.

PATHOPHYSIOLOGY OF LOW-LYING PLACENTA AND PLACENTA PRAEVIA

The aetiology is not fully understood, but it is theorised that the factors that influence implantation, placental growth and migration play a role in the condition (Figure 4.2).

The blastocyst usually implants into the endometrium in the fundal area where there is a good blood supply and a better chance of growth and survival.[47] It is not clear why some implant nearer to the internal cervical os than the upper section of

Table 4.4 Placenta praevia classification (Royal College of Obstetricians and Gynaecologists and The American Institute of Ultrasound in Medicine[19,43]

Terminology	Previous classification	Position of placenta
Low-lying placenta	Previously Type I (minor placenta praevia)	Lateral or low-lying: the placenta encroaches on the lower uterine segment and ends within 20mm of, but does not reach, the cervical os.
	Previously Type II (minor placenta praevia)	Marginal: the edge of the placenta extends to the internal cervical os but does not cover it.
Placenta praevia	Previously Type III (major placenta praevia)	Partial: the placenta mostly covers the internal cervical os.
	Previously Type IV (major placenta praevia)	Central: the placenta completely covers the internal cervical os.

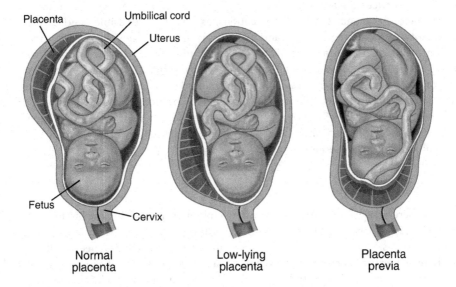

Normal placenta

Low-lying placenta

Placenta previa

Figure 4.2 Placenta praevia

BOX 4.2: Placenta accreta spectrum (PAS)

This term refers to a spectrum of abnormal adherence or invasion of the placental tissue into the myometrium.[19, 55] The depth can vary throughout the placental site and typically occurs when the placenta implants where there is an area of scar tissue.[56] Uterine scarring may lead to the residual myometrium being thinner and to the absence or defective formation of the decidua and spiral arteries.[56] Therefore, the chorionic villi attach directly to the myometrium and/or may infiltrate further into the myometrium and embed closer to the serosal lining of the uterus in order to access the larger arteries beyond the area damaged by scar tissue.[56]

The spectrum ranges from placenta *accreta* or *'creta'* (where the chorionic villi attach superficially to the inner myometrium) to the more invasive placenta *increta* (where the villi deeply infiltrate the myometrium) and placenta *percreta* (where the villi penetrate the myometrium and through the serosa layer of the uterus, reaching adjacent organs, for example, the bladder).[55] With placenta percreta, ultrasound imaging shows that instead of the villi being overly invasive, involvement of the serosa and external organs appears to occur when there is extended damage to the uterine wall and adjacent tissues from uterine rupture, dehiscence or adhesions, leaving excessive scarring and little or no myometrium at the site of placentation.[56]

The incidence of PAS is increasing worldwide. This is most likely due to increasing CS rates, which is the most common risk factor for PAS.[55] Furthermore, the PAS risk increases relative to the number of previous CS births. PP and an anterior low-lying placenta are also important risk factors for PAS. Therefore, PAS should be suspected if a woman presents with these coexisting factors at the mid-pregnancy fetal anomaly scan. Although uncommon, a primiparous woman with previous uterine scarring from artificial reproductive technologies, uterine scarring or uterine abnormalities may also be at risk.

When the placenta is abnormally adherent, it does not spontaneously separate at birth, causing severe and sometimes life-threatening bleeding when manual removal is attempted. If the placenta is not easily removed within 30 minutes after the birth and remains attached (and not entrapped), PAS may be suspected, especially if manual removal is difficult to perform.[55]

More than half the cases are not recognised antenatally, markedly increasing maternal morbidity and mortality.[46] Antenatal identification is important to ensure that appropriate care and a plan for CS birth take place in a maternity unit where multidisciplinary expertise, transfusion and critical care services are available. Pre-birth counselling should include discussions about the risk of haemorrhage and surgical complications, as well as the possible need for blood transfusion, interventional radiography and cell salvage. It is also likely that peripartum hysterectomy with the placenta insitu will be needed. If the woman declines an elective peripartum hysterectomy, or PAS is diagnosed following a vaginal birth, then in the absence of bleeding, leaving the placenta in place may be considered with appropriate care and follow-up.[19]

Antenatal care is otherwise similar to the care received by women with PP and/or APH (see what follows for related care). Birth by CS will be planned for 35 to 36 weeks.[19] For women who request elective non-medical CS, there needs to be a discussion about the risk of PAS and related complications in subsequent pregnancies.[19]

the uterus, but there are several associations with the maternal risk factors discussed in what follows that may influence this.

Where there is uterine scarring, as with previous caesarean section or endometriosis, there may be changes in the peristaltic movement of the endometrium, forcing the blastocyst to move lower in the uterus rather than implant nearer the fundus.[48] As the blastocyst needs collagen for implantation, adherence to uterine scarring is still possible as the scar tissue is rich in collagen. This environment enables it to proliferate even though the scar tissue is less vascularised and hypoxic.[49] Where the trophoblastic cells of the blastocyst implant into a scarred or hypoxic area of the uterus, they are more likely to invade deeply into the decidua and myometrium to access the richer blood supply below.[47] This will result in the developing placenta becoming adherent as with the placenta accreta spectrum. See Box 4.2 for further details.

Placental hypertrophy, where the placenta grows abnormally large in response to adverse conditions within the uterus, may result in part of the placenta inhabiting the lower segment of the uterus. This may occur where there is hypoxia from smoking or in the case of multiparity or advanced maternal age.[47]

In early pregnancy, it is more common for the placenta to be low-lying as the lower uterine segment has not yet developed. As the uterus grows and the lower segment lengthens and stretches, the placenta appears to 'migrate' upwards and away from the os and the developing lower uterine segment.[3] During this process, the placenta itself does not move but grows towards an area of the uterus that is better vascularised, and the part of the placenta lying over the less vascularised area in the lower segment will atrophy and regress, in a process called trophotropism.[50] Occasionally, blood vessels may be left behind causing a vasa praevia, or if the atrophy is incomplete a succenturiate lobe may be left behind.[51] Velamentous cord insertion is also more likely when placental migration has occurred.[52]

Approximately 90% of low-lying placentas in early to mid-pregnancy will 'migrate' to a normal location by term. However, when the placental edge extends over the os, migration is less likely. The more the placental edge overlaps the os, the less likely it is to migrate. Where the placenta does not migrate, it is known as a persisting low-lying placenta or placenta praevia[19,51] This is associated with a posterior placenta, a history of previous CS, other uterine procedures or damage to the endometrium or myometrium.[53]

Antenatal bleeding from placenta praevia occurs as a result of placental separation during the formation of the lower uterine segment or when cervical effacement occurs. It follows that initial episodes of antenatal bleeding or 'warning bleeds' are more likely after 26–28 weeks' gestation, and torrential haemorrhage will occur when labour begins.[54] Vaginal examination and sexual intercourse may also cause bleeding.

CLINICAL FEATURES OF LOW-LYING PLACENTA AND PLACENTA PRAEVIA

Diagnosis of low-lying placenta and placenta praevia

Routine mid-pregnancy ultrasound at approximately 20 weeks will include screening for placental localization.[57] If the placenta is found to be low-lying or covering the cervical os, then ultrasound scanning, including a transvaginal scan, will be offered at 32 weeks. Transvaginal scanning is safe and more accurate than transabdominal scanning and allows the precise location of the placental edge and distance from the os to be measured, thereby accurately diagnosing a persisting low-lying placenta or placenta praevia.[19] The length of the cervix can also be measured to predict the likelihood of preterm birth. If the placenta is still low-lying or covering the os at 32 weeks, a further transvaginal scan will be offered at 36 weeks to confirm the diagnosis of either a low-lying placenta or PP.[19]

For women with an anterior placenta praevia and who have had a previous caesarean section, placenta accreta should be suspected. In this situation, expert ultrasound imaging is recommended. Magnetic resonance imaging (MRI) may be used to assess the depth of placental invasion.

Signs and symptoms of placenta praevia

Although a definitive diagnosis of a low-lying placenta or placenta praevia is almost always made with ultrasound scanning, if any woman presents with painless bleeding, a high presenting part and an abnormal lie at any stage of pregnancy, placenta praevia must be suspected. Only about 10% of women diagnosed with placenta praevia will reach term without bleeding.[38] The initial bleeds do not normally compromise the woman or fetus and are sometimes referred to as 'warning bleeds'. More severe bleeding usually occurs after the 34th week of pregnancy. For more detail on the signs and symptoms of placenta praevia, see Table 4.3.

SPECIFIC CARE FOR WOMEN WITH LOW-LYING PLACENTA AND PLACENTA PRAEVIA

Once a confirmed diagnosis is made on ultrasound, an appointment with the obstetric consultant is recommended to discuss the mode of birth. The discussion should include the need for a caesarean section in the case of a persisting placenta praevia or with a low-lying placenta where there are other associated risk factors or bleeding. A vaginal birth may be possible in the case of an asymptomatic low-lying placenta.[19] The decision will be based on the woman's preferences and further ultrasound scanning. The birth should take place in a maternity unit where there is access to critical care and blood transfusion services.

A sensitive explanation of the risks associated with placenta praevia needs to take place once a diagnosis has been made. This should include the risk of haemorrhage, preterm birth, the need for hospitalisation and the possibility of blood transfusion and hysterectomy.

Most women who are diagnosed with a low-lying placenta or placenta praevia who remain asymptomatic will continue with outpatient care. This will depend on their individual circumstances and proximity to the hospital. In this situation, it is important that women and their partners are advised about safety precautions to ensure that there is continuous support at home and the means for immediate transfer to hospital should any signs of bleeding, pain or contractions become apparent. The woman should also be advised that sexual intercourse should be avoided.

Women who are likely to refuse blood products should already have been identified routinely.[58] Following diagnosis of a low-lying placenta or placenta praevia additional discussion and planning will be needed, following the specific Trust protocols. Staff need to be aware that there will be variations in products and techniques that are acceptable and the woman should always be given the opportunity to change her mind if the need arises.

Antenatal care includes correction of anaemia and serial ultrasound scans for fetal wellbeing. Anti-D should be administered as appropriate (as in PA discussed previously). A course of antenatal corticosteroids may be offered between 34 and 35 + 6 weeks, which will improve neonatal outcome.[42] Corticosteroids can be given prior to this if preterm birth is expected. If the woman and baby are stable, tocolytics may be used to allow time for the corticosteroids to work.[19] However, the birth should not be delayed to allow time for the corticosteroids to be effective if the wellbeing of the woman or baby are at risk.[42]

Psychological care must be considered, particularly as the woman is likely to stay in hospital for the whole of the third trimester if any bleeding has occurred. Prolonged hospitalisation and separation from family and other children may have a negative effect on the woman's mental health. Support and sensitive discussion are needed, and a visit to the neonatal unit can be organised.

The timing of the birth will depend on whether any symptoms are present. With asymptomatic placenta praevia, the optimal time for the birth of the baby is between 36 and 37 weeks.[19] If the woman is symptomatic or has any risk factors for preterm birth, then it is suggested that the birth should take place between 34 and 36 + 6 weeks if possible.[19]

The mode of birth will be by CS, which must be performed by a consultant or experienced senior obstetrician and anaesthetist due to the likelihood of a major haemorrhage as the lower uterine segment is unable to contract and there may be the need to incise through the placenta.[23] Cell salvage should be discussed with the woman prior to a planned CS where massive haemorrhage is anticipated.[19]

Although a CS is always indicated for women with placenta praevia, when the placenta is low-lying, a vaginal birth is possible as long as there are no contraindications and the woman remains asymptomatic.[59] In-depth discussion and joint decision-making are needed, and the birth should take place within a consultant-led maternity unit. Should any complications or bleeding occur, the procedure should be immediately abandoned and an emergency CS should be performed.

CARE FOR ALL WOMEN WITH APH (PLACENTAL ABRUPTION AND PLACENTA PRAEVIA)

It is important to remember that every woman who experiences an antepartum haemorrhage is different and should be treated sensitively and individually. A calm attitude and continual explanation of procedures are paramount to instil trust and confidence in the woman and her family.

Care prior to hospital admission

Should a woman call the maternity unit from home with signs and symptoms of bleeding or other related complications, she must be asked to come to triage or labour ward immediately. If the signs and symptoms are severe, emergency services will be required to ensure a timely transfer to the nearest consultant-led maternity unit, ideally one with appropriate neonatal, transfusion and critical care facilities.

If the midwife is attending to the woman at home or a free-standing birth unit, the priority is arranging the transfer, as mentioned previously. Intravenous access must be gained and fluid replacement initiated. The woman should be positioned in a left lateral position to avoid supine hypotension, which could exacerbate her state of shock and compromise the fetus. Blood pressure, heart rate, respirations, oxygen saturations and temperature should be taken and recorded. The presence and location of pain and the amount and nature of the blood loss must be noted. Any blood-stained sanitary pads, sheets or clothing should be kept to assist with accurate blood loss estimation.[60,61]

Accurate and thorough history-taking will give the team information on the amount of blood loss, any associated pain, trauma, recent sexual intercourse, any previous episodes of bleeding and fetal wellbeing/movement. This will help determine the cause of the bleeding. The woman may have had a recent scan indicating placental location, or she may have had previous hospital admissions with bleeding or other risk factors for APH. Hence, it is important that the maternity notes accompany the woman to hospital.

A vaginal examination must not be undertaken, as this may cause heavy bleeding in the case of a placenta praevia.[19] An abdominal examination should be avoided prior to admission as this may cause uterine irritability, which may exacerbate bleeding.[61]

Care in the hospital setting

On arrival in hospital, or at any time if already hospitalised, if signs and symptoms of an APH are recognised, immediate escalation and a multidisciplinary approach are essential. Any amount of bleeding could be serious, and the condition of the woman and fetus may deteriorate rapidly. Treatment will depend on the severity of the haemorrhage (see Table 4.5), the gestation and the condition of the woman and fetus. As blood loss may be concealed or underestimated, it is essential that frequent and thorough assessment for maternal and fetal compromise is undertaken and repeated as appropriate.

Once in hospital, careful abdominal palpation can help to determine the cause of haemorrhage according to whether or not the abdomen is soft, tender or 'board-like'. However, it should be performed gently to avoid pain or further bleeding. Abdominal palpation will also indicate the size of the baby. A history of repeated small bleeds during the pregnancy may be linked to placental insufficiency, which can lead to associated fetal growth restriction.[11] If the presenting part is found to be high, placenta previa may be suspected.

Vaginal and/or rectal examinations must not be performed as this could aggravate the bleeding. A scan is necessary in most cases to determine the location of the placenta to exclude placenta praevia. Even if this has been done previously in pregnancy, it should be repeated as routine pregnancy ultrasounds may not always accurately identify placental localisation. A placenta that is normally sited will indicate that the APH is probably due to PA. Separation may occasionally be seen on ultrasound if there is a particularly large retroplacental clot, although this is not usually the case.[25] The fetal condition is assessed by initial auscultation, followed by a CTG and a description of the nature of recent fetal movements. A speculum examination may be carried out to exclude cervical or

Table 4.5 The Royal College of Obstetricians and Gynaecologists definitions used for assessing the severity of an APH[1]

Spotting	Staining, streaking or blood spotting noted on underwear or sanitary towels
Minor haemorrhage	Blood loss of less than 50 ml that has settled
Major haemorrhage	Blood loss of 50–1000 ml with no signs of clinical shock
Massive haemorrhage	Blood loss of greater than 1000 ml and/or signs of clinical shock

vaginal lesions as a cause for the bleeding once placenta praevia has been excluded.[1]

After 37 weeks and if the woman and fetus are stable (or indeed before 37 weeks if the baby has died), induction of labour may be considered if the woman has experienced an APH of less than 1000mls with no further complication or PP (see Table 4.5).[1] Careful assessment of labour progress, maternal wellbeing and continuous CTG monitoring must be undertaken.

At any stage, should any maternal compromise occur, despite the estimated blood loss, a major obstetric haemorrhage (MOH) protocol should be initiated, and the birth of the baby expedited.

Immediate care of a major/massive APH

Once the emergency is recognised, the initial call for assistance is made and a multidisciplinary approach is taken for optimum care. See Box 4.3 for a list of experienced personnel who may be involved. One team member must be identified as the team leader and maintain a helicopter view of the management of the emergency. This will involve standing back and observing the emergency, delegating tasks and communicating clearly and calmly.[6] Another member of the team must take responsibility for recording events, fluids, drugs and vital signs in chronological order and

---

BOX 4.3: Team members for managing a massive APH

- Labour ward coordinator
- Consultant obstetrician
- On-call obstetric team
- Midwives
- Senior anaesthetist
- Haematologist
- Blood transfusion service
- Porters to expedite specimens and blood product delivery
- Operating theatre staff
- Neonatologist
- Neonatal unit nursing staff
- An identified scribe to document events, fluids, drugs and vital signs.
- Any other staff to assist

---

completing the proforma, MEOWS/HDU and fluid balance charts.

All actions undertaken from the time the emergency has been recognised should be taken simultaneously where possible, with priority given to resuscitating and stabilising the woman before delivering the baby. The initial management of the haemorrhage will be the same irrespective of the cause. Once the woman and fetus are stabilised, specific treatment will be considered.

The compromised pregnant woman needs to be positioned in a left lateral position to avoid aortocaval compression. Should cardiopulmonary resuscitation be necessary, the woman should be moved back into a supine position and manual uterine displacement to the left should be used[39] (see Chapter 3). The airway must be kept patent and breathing assessed and assisted if necessary. High-flow oxygen must be administered via a mask at 15L/minute, and the circulation must be continuously evaluated and maintained.

Early intravenous access with two wide-bore canulae is essential so that fluid replacement can be commenced to maintain blood pressure and circulating volume. A blood transfusion may be needed, and O-negative blood (usually kept in the labour ward fridge) may be used while waiting for cross-matched blood to arrive if the haemorrhage is life-threatening. The woman must be kept warm, and all fluids must be warmed to avoid hypothermia, which exacerbates maternal shock and also increases the risk of coagulopathy.[6] Should coagulopathy arise, it will need to be corrected promptly by the medical team.[62]

An arterial line and ECG monitoring may be necessary, and a central venous line may be needed to monitor fluid levels. Bloods will be taken and sent for urgent analysis (see Box 4.4). Analgesia must be administered, and an in-dwelling urinary catheter with a urometer should be inserted to monitor the urine output hourly for inclusion in detailed fluid balance records.

Vital signs and ongoing assessment for other signs of shock must be carried out. These include poor peripheral perfusion (reduced capillary refill time, clammy skin, pallor), air hunger, oliguria and changes in alertness. The vital signs may show rising heart rate and respirations and lowered blood pressure, although low blood pressure is often a late sign of shock in the pregnant woman.[6] The blood pressure may not be

BOX 4.4: Blood tests

- Full blood count
- Group and screen/cross-match group specific blood
- Coagulation screen
- Urea and electrolytes
- Baseline liver function
- Kleihauer test (if the woman is rhesus negative)
- Venous and arterial blood gasses
- Near bedside testing for haemoglobin and coagulation
- Biochemistry screen in cases of hypertension (see Chapter 7 for details of the pre-eclampsia blood tests)

particularly low in the early stages of shock for women with underlying hypertension alongside an APH, thus further masking the clinical signs of shock. Women who are taking beta-blockers for high blood pressure may not become tachycardiac. Midwives must also be aware that paroxysmal bradycardia may occur when there is peritoneal irritation.[39]

The fetal heart rate must be continuously monitored and is also indicative of maternal shock. An emergency CS will be performed if vaginal birth is not imminent/possible. The birth should not be delayed for fetal reasons, for example, waiting for steroids to take effect,[6,42] as the woman's wellbeing must take precedence.[6] The neonatal team must be notified early in the emergency so that they can prepare for imminent resuscitation of the baby.

The birth of the baby and placenta may assist in controlling the bleeding by allowing the uterus to contract, thereby ensuring a more favourable outcome for the woman. However, uterine contraction following a PP may be less effective due to fewer muscle fibres at the placental site in the lower uterine segment.[62] The birth of the baby and placenta will also improve the maternal circulation by relieving aortocaval compression and increasing maternal oxygen consumption.[63] Removal of the placenta may also assist in avoiding further complications, as placental tissue factors can exacerbate any developing coagulation disorders.[1]

Once the birth has taken place, an actively managed third stage is essential and PPH is anticipated.

Following a massive APH, the woman is likely to need to be cared for in a critical care setting, requiring further treatment of shock, close monitoring and observation of blood loss.[64] The baby may need to be transferred to the neonatal intensive care unit due to prematurity and/or the effects of hypoxia. Postnatal care will be the same as that discussed in Chapter 12 on PPH.

POTENTIAL OUTCOMES OF APH

Maternal outcomes

Postpartum haemorrhage: This is to be anticipated, and an actively managed third stage is recommended. However, following the birth, uncontrollable bleeding may occur despite the administration of oxytocics[40] (also see Chapter 12 on PPH). The presence of an adherent placenta and coagulopathy will exacerbate the haemorrhage. Blood transfusion may be required.

Hysterectomy: This may be necessary to control a massive haemorrhage, particularly as a result of a Couvelaire uterus, placenta accreta spectrum, uterine rupture or coagulation defects.

Disseminated intravascular coagulation (DIC): DIC can arise secondary to APH and hypovolaemic shock and is triggered when thromboplastins enter the circulation, inducing the coagulation cascade. This results in the formation of intravascular thrombi and depletion of fibrinogen, coagulation factors and circulating platelets. Haemorrhage and thrombosis thus occur simultaneously. The thrombi obstruct the smaller blood vessels leading to ischaemia and organ failure. The damaged tissue releases thromboplastins once more, and the cycle is repeated, causing further damage. At the same time, uncontrolled bleeding will continue due to the depletion of the clotting factors. The midwife must observe the nature of the blood loss and clot formation, whether there is spontaneous bleeding from venepuncture and epidural sites, wounds or from the mucosa of the mouth or nose. There may also be haematuria and/or petechiae. Prompt escalation and treatment with haematology, senior obstetric and anaesthetic input is needed.[6] See Chapter 12, Box 12.11 for further information on diagnosis and management.

Acute kidney injury: Deterioration of renal function can occur as a result of hypovolaemic shock, resulting in poor kidney perfusion and damage. The midwife should monitor fluid balance and urine output hourly, reporting if it falls below 30mls/hour. Fluid restriction will be required.[65] If the condition does not resolve, renal dialysis will be implemented at the instruction of the nephrologist.

Thromboembolism: Due to the increased risk, thromboprophylaxis should be commenced as soon as the immediate risk of haemorrhage is reduced. See Chapter 6 for further discussion.

Anaemia: A result of excessive blood loss or underlying disease, anaemia may require correction by blood transfusion or oral/intravenous iron therapy as appropriate.

Infection: Infection may be acquired through low resistance caused by shock and/or anaemia or through increased interventions. Signs and symptoms of sepsis will ensue if left untreated. See Chapter 14 for further information on serious infection.

Maternal mortality: With PA, the maternal outcome is related to the extent of the placental separation, and therefore, maternal death is more likely with a severe abruption and massive haemorrhage. Maternal mortality rates are low in resource-rich countries but high in resource-poor areas where maternal anaemia is more common and there is a lack of medical expertise and resources.[38]

Fetal/Baby outcomes

Fetal hypoxia: Fetal hypoxia may occur as a result of premature placental separation. In the case of chronic PA, the fetus may already have been growth-restricted and compromised due to poor placental perfusion. This is likely to result in the need for assistance at birth, apnoea and respiratory distress syndrome.[22] The neonatal outcomes for PP are less severe, possibly owing to complex physiological changes in the placental circulation, which maintain placental perfusion and prevent hypoxia.[52]

Preterm birth and resulting sequelae: Any birth occurring between 24 and 36 + 6 weeks' gestation as a result of PA or PP will require varying degrees of input from the neonatal team.

Fetal death: Death of the fetus is rare but more common where there has been an acute PA than where there is a PP.

FOLLOW-UP/LONG-TERM ISSUES

Postpartum hypopituitary (Sheehan's) syndrome: Anterior pituitary necrosis or Sheehan's syndrome is a rare complication of prolonged shock. It can occur immediately postpartum or manifest later in life.[66] The damage can result in poor lactation due to insufficient prolactin secretion, amenorrhoea, infertility, hypothyroidism and adrenocortical insufficiency.

Coping with the preterm or sick infant: If separated from her baby, the woman may feel more vulnerable. The midwife needs to ensure that information about the baby's condition is explained and there is sufficient opportunity to be involved in the care and bond with the baby. Breastfeeding difficulties are likely; therefore, the midwife will need to provide enhanced breastfeeding support.

Adverse psychological effects: Postnatal depression or post-traumatic stress syndrome (see Chapter 16 for additional discussion of these issues) may occur as a result of prolonged periods of hospitalisation, a traumatic birth or life-changing outcomes. Information about what has happened needs to be given, and the woman should be encouraged to ask questions about her condition, the immediate and long-term effects of her condition and her physical recovery and subsequent pregnancies and fertility. Information concerning 'birth reflections' or other similar services may be useful for the woman, as she can access this at her convenience. It may also be necessary to refer the woman and family for bereavement counselling.

Recurrence: Traumatic PA is unlikely to recur. However, even though abruption may not be preventable, women who have chronic underlying causes can be advised on various lifestyle behaviours to lessen the risk.[36] This can include encouraging the cessation of smoking, drug and alcohol abuse and measures to control hypertension and obesity.

PP is likely to recur in approximately 5% of subsequent pregnancies.[67]

SUMMARY OF MIDWIFERY RESPONSIBILITIES

- Awareness of unit protocols and participation in skills drills training
- Maintain good communication with the multi-disciplinary team
- Risk assessment
- Antenatal correction of anaemia
- Accurate recognition and diagnosis of APH
- Appropriate and timely referral and escalation
- APH immediate management (some actions will take place simultaneously):
  - Call for appropriate help immediately/transfer to hospital if at home
  - Continuously assess clinical situation
  - Do not perform a vaginal examination
  - Left lateral tilt and oxygen therapy (15L/min)
  - Commence resuscitation (with manual uterine displacement to the left) if necessary
  - Establish venous access and administer warmed blood and fluids (crystalloids, colloids) as directed
  - Collect, label and dispatch blood samples
  - Continuous assessment of maternal and fetal condition
  - Monitor and record blood loss
  - Accurately take and record vital signs (pulse, BP, respirations, O_2 saturations and temperature) on a MEOWS chart and note any changes in trends
  - Monitor and record fluid balance
  - Administer analgesia as necessary
- Assist with the birth of the baby (if necessary) once the woman is stabilised
- Actively manage third stage
- Maintain documentation: personnel, times, actions, reactions
- Administration of anti-D when needed
- Provision of accurate information, continual discussion and reassurance for the woman and family
- Maintain a calm and professional attitude
- Appropriate postnatal care, recognise and minimise complications
- Consideration of long-term psychological complications (also see Chapter 16)
- Clinical incident reporting, review of care and information sharing with the multidisciplinary team

FURTHER READING AND RESOURCES

- PRompt Maternity Foundation. Management of APH interactive video.
  www.youtube.com/watch?v=NVnUpMj-iVs
  PRompt (Practical Obstetric Multi-Professional Training) is a multi-professional training programme for the management of obstetric emergencies. *This video demonstrates the importance of interprofessional teamworking and communication during a simulated APH scenario.*
- Royal College of Obstetrics and Gynaecology. Placenta Praevia and Placenta Accreta: Diagnosis and Management. Green-top Guideline No. 27.
  This document provides a guideline and explanation of placenta praevia and placenta accrete.
- Royal College of Obstetrics and Gynaecology Placenta Praevia, placenta accreta and vasa praevia. Information for you. Published September 2018. London: RCOG.
  This is a leaflet to explain conditions and the guidelines to women and their families.
- Tommy's pregnancy Hub: Information and support for women with pregnancy complications.
  Placental abruption: www.tommys.org/pregnancy-information/pregnancy-complications/placenta-complications/placental-abruption
  Low-lying placenta and placenta praevia: www.tommys.org/pregnancy-information/pregnancy-complications/low-lying-placenta-placenta-praevia

REFERENCES

1. Royal College of Obstetricians and Gynaecologists (RCOG). Antepartum haemorrhage. Green-top guideline no. 63. London: RCOG; Nov 2011.
2. Tuffnell D, Knight M, On Behalf of the MBRRACE-UK. Haemorrhage and AFE chapter-writing group lessons for care of women with haemorrhage or amniotic fluid embolism. In Knight M, Bunch K, Tuffnell D, Shakespeare J, Kotnis R, Kenyon S, Kurinczuk JJ, On Behalf of MBRRACE-UK, editors. Saving lives, improving mothers' care – lessons learned to inform maternity

care from the UK and Ireland confidential enquiries into maternal deaths and morbidity 2016–18. Oxford: National Perinatal Epidemiology Unit, University of Oxford; 2020. p. 58–63.

3. Navti OB, Konje JC. Bleeding in late pregnancy. In: James D, Steer PJ, Weiner CP, Gonik B, Robson SCE, editors. High risk pregnancy: management options. Cambridge: Cambridge University Press; 2017. p. 1557–1580.

4. Bhandari S, Raja E, Shetty A, Bhattacharya S. Maternal and perinatal consequences of antepartum haemorrhage of unknown origin. BJOG: An International Journal of Obstetrics and Gynaecology. 2014;121(1):44–52. Available from: <doi:10.1111/1471-0528.12464>

5. Jauniaux ERM, Alfirevic Z, Bhide AG, Burton GJ, Collins SL, Silver R, On Behalf of the Royal College of Obstetricians and Gynaecologists. Vasa praevia: diagnosis and management RCOG green top guideline no. 27b. 2018. Available from: https://obgyn.onlinelibrary.wiley.com/doi/full/10.1002/uog.21953

6. Winter C, Crofts J, Draycott T, Muchatuta N. Practical obstetric multi-professional training (PROMPT) course manual. 3rd ed. Cambridge: Cambridge University Press; 2017.

7. Yang Q, Wen SW, Phillips K, Oppenheimer L, Black D, Walker MC. Comparison of maternal risk factors between placental abruption and placental praevia. American Journal of Perinatology. 2009;26(4):279–286. Available from: <doi:10.1055/s-0028-1103156>

8. Boisramé T, Sananès N, Fritz G, Boudier E, Aissi G, Favre R, Langer B. Placental abruption: risk factors, management and maternal-fetal prognosis: cohort study over 10 years. European Journal of Obstetrics & Gynecology and Reproductive Biology. 2014;179:100–104. Available from: <doi:10.1016/j.ejogrb.2014.05.026>

9. Tikkanen M. Placental abruption: epidemiology, risk factors and consequences. Acta Obstetrica et Gynaecology Scandenavica. 2011;90:140–149. Available from: <doi:10.11 1/j.1600-0412.10.01030>

10. Ananth CV, Lavery JA, Vintzileos AM, Skupski DW, Varner M, Saade G, et al. Severe placental abruption: clinical definition and associations with maternal complications. Am J Obstet Gynecol. 2016;214:272, e1–e9. ISSN:0002-9378. Available from: <doi:10.1016/j.ajog.2015.09.069>

11. Brandt JS, Ananth CV. Placental abruption at near-term and term gestations: pathophysiology, epidemiology, diagnosis, and management. Am J Obstet Gynecol. 2023;228(Suppl 5):S1313–S1329. ISSN:0002-9378. Available from: <doi:10.1016/j.ajog.2022.06.059>

12. Jenabi E, Salimi Z, Ayubi E, Bashirian S, Salehi AM. The environmental risk factors prior to conception associated with placental abruption: an umbrella review. Syst Rev. 2022;11:55. Available from: <doi:10.1186/s13643-022-01915-6>

13. Yeo L, Ananth CV, Vintzileoa AM. Placental abruption. Global Library of Women's Medicine; 2008. ISSN:1756-2228. Available from: <doi:103843/GLOWM.10122>

14. Anderson E, Raja EA, Shetty A, Gissler M, Gatt M, Bhattacharya S, et al. Changing risk factors for placental abruption: a case crossover study using routinely collected data from Finland, Malta and Aberdeen. PLOS One. 2020;15(6):e0233641. Available from: <doi:10.1371/journal.pone.0233641>

15. Goldbart A, Pariente, G, Sheiner E, Wainstock T. Identifying risk factors for placental abruption in subsequent pregnancy without a history of placental abruption. Int J Gynaecol Obstet. May 2023;161(2):406–411, 6. Available from: <doi:10.1002/ijgo.14446>

16. Jenabi E, Salimi Z, Bashirian S, Khazaei S, Ayubi E. The risk factors associated with placental previa: an umbrella review. Placental. 2022;117:21–27. ISSN:0143-4004. Available from: <doi:10.1016/j.placenta.2021.10.009>

17. Martinelli KG, Garcia EM, Dos Santos Neto ET, Nogueira de Gama SG. Advanced maternal age and its association with placenta praevia and placenta abruption: a meta-analysis, Cad. Saúde

Pública. 2018;34(2). Available from: <doi:10.1590/0102-311X00206116>

18. Zhou C, Zhao Y, Li Y. Clinical analysis of factors influencing the development of placenta praevia and perinatal outcomes in first-time pregnant patients. Front Surg. 2022 Mar 22;9:862655. Available from: <doi:10.3389/fsurg.2022.862655>

19. Jauniaux ERM, Alfirevic Z, Bhide AG, Belfort MA, Burton GJ, et al. On behalf of the royal college of obstetricians and gynaecologists. Placenta praevia and placenta accreta: diagnosis and management. Green-top guideline. BJOG. 2018;27a.

20. Lao TT, Hui SYA, Wong LL, Sahota DS. Iron deficiency anaemia associated with increased placenta praevia and placental abruption: a retrospective case-control study. Eur J Clin Nutr. 2022;76:1172–1177. Available from: <doi:10.1038/s41430-022-01086-6>

21. Ananth C, Keyes K, Hamilton A, Gissler M, Wu C, Liu S, et al. An international contrast of rates of placental abruption: an age-period-cohort analysis. PLOS One. 2015;10(5):e0125246. Available from: <doi:10.1371/journal.pone.0125246,26018653>

22. Downes KL, Shenassa ED, Grantz KL. Neonatal outcomes associated with placental abruption. American Journal of Epidemiology. 2017 Dec 15;186(12):1319–1328. Available from: <doi:10.1093/aje/kwx202>

23. Nugent F, Thomson A. Obstetric haemorrhage. In: Layden EA, Thomson, A, Owen P, Madhra, M, Magowan, BA, editors. Clinical obstetrics and gynaecology. 5th ed. London: Elsevier; 2023. p. 314–323.

24. Ananth CV, Oyelese Y, Prasad V, Getahun D, Smulian JC. Evidence of placental abruption as a chronic process: associations with vaginal bleeding early in pregnancy and placental lesions. European Journal of Obstetrics & Gynecology and Reproductive Biology. 2006;128(1–2):15–21 Available from: <doi:10.1016/j.ejogrb.2006.01.016>

25. Ananth CV, Kinzler WL. Acute placental abruption: pathophysiology, clinical features, diagnosis and consequences. In: Lockwood CJ, editor. UpToDate. Waltham, MA: UpToDate.com; 2023. [Accessed 1 June 2023].

26. Cheng HT, Wanf YC, Lo HC, Sung FC, Hsieh CH. Trauma during pregnancy: a population based analysis of maternal outcome. World Journal of Surgery. 2012;36(12):2767–2775. Available from: <doi:10.1007/s00268-012-1750-6>

27. Leone JM, Lane S, Koumans EH, DeMott K, Wojtowycs MA, Jensen J, et al. Effects of intimate partner violence on pregnancy trauma and placental abruption. Journal of Women's Health. 2010;19(8):1501–1509. Available from: <doi:10.1089/jwh.2009.1716>

28. Grootscholten K, Kok M, Oei S, Mol B, van der Post, JA. External cephalic version – related risks: a meta-analysis. Obstetrics and Gynecolgy. 2008;112(5)1143–1151. Available from: <doi:10.1097/AOG.0b013e31818b4ade>

29. Blackburn ST. Maternal, fetal, & neonatal physiology: a clinical perspective. 5th ed. Missouri: Elsevier; 2017.

30. Kovo M, Gonen N, Schreiber L, Hochman R, Noy LK, Levy M, Bar J, Weiner E, Histologic chorioamnionitis concomitant placental abruption and its effects on pregnancy outcome. Placenta. 2020;94:39–43. ISSN:0143-4004. Available from: <doi:10.1016/j.placenta.2020.03.012>

31. de Moreuil C, Hannigsberg J, Chauvet J, Remoue A, Tremouilhac C, et al. Factors associated with poor fetal outcome in placental abruption. Pregnancy Hypertension. 2021;23:59–65. ISSN:2210-7789. Available from: <doi:10.1016/j.preghy.2020.11.004>

32. Ananth CV, Kioumourtzoglou MA, Huang Y, Ross Z, Friedman AM, Williams MA, et al. Exposures to air pollution and risk of acute-onset placental abruption: a case-crossover study. Epidemiology. 2018;29:631–638. Available from: <doi:10.1097/EDE.0000000000000859>

33. Chahal HS, Gelaye B, Mostofsky E, Salazar MS, Sanchez SE, Ananth CV, et al. Relation of outbursts of anger and the acute risk of placental abruption: a case-crossover study. Paediatr Perinat Epidemiol. 2019;33:405–411. Available from: <doi:10.1111/ppe.12591>

34. Ananth CV, Lavery JA, Vintzileos AM, Skupski DW, Varner M, et al. Severe placental abruption: clinical definition and associations with maternal complications. Am J Obstet Gynecol. 2016;214(2):272. e1–272.e9. ISSN 0002-9378. Available from: <doi:10.1016/j.ajog.2015.09.069>

35. Pariente G, Shoham-Vardi I, Kessous R, Sherf M, Sheinera E. Placental abruption as a significant risk factor for long-term cardiovascular mortality in a follow-up period of more than a decade 2013 John Wiley & Sons Ltd. Paediatric and Perinatal Epidemiology. 2014;28:32–38. Available from: <doi:10.1111/ppe.12089>

36. Ananth CV, Patrick HS, Ananth S, Zhang Y, Kostis WJ, Schuster M. Maternal cardiovascular and cerebrovascular health after placental abruption: a systematic review and meta-analysis (CHAP-SR). Am J Epidemiol. 2021 Dec 1;190(12):2718–2729. Available from: <doi:10.1093/aje/kwab206>

37. Matsuzaki S, Ueda Y, Matsuzaki S, Sakaguchi H, Kakuda M, Lee M, et al. Relationship between abnormal placenta and obstetric outcomes: a meta-analysis. Biomedicines. 2023;11(6):1522. Available from: <doi:10.3390/biomedicines11061522>

38. Lockwood CJ, Russo-Stieglitz K. Placenta previa: epidemiology, clinical features, diagnosis, morbidity and mortality. UpToDate, Wolters Kluwer; 2023. [online]. [Accessed May 2023]. Available from: www.uptodate.com

39. Burns R, Dent K, editors. On behalf of the advanced life support group: managing medical and obstetric emergencies and trauma: a practical approach. 4th ed. Oxford: John Wiley & Sons; 2022.

40. Oats J, Boyle J. Llewellyn-Jones fundamentals of obstetrics and gynaecology. 11th ed. Chapter 13 Antepartum Haemorrhage. London: Elsevier; 2023.

41. Schmidt P, Skelly CL, Raines DA. Placental abruption. Treasure Island, FL: StatPearls Publishing; 2023 Jan. [Updated 2022 Dec 19]. Available from: www.ncbi.nlm.nih.gov/books/NBK482335/

42. Stock SJ, Thomson AJ, Papworth S, The Royal College of Obstetricians, Gynaecologists. Antenatal corticosteroids to reduce neonatal morbidity and mortality. BJOG. 2022;129:e35–e60. Available from: <doi:10.1111/1471-0528.17027>

43. Reddy UM, Abuhamad AZ, Levine D, Saade GR, Fetal Imaging Workshop Invited Participants. Fetal imaging: executive summary of a joint Eunice Kennedy Shriver national institute of child health and human development, society for maternal-fetal medicine, American institute of ultrasound in medicine, American college of obstetricians and gynecologists, American college of radiology, society for pediatric radiology, and society of radiologists in ultrasound fetal imaging workshop. J Ultrasound Med. 2014;33:745–757. Available from: <doi:10.1016/j.ajog.2014.02.028>

44. Liu B, Deng S, Lin M, Chen Y, Cai J, Yang J, et al. Prediction of cesarean hysterectomy in placenta previa complicated with prior cesarean: a retrospective study. BMC Pregnancy Childbirth. 2020 Feb 7;20(1):81. Available from: <doi:10.1186/s12884-020-2790-9>

45. Fan D, Wu S, Liu L, Xia Q, Wang W, Guo X, et al. Prevalence of antepartum hemorrhage in women with placenta previa: a systematic review and meta-analysis. Sci Rep. 2017;7:40320. Available from: <doi:10.1038/srep40320>

46. Jauniaux E, Grønbeck L, Bunce C, Langhoff-Roos J, Collins SL. Epidemiology of placenta previa accreta: a systematic review and meta-analysis BMJ Open. 2019;9:e031193. Available from: <doi:10.1136/bmjopen-2019-031193>

47. Jansen CHJR, Kastelein AW, Kleinrouweler CE, Van Leeuwen E, De Jong KH, Pajkrt E, et al. Development of placental abnormalities in location and anatomy – a narrative review. Acta Obstet Gynecol Scand. 2020;99:983–993. Available from: <doi:10.1111/aogs.13834>

48. Jordans IP, Vissers J, Huang Y, Mischi M, Schoot D, Huirne JA. Increased amplitude of subendometrial contractions identified by ultrasound speckle tracking in women with a caesarean scar defect. Reproductive BioMedicine Online. 2023;46(3):577–587. ISSN:1472-6483. Available from: <doi:10.1016/j.rbmo.2022.12.002>

49. Macklin PS, McAuliffe J, Pugh CW, Yamamoto A. Hypoxia and HIF pathway in cancer and the placenta. Placenta. 2017;56:8–13. ISSN:0143-4004. Available from: <doi:10.1016/j.placenta.2017.03.010>

50. Silver RM. Abnormal placentation: placenta previa, vasa previa, and placenta accreta. Obstetrics & Gynecology. 2015 Sep;126(3):654–668. Available from: <doi:10.1097/AOG.0000000000001005>

51. Oyelese Y, Smulian JC. Placenta previa, placenta accreta and vasa previa. Obstetrics and Gynaecology. 2006;107(4):927–941. Available from: <doi:10.1097/01.AOG.0000207559.15715.98>

52. Jung EU, Cho HJ, Byun JM, Jeong DH, Lee KB, Sung MS, et al. Placental pathologic changes and perinatal outcomes in placenta previa. Placenta. 2018;63:15–20. ISSN:0143-4004. Available from: <doi:10.1016/j.placenta.2017.12.016>

53. King LJ, Mackeen AD, Nordberg C, Paglia MJ, Maternal risk factors associated with persistent placenta previa. Placenta. 2020;99:189–192. ISSN:0143-4004. Available from: <doi:10.1016/j.placenta.2020.08.004>

54. Symonds I, Arulkumaran S. Antepartum haemorrhage. In: Essential obstetrics and gynaecology. 5th ed. London: Churchill; 2013.

55. Jauniaux E, Chantraine F, Silver RM, Langhoff-Roos J. FIGO consensus guidelines on placenta accreta spectrum disorders: epidemiology. Int J Gynecol Obstet. 2018;140(3):265–273. Available from: <doi:10.1002/ijgo.12407>

56. Jauniaux E, Jurkovic D, Hussein AM, Burton GJ, New insights into the etiopathology of placenta accreta spectrum. Am J Obstet Gynecol. 2022;227(3):384–391. ISSN:0002-9378. Available from: <doi:10.1016/j.ajog.2022.02.038>

57. National Institute for Health and Care Excellence (NICE). Clinical guideline NG201: antenatal care. London: NICE Publications; 2021.

58. Royal College of Obstetricians and Gynaecologists (RCOG). Blood transfusions in obstetrics: green-top guideline no. 47. London: RCOG; May 2015.

59. Jansen CHJR, de Mooij YM, Blomaard CM, Derks JB, van Leeuwen E, Limpens J, et al. Vaginal delivery in women with a low-lying placenta: a systematic review and meta-analysis. BJOG. 2019;126:1118–1126. Available from: <doi:10.1111/1471-0528.15622>

60. Needham J. Antepartum haemorrhage. In: Bates K, Crozier K, editors. Managing childbirth emergencies in the community and low tech settings. 2nd ed. London: Palgrave; 2015.

61. Hutcherson A. Bleeding in pregnancy In: MacDonald S, Johnson G, editors. Mayes midwifery. 16th ed. Chapter 55. London: Elsevier; 2023.

62. Carillo AP, Chandraharan E. Management of massive obstetric haemorrhage: antepartum, intrapartum and postpartum. In: Chandraharan E, Arulkumaran S, editors. Obstetric and intrapartum emergencies: a practical guide to management. 2nd ed. Chapter 5. Cambridge: Cambridge University Press; 2021.

63. Chu, J, Johnston, TA, Geoghegan, J, On Behalf of the Royal College of Obstetricians and Gynaecologists. Maternal collapse in pregnancy and the puerperium. BJOG. 2020; 127: e14–e52.

64. Boyle M, Bothamley J. Critical care assessment by midwives. London: Routledge; 2018.

65. Bothamley J, Boyle M. Medical conditions affecting pregnancy and childbirth. 2nd ed. London: Routledge; 2021.

66. Matsuzaki S, Endo M, Ueda Y, Mimura K, Kakigano A, Egawa-Takata T. A case of acute Sheehan's syndrome and literature review: a rare but life-threatening complication of postpartum hemorrhage. BMC Pregnancy Childbirth. 2017;17:188. Available from: <doi:10.1186/s12884-017-1380-y>

67. Roberts CL, Algert CS, Warrendorf J, Olive EC, Morris JM, Ford JB. Trends and recurrence of placenta praevia: a population-based study. Aust NZ J Obstet Gynaecol. 2012;52:483–486. Available from: <doi:10.1111/j.1479-828X.2012.01470.x>

5

Cardiac conditions

MAUREEN BOYLE

Introduction	76	Long term issues	83
Pathophysiology	77	Summary of midwifery responsibilities	84
Pre-disposing/risk factors	78	Further reading and resources	84
Clinical features	78	References	85
Specific care	80		
Common cardiac conditions complicating pregnancy	83		

BOX 5.1: Definition

Women in pregnancy can be affected by two types of cardiac disease:

Congenital: abnormalities of the heart present at birth, which may or may not have previously been identified and treated.

Acquired: largely ischaemic and related to lifestyle/family history, although women who have had limited access to health care may present with untreated heart disease damage.

In many cases, a cardiac condition may be undiagnosed and relatively symptom-free, and it is usually the increasing circulation of pregnancy that provides the stress on the heart that makes the condition apparent and potentially lethal.

INTRODUCTION

Cardiac conditions have long been the leading cause of death among pregnant women and those who have recently given birth.[1] Overall, this has significantly increased over the last three decades, with deaths from ischaemic heart disease, myocardial infarction and peripartum cardiomyopathy responsible.[2]

In the most recent Confidential Enquires Report,[1] 90% of women who died from cardiac conditions had undiagnosed cardiac disease, and many had not been identified as being at risk before late pregnancy/labour. This presents a particular challenge for midwives, as the initial symptoms may arise unheralded due to the physiological changes in pregnancy, and therefore midwives may be the first health professionals to be in a position to recognise these new symptoms. In a recent French study, where more than two-thirds of the women had unknown cardiac conditions, it was suggested that most maternal cardiac deaths were potentially preventable, and the main factor was inadequate pre-hospital care, in particular underestimation of the severity and inadequate investigation of dyspnoea.[3]

Outside of pregnancy, there have been significant improvements to cardiovascular outcomes (particularly in acute coronary syndrome: ACS), but this has not been reflected in the maternity population.[4] In the USA, a new multidisciplinary speciality has been identified: cardio-obstetrics.[5] This underlines the importance of experts in this

DOI: 10.4324/9781003382195-5

field to improve the outcomes of cardiac disease in pregnant women.

It has been identified that the number of pregnant women with cardiac disease is growing.[2] Women with a known cardiac condition have been able to increasingly benefit from on-going advances in medical/surgical treatment, which ensures they are able to live healthy lives and consider becoming pregnant. There is also generally in the population an increase in lifestyle issues, such as increased maternal age, obesity and other co-morbidities, which impact poorly on cardiac and circulation systems, and women during pregnancy may be subject to these.[1]

PATHOPHYSIOLOGY

Pregnancy involves many physiological adaptations, and these are usually well tolerated. However, for those women with an underlying cardiac disease, these changes, and in particular the increase in cardiac output, may have a considerable effect. The considerable rise in cardiac output in pregnancy is caused by an increase in blood volume and heart rate.[6]

Box 5.2 gives a summary of the key cardiovascular changes in pregnancy.

Changes to the cardiovascular systems in the labour and postnatal period

In labour and the postnatal period, there are increases in cardiac output, which make this a vulnerable time for women with cardiac disease. Compared with prelabour, cardiac output rises around 15% in early labour, increasing by approximately 25% during contractions and by approximately 50% during active pushing.[10] Sympathetic nervous system response to pain and anxiety further elevates heart rate and blood pressure at this time. This increase may be significantly reduced by regional analgesia.[11]

However, the biggest rise occurs immediately after the birth when cardiac output increases by 60–80%.[12] This rise is due to a number of factors, including:

- relief in pressure from the gravid uterus with subsequent improvement in venous return,
- transfusion of blood from the placental bed now going back into the maternal circulation.

Excess blood loss leads to a reduction in cardiac output, and the use of oxytocic drugs such as ergometrine, which increase BP, further complicates haemodynamic shifts affecting the heart at this time. Therefore, careful observation needs to be

---

BOX 5.2: Changes to the cardiovascular system in pregnancy[7,8,9]

- Oxygen consumption increases.

- Plasma volume increases (up to 50% extra blood volume).

- Peripheral vasodilation leads to a fall in systemic vascular resistance.

- Cardiac output increases: about 20% greater by eight weeks gestation, reaching pregnancy maximum by 20–28 weeks. Rises further in labour and is highest immediately after birth.

- The heart is physiologically dilated, and myocardial contractility increases.

- Stroke volume increases.

- Heart rate increases by about 10–20 beats per minute.

- Development of placental circulation and extra blood flow to the uterus and kidneys.

- Reduced colloid osmotic pressure, therefore, oedema and pulmonary oedema are more likely.

- Procoagulant changes of pregnancy pre-dispose to venous thromboembolism.

- Supine hypotension occurs when lying flat due to the vena cava becoming compressed by the growing uterus.

made of women who may be compromised by fluid swings.

Hypoxia, by causing a constriction in small pulmonary arteries and dilatation in the systemic arteries, increases pulmonary vascular resistance,[13] so oxygen administration may be required. Between days two and five, diuresis occurs to get rid of extracellular fluid. Without this diuresis, pulmonary oedema can develop in women with cardiac disease. Careful assessment of oxygen saturation and fluid balance will monitor these changes.

The cardiac output and stroke volume may still be elevated for several days postnatal, and there is evidence that changes in the haemodynamic status can persist for some time into the puerperium.[14]

PRE-DISPOSING/RISK FACTORS

Identification of pre-existing risk factors (see Box 5.3) may be important when assessing signs and symptoms that present during pregnancy, so it is essential that this information is documented clearly by the midwife, alongside any developments during pregnancy.

CLINICAL FEATURES

It can often be very challenging to differentiate between the physiological effects of pregnancy and the pathological signs and symptoms of a developing cardiac condition (see Box 5.4). For many of these, there may be other diagnoses, or indeed, may be only symptomatic of being pregnant. The midwife needs to be aware of individual risk factors for the woman (see Box 5.3) and evaluate signs and symptoms carefully to ensure appropriate investigations and referrals are made when necessary.

Because many signs and symptoms that could indicate cardiac or respiratory disease overlap with common normal pregnancy signs and symptoms, assessment of pregnant women may be challenging – see Table 5.1 for some of the characteristics that may show normalcy or not. However, it is important that if there is any doubt, it is safest to investigate the findings. Also, if there is more

---

BOX 5.3: Pre-disposing/Risk Factors

General

- Smoking history
- Obesity
- Family history of cardiac disease (sudden death of a young relative may be significant)
- Hypercholesterolemia
- Other pre-existing medical conditions, especially diabetes, respiratory conditions
- Risk increases with age

Pregnancy-related

- Pre-eclampsia
- Thrombophilia
- Multiparity
- Postpartum haemorrhage

BOX 5.4: Signs and Symptoms of cardiac disorders[1,15,16]

- Shortness of breath (SOB) or breathlessness, especially when at rest and/or lying down (orthopnoea)
- Paroxysmal nocturnal dyspnoea
- Chest pain
- Palpitations – although common in pregnancy and frequently benign, some will be caused by a significant arrhythmia
- Irregular pulse
- Tachycardia, especially isolated tachycardia at rest
- Isolated systolic hypertension
- Syncope/collapse – syncope during exertion is not physiological and should not be attributed to pregnancy; instead, it suggests an inability to increase cardiac output
- Peripheral oedema
- Unexplained cough, especially with pink, frothy sputum
- Wheeze not associated with asthma
- Cyanosis
- Reduced level of consciousness and behaviour changes

Unexplained SOB should always be investigated, especially if increasing, leading to a decreased effort tolerance or involves orthopnoea, paroxysmal nocturnal dyspnea, chest pain or syncope.

Table 5.1 Cardiac/respiratory signs and symptoms

SIGN/SYMPTOM	PHYSIOLOGICAL	PATHOLOGICAL
Shortness of breath	Gradually increases with increasing gestation, as the uterus/fetus grows	Sudden onset, or worsens quickly and/or before the uterus becomes enlarged. Associated with a decreased effort tolerance or involves orthopnoea, paroxysmal nocturnal dyspnea or syncope.
Chest pain	Reflux that comes on when laying down/leaning forward and responds to treatment	At rest or with minimal exertion or associated with syncope or light-headedness.
Syncope (fainting)	Associated with prolonged standing, dehydration or briefly occurring when standing up suddenly.	Exertional or unprovoked
Fatigue	Mild and/or can be explained by high activity or a lack of sleep.	Moderate/extreme with no explanation
Palpitations	Lasting only a short time, no light-headedness or syncope.	Prolonged and/or associated with syncope or light-headedness.
Blood pressure	<140/90 mm/Hg	>140/90 mm/Hg
Heart rate	<90bpm	>90bpm and rising Weak, thready pulse
Respiration rate	12–18/20 per minute	>20 per minute Respiratory symptoms such as wheeze, air hunger
Oxygen saturation	>95 on room air	<95% on room air Respiratory symptoms such as wheeze, air hunger

than one sign/symptom that is being queried, investigation is even more important.

Shortness of breath (SOB) is one of the most common presenting symptoms for those with cardiac disease. However, it is also a common presenting symptom for many other conditions, including respiratory disease and sepsis, as well as being a normal pregnancy symptom. Cardiac causes may result in breathlessness from pulmonary congestion, oedema or reduced cardiac output.[17]

Chest pain (and pain in other potentially related sites, such as upper back, arms and neck) is a common presenting symptom for those with cardiac disease. Care needs to be taken in assessing specific sites, the degree and type of pain, what worsens or improves it and any other relevant information. See Box 5.5 for 'red flags' in pregnant women presenting with chest pain.

BOX 5.5: Red flags in a pregnant woman presenting with chest pain[1,18]

- Pain requiring opioids
- Pain radiating to arm, shoulder, back or jaw
- Sudden onset, tearing or exertional chest pain
- Breathlessness (including orthopnoea)
- Persistent tachycardia
- Wheeze (when asthma is ruled out)
- Haemoptysis
- Exertional syncope
- Abnormal neurology
- Abnormal vital signs (especially persistent tachycardia)

Level of consciousness and mood state can be a sensitive indicator of cardiac function. Alternation of cardiac output will influence cerebral perfusion, and a reduction in cerebral perfusion can lead to drowsiness, confusion, agitation and reduced level of consciousness – and finally to unconsciousness.[6]

Alternatively, the woman may feel anxious and frightened but not be hypoxic.[19]

SPECIFIC CARE

Preconception care

It is important that all women with known cardiac disease access preconception care before getting pregnant. All cardiac diseases have the potential to be progressive, and an assessment is even more necessary if the woman is taking medication, as this may need to be reviewed to ensure it is the optimum prescription and is safe in pregnancy. Although the midwife does not normally undertake preconception care, it would be appropriate to remind a woman in the postnatal period that a preconception assessment would be important when planning another pregnancy.

Actions when cardiac conditions are suspected

Although it is much more likely a woman with previously unknown cardiac compromise will present with signs and symptoms in the latter half of pregnancy, it is possible that first identification could happen during labour or in the early postnatal period. Pre-disposing and/or risk factors (see Box 5.3) are usually identified at booking by the midwife, and the knowledge of these can underpin suspicion of heart involvement if the woman presents with symptoms.

When diagnosed with a cardiac condition in the antenatal period, a plan must be made concerning labour and a written copy of this should be available for the woman in case admission to another hospital is unexpectedly needed.[20] See Box 5.6 for suggested initial care of a woman with suspected cardiac complications.

BOX 5.6: Initial care of a woman with suspected cardiac complications

The urgency, site and investigations will depend on the woman's condition but may involve:

- *Transfer*: if not in a clinical setting, transfer to A&E, delivery suite triage, or any other appropriate site.
- *Referral*: immediate referral to the obstetric/cardiac team.
- *On-going assessment* by the midwife; see Box 5.7 for details of possible assessments
- *Cannulation* (although fluid administration needs to be prescribed and careful fluid balance records maintained. Fluid overload may be dangerous).
- *Blood tests*: see Box 5.8 for some suggested tests.
- *Specific cardiac assessment/monitoring*: a 'bedside' three-lead cardiac monitor (oscilloscope), a 12-lead ECG (electrocardiogram), an echocardiogram and a chest X-ray.

Labour care

- As many women with known cardiac disease are receiving anti-coagulants, consideration of this needs to be made when IOL or CS is planned.
- Regional anaesthesia is usually recommended as it can blunt the cardiovascular response to pain.[21]
- On-going maternal monitoring throughout labour will depend on the woman's condition, but continuous three-lead cardiac monitoring, continuous pulse oximetry and frequent BP assessment are common.[21]
- There may be a decision to limit the time spent pushing in the second state in order to restrict any adverse effect on the heart.[22,23]
- Third-stage management should be planned prior to the birth and will depend on the woman's condition; however, ergometrine should be avoided.[8,21]
- As the baby may have some growth restrictions, close attention to fetal monitoring throughout labour is necessary.

BOX 5.7: Midwifery assessment and care of a woman with suspected cardiac issues[6]

- Respirations: observation of features of breathing, respiratory rate and usually continuous pulse oximetry for O_2 saturation levels. Note that some oximeters can under/over-estimate levels,[15] and over-estimation has been reported in people with dark skin (see Chapter 14; Box 14.4).
- Heart rate: continuous pulse oximetry reading for on-going assessment of heart rate – a manual pulse should also be done to assess the quality of the pulse: a 'thready' pulse can indicate poor cardiac output.
- Blood pressure: regular and frequent blood pressure assessment: a narrow pulse pressure, i.e., the difference between systolic and diastolic pressure (normal is 35–45 mmHg) suggests arterial vasoconstriction, potentially from cardiogenic shock or hypovolaemia.
- Temperature: bacterial endocarditis and myocarditis may occur when there is damage to the cardiovascular system from any complications, and it has been suggested that these conditions should always be considered when a cause of pyrexia is not immediately obvious.
- Fluid Balance: when cannulating, the state of the veins should be assessed, as under-filled or collapsed veins could indicate hypovolaemia. As it is possible the heart may not be working efficiently, the dangers of overload are clear. Fluid administration will depend on individual conditions and the physical state of the woman, but the midwife must ensure accurate fluid balance records are maintained, and hourly urine measurements are particularly important at this time.
- Cardiac monitoring: it is not within the scope of midwifery care to evaluate cardiac monitoring; however, when a woman has a three-lead continuous monitor in place, the midwife should be able to recognise a deviation from the normal to enable timely referral. See Figure 5.1 for an example of normal sinus rhythm.
- Fetal assessment: depending on the woman's condition and gestation, a continuous CTG may be used. Changes in the fetal trace can often be the first indication of a change in the woman's condition.

BOX 5.8: Blood tests

- Troponin levels (a diagnostic marker of damage to the heart) – serial measurements may be necessary
- N-terminal pro-brain natriuretic peptide (NT-proBNP) for assessment of suspected heart failure
- FBC (Hb for anaemia/WBC for infection)
- U&Es (electrolyte imbalance can cause arrhythmias)
- Renal function tests (abnormalities could indicate poor cardiac output)
- Clotting times
- Lipids (cardiovascular risk factor)
- Amylase (rule out acute pancreatitis)
- CRP (assess inflammatory process)
- Capillary glucose assessment
- VBGs/ABGs if necessary

All cases of documented sinus tachycardia, SVT (supraventricular tachycardia) or atrial fibrillation or flutter should have thyroid function measured.[8]

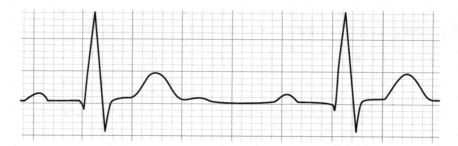

Figure 5.1 Normal Sinus Rhythm

Postnatal care

The immediate postnatal period is the time of highest risk for a woman with heart disease, as many haemodynamic changes can occur at the same time. After the birth, a woman with cardiac disease, whether newly diagnosed or previously treated, needs careful, attentive care. Most deaths from cardiac disease occur in the early postnatal period,[24] and fluid balance is particularly important at this time. High dependency care should continue for 24–72 hours after the birth as significant fluid shift can lead to congestive cardiac failure and if spontaneous diuresis does not occur, pulmonary oedema may result. Very careful monitoring should be on-going, and in some cases, may involve the transfer of the woman to critical care facilities.

For a woman previously undiagnosed, it is also possible that cardiac disease may present for the first time in the postnatal period. Aortic dissection and acute coronary syndromes may manifest early postpartum and, by definition, peripartum cardiomyopathy occurs between the last month of pregnancy and the first few months of the puerperium. The risk of cardiac disease is compounded by common complications such as postpartum haemorrhage, hypertensive disorders and infection. The midwife should, therefore, not relax her normal observation of the woman and must maintain suspicion of any relevant signs or symptoms, prompting appropriate referrals.

Treatment of most women with heart disease includes anti-coagulant therapy, and this may have been discontinued prior to the birth. When prescribed to recommence, the midwife should ensure this takes place (teaching the woman to give themselves LMWH injections if this is a new procedure). Meanwhile, the midwife needs to ensure

that preventative measures are encouraged, as listed here. Although early mobilization would be ideal, it may not be possible initially, and therefore, it is important to ensure:

- Wearing of correctly fitting anti-embolic stockings (AES)
- Deep-breathing exercises to encourage venous return
- Effective postpartum pain relief to enable mobility
- Intermittent pneumatic compression devices used during operative procedures and whilst immobile
- Adequate hydration (although with any necessary monitoring of fluid balance as fluid overload may continue to be a risk)

Infection rates in the puerperium are directly related to the length and the number of interventions during labour, and a woman with cardiac disease may have received many interventions. Besides making sure strict asepsis is followed wherever appropriate, the midwife could also ensure the woman understands the importance of sleep and nutrition to efficient healing and building a healthy immune system.[25]

Any cardiac medication the woman is taking should be assessed for breastfeeding safety. A neonatologist review of the baby is recommended, as there may be potential for the baby to inherit a cardiac condition.

If the woman was newly diagnosed with cardiac disease during pregnancy or postnatally, she will need to be made aware of how to access appropriate on-going care and the importance of preconception care if she plans another pregnancy.

For those women with cardiac conditions already diagnosed, preconception care by a cardiologist is important, even if a previous pregnancy was uncomplicated, as cardiac conditions are known to be progressive. Since midwives are rarely involved in preconception care, it would be opportune to remind the woman, during postnatal contact, of the importance of regular cardiac assessments, particularly when she is planning another pregnancy.

Since many general pre-disposing factors for cardiac disease may be reduced by improvements in general health, these issues should be addressed by every professional undertaking preconception care for all women.

COMMON CARDIAC CONDITIONS COMPLICATING PREGNANCY

For a summary of some common conditions which may be seen by midwives, see Boxes 5.9–5.12.

LONG TERM ISSUES

If the woman was newly diagnosed with cardiac disease during pregnancy, she will need to be made aware of how to access appropriate on-going care and the importance of preconception care if she plans another pregnancy.

BOX 5.9: Cardiac Failure

Heart failure is usually caused by another cardiac condition, commonly in maternity situations a cardiomyopathy (specifically peripartum cardiomyopathy):

Signs and Symptoms: pale, sweaty, agitated, cool peripheries, HR >110 persistently, palpitations, hypotension, breathlessness, O_2 saturations <95%.
Actions: immediate referral, review by cardiologist, cannulation.
Specific Investigations: ECG, echocardiogram, X-ray, U&Es, FBC and measurement of NT-proBNP levels.
Care: following stabilization, immediate delivery of the baby if still pregnant and supportive care, usually in ITU.

BOX 5.10: Acute coronary syndrome/ischemic heart disease/Myocardial Infarction (MI)/Spontaneous Coronary Artery Dissection (SCAD)

Commonly referred to as 'heart attacks', these conditions are growing more common in the maternity population but continue to be not suspected and therefore diagnosed late in young women.[1] Pregnancy may cause differences in the pathophysiology of acute coronary syndrome as SCAD and coronary thrombosis may occur more frequently due to specific physiological adaptations to pregnancy such as a more hypercoagulable state, increase in stroke volume and increase in cardiac output.
Signs and Symptoms: 'crushing' chest pain which could radiate to the arm (frequently left side), shoulder, back or jaw (although note many women do not experience these traditional male symptoms) and a history of angina may be reported. May be associated with sweating, nausea, haemoptysis, breathlessness and epigastric pain.
Actions: immediate referral, review by cardiologist, cannulation.
Specific Investigations: ECG, echocardiogram, coronary angiography, cardiac MRI, cardiac enzymes (troponin levels), U&Es, FBC.
Care: drug treatment, in particular antiplatelets (aspirin) is usual, and stents may be used.
Midwifery care will involve monitoring vital signs, fluid balance and fetal wellbeing at a frequency appropriate to the woman's condition.

BOX 5.11: Aortic Dissection (AD)

Cardiovascular changes associated with pregnancy (hormonal and biochemical changes that may modify the ability of the aorta to withstand the haemodynamic effects placed on it – may be weakening of elastic fibres)[26] as well as inheritable conditions, including connective tissue disorders such as Marfan syndrome, may be a factor in aortic dissections. The most common time for presentation is late pregnancy and early postpartum.[8]

Signs and Symptoms: sudden onset, severe 'tearing' chest pain possibly radiating to interscapular area and may be associated with haemoptysis, breathlessness, syncope or abnormal neurology.

Actions: immediate referral, review by cardiologist, cannulation.

Specific Investigations: ECG, echocardiogram, chest X-ray, MRI, cardiac enzymes (troponin levels), U&Es, FBC.

Care: care of aortic dissection is usually surgical, and transfer to ITU following would be normal.

BOX 5.12: Cardiac Valve Compromise

Women can present during pregnancy with new cardiac symptoms from an undiagnosed heart valve issue (frequently mitral stenosis resulting from rheumatic fever with no medical involvement) or start pregnancy following valvular surgery.

Both women will probably need anticoagulation treatment (not usually necessary in grafted-tissue heart valves), and during pregnancy, this is known to be complex[1] and is associated with a high risk of maternal and fetal complications.[27]

Signs and Symptoms: dyspnoea, orthopnoea, paroxysmal nocturnal dyspnoea, cough/haemoptysis, tachycardia, signs of pulmonary oedema.

Actions: immediate referral, review by cardiologist, cannulation.

Care: Midwifery care will involve monitoring vital signs, fluid balance and fetal wellbeing at a frequency appropriate to the woman's condition. Any change in a woman with a known artificial heart valve must be immediately investigated in case of infective endocarditis.

There is some data that suggests pregnancy in women with heart disease may accelerate lesion progression.[28] This means that midwives must remind women to access regular cardiology checks in the future and, in particular, before they plan another pregnancy.

SUMMARY OF MIDWIFERY RESPONSIBILITIES

Maintain the awareness that young women with no risk factors can present with an undiagnosed cardiac condition during pregnancy, and ensure they have appropriate assessment.

Ensure all women with a cardiac condition understand the importance of accessing preconception care before planning another pregnancy.

Women with cardiac conditions should have regular assessments, and the midwife should make sure they know (especially if they are newly diagnosed) where and how to access these.

Maintain an up-to-date knowledge of care for women with unexpected collapse, including where and how to access specialized equipment and drugs.

FURTHER READING AND RESOURCES

Royal College of Physicians (RCP). Acute care toolkit 15: managing acute medical problems in pregnancy. London: RCP; 2019.

Burns R, Dent K, editors. Managing medical and obstetric emergencies and trauma. Cambridge: Wiley Blackwell; 2022.
  Chapter 9: acute cardiac disease in pregnancy.

Regitz-Zagrosek V, Lundqvist C, Borghi C, et al., European Society of Gynecology (ESG), the Association for European Paediatric Cardiology (AEPC), the German Society for gender medicine (DGesGM), et al. Guidelines on the management of cardiovascular diseases during pregnancy: the task force on the management of cardiovascular diseases during pregnancy of the European Society of Cardiology (ECS). 2018. Available from: <doi:10.1093/eurheartj/ehy340>

REFERENCES

1. Engjom H, Clarke B, Girling J, Hillman S, Holden S, Lucas S, et al. Messages on caring for women with multiple morbidities. In: Knight M, Bunch K, Patel R, Shakespeare J, Kotnis R, Kenyon S, Kurinczuk JJ, On Behalf of MBRRACE-UK, editors. Saving lives, improving mothers' care core report – lessons learned to inform maternity care from the UK and Ireland confidential enquiries into maternal deaths and Morbidity 2018–20. Oxford: National Perinatal Epidemiology Unit, University of Oxford; 2022. p. 34–44.

2. Zacharzewski A, Macnab R. Cardiac disease in pregnancy. Anaesthesia and Intensive Care Medicine. 2019;23(8):448–454. Available from: <doi:10.1016/j.mpaic.2019.07.002>

3. Diguisto C, Choinier P-M, Saucedo M, Bruyere M, Verspyck E, Morau E, et al. Timing and preventability of cardiovascular-related maternal death. Obstetrics & Gynecology. 2023;141(6):1190–1198.

4. Freeman A, Squire G, Herrey A, Hogrefe K, Allen R. Acute coronary syndromes in pregnancy: a literature review. The Obstetrician and Gynaecologist 2023;25(2):101–109.

5. Mehta L, Warner's C, Bradley E, Burton T, Economy K, Mahran R, Sandra B, Sharla G, On Behalf of the American Heart Association Council on Clinical Cardiology, Council on Arteriosclerosis, Thrombosis and Vascular Biology; Council on Cardiovascular and Stroke Nursing; and Stroke Council. Cardiovascular consideration in caring for pregnant patients: a scientific statement from the American Heart Association. Circulation. 2020;141:e884–e903. Available from: <doi:10.1161/CIR.0000000000000772>

6. Boyle M, Bothamley J. Critical care assessment by midwives. Abington: Routledge; 2018.

7. Bothamley J, Boyle M. Medical conditions affecting pregnancy and childbirth. 2nd ed. Abington: Routledge; 2021.

8. Nelson-Piercy C. Handbook of obstetric medicine. 6th ed. London: CRC Press; 2021. ISBN:9780367541026.

9. Blackburn ST. Maternal, fetal and neonatal physiology, 4th ed. London: Saunders; 2013.

10. Soma-Pillay P, Nelson-Piercy C, Tolppanen H, Mebazaa A. Physiological changes in pregnancy. Cardiovasc J Afr. 2016 Mar-Apr;27(2):89–94. Available from: <doi:10.5830/CVJA-2016-021>. PMID: 27213856; PMCID:PMC4928162.

11. Johnson M, von Klemperer K 2016 cardiovascular changes in pregnancy chapter 3 in Steer P, Gatoulis M, editors. Heart disease and pregnancy 2nd ed. Cambridge university press pp. 19–28.)

12. Schaufelberger M. Cardiomyopathy and pregnancy. Heart. 2019;105:1543–1551. Available from: http://orcid.org/0000-0002-0611-0863

13. Tarry D, Powell M. Hypoxic pulmonary vasoconstriction. BJA Education. 2017;17(6): 208–213. Available from: <doi:10.1093/bjaed/mkw076>

14. Ramsay M. Management of the puerperium in women with heart disease. In: Steer P, Gatzoulis M, editors. Heart disease and pregnancy. 2nd ed. London: RCOG; 2016. p. 218–226.

15. NICE Guideline. Intrapartum care for women with existing medical conditions or obstetric complications and their babies. 2019. Available from: http://nice.org.uk/guidance/ng121

16. Moran N, Khaliq O, Ngene N et al. Persistent maternal tachycardia: a clinical alert for healthcare professionals providing maternity care in South Africa. South African Medical Journal. 2022;112(6):403–404.

17. Burns R, Dent K, editors. Managing medical and obsetric emergencies and trauma. Chapter 9: acute cardiac disease in pregnancy. Cambridge: Wiley Blackwell; 2022. p. 73–86.

18. Royal College of Physicians. RCP acute care toolkit 15: managing acute medical problems in pregnancy. London: RCP; 2019.

19. Burtscher J, Niedermeier M, Hufner K et al. The interplay of hypoxic and mental stress: implications for anxiety and depressive disorders. Neuroscience & Biobehavioral Reviews 2022;138:104718. Available from: <doi:10.1016/j.neubiorev.2022.104718>

20. Elkayam U, Goland S, Pieper PG, Silverside CK. High-risk cardiac disease in pregnancy: part I. J Am Coll Cardiol. 2016 Jul 26;68(4):396–410. Available from: <doi:10.1016/j.jacc.2016.05.048> PMID: 27443437.

21. Caldwell M, Dos Santos F, Steer P, Swan L, Gatzoulis M & Johnson M. Pregnancy in women with congenital heart disease. BMJ 2018;360:k478 Available from: <doi:10.aa36/bmj.k478>

22. Burt C & Durbridge J. Management of cardiac disease in pregnancy. Continuing Education in Anaesthesia, Critical Care and Pain. 2009;9(2):44–47. Available from: <doi:10.1093/bjaceaccp/mkp005>

23. Ashrafi R, Curtis SL. Heart Disease and Pregnancy. Cardiol Ther. 2017 Dec;6(2): 157–173. Available from: <doi:10.1007/s40119-017-0096-4>. Epub 2017 Jul 5. PMID: 28681178; PMCID:PMC5688973.

24. Kotit S & Yacoub M. Cardiovascular adverse events in pregnancy: a global perspective. Glob Cardiol Sci Pract 2021;1:e202105. Available from: <doi:10.21542/gcsp.2021.5>

25. Bothamley J, Boyle M. Infections affecting pregnancy and childbirth. London: Radcliffe; 2015.

26. Kamel H, Roman M, Pitcher A & Devereux R. Pregnancy and the risk of aortic dissection or rupture. Circulation. 2016;134(7): 527–533. Available from: <doi:10.1161/CIRCULATIONAHA.116.021594>

27. Vahanian A, Beyersdorf F, Praz F, Milojevic M, Baldus S, Bauersachs J, Capodanno D, Conradi L, De Bonis M, De Paulis R, Delgado V, Freemantle N, Gilard M, Haugaa KH, Jeppsson A, Jüni P, Pierard L, Prendergast BD, Sádaba JR, Tribouilloy C, Wojakowski W; ESC/EACTS Scientific Document Group. 2021 ESC/EACTS Guidelines for the management of valvular heart disease. Eur Heart J. 2022 Feb 12;43(7):561–632. Available from: <doi:10.1093/eurheartj/ehab395>. Erratum in Eur Heart J. 2022 Feb 18;: PMID: 34453165.

28. Siu S, Lee D, Rashid M, Fang J et al. Long-Term Cardiovascular Outcomes After Pregnancy in Women With Heart Disease. Journal of the American Heart Association. 2021;10:e020584 Available from: <doi:10.1161/JAHA.120.020584>

6

Thromboembolism in pregnancy

JUDY BOTHAMLEY

Introduction	87	Clinical features	94
Pathophysiology	88	Care	94
Pre-conception care	88	Further reading and resources	99
Risk assessment	89	References	99
Antenatal care	93		

BOX 6.1: Definitions

Venous thromboembolism (VTE) refers to blood clots that develop in veins.

Deep vein thrombosis (DVT) occurs when a blood clot forms in a deep vein of the lower leg, thigh, or pelvis.

Pulmonary embolism (PE) is the most common cause of death associated with VTE. It occurs when a clot from a deep vein, commonly in the leg, detaches itself and travels to the lungs, where it lodges in a pulmonary blood vessel. Collapse and death will occur if the clot is large enough to compromise the pulmonary circulation.

Cerebral vein thrombosis (CVT) is a blood clot in a cerebral vein in the brain. It causes a severe headache, can lead to stroke and is a rare cause of maternal death.

INTRODUCTION

Pregnant and postpartum women, when compared with non-pregnant women of the same age, are at significantly increased risk of developing venous thromboembolism (which includes DVT and PE).[1] PE has been the leading direct cause of maternal deaths in the UK for over 20 years.[2] It is estimated that for every woman who has died of pulmonary embolism, a further 50 women have a pulmonary embolism, many of whom are left with long-term complications.[3]

The pro-coagulant changes that underlie the development of VTE in pregnancy start early in gestation, and a number of VTEs occur in early pregnancy.[4] However, the greatest risk of VTE is in the period immediately following birth.[1,4] Of VTE events that occur in association with child-bearing, about 75% are DVT and 25% are PE.[5] If a DVT is not recognised and treated, up to a quarter of women will develop a PE.[6]

Detailed risk assessment and timely and effective prophylaxis both in the antenatal and postnatal period have been noted as effective measures to prevent deaths, but challenges remain. The rise in rates of obesity, advanced maternal age, caesarean section and medical co-morbidities among pregnant women are contributing to persistent rates of women dying from this complication,[2] and midwives need to remain knowledgeable in identifying both those at risk and those showing symptoms of a VTE.

DOI: 10.4324/9781003382195-6

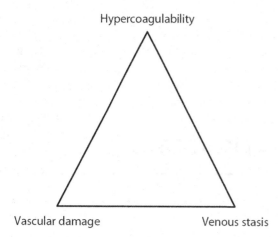

Figure 6.1 Triad of factors associated with venous thrombosis

PATHOPHYSIOLOGY

Clot formation normally occurs in response to injury in a vessel wall and is an important mechanism to prevent blood loss. A DVT will develop when clots collect in a vein (often iliofemoral, thigh or calf veins) because of slow blood flow. They may occur around the cusp of a venous valve, which can cause irreversible valve damage, resulting in chronic valve insufficiency and a condition known as post-thrombotic syndrome. A PE will arise when clots travel to the pulmonary circulation, impairing oxygenation.

Rudolf Virchow (1821–1902) first described the triad of factors that are associated with venous thrombosis, all of which are present during pregnancy and the puerperium (see Figure 6.1).

Hypercoagulability

Normal pregnancy is associated with alterations in the proteins of the coagulation and fibrinolytic systems, resulting in a relative state of hypercoagulability.[7] These changes ensure the effective control of bleeding in the third stage of labour. Pro-coagulant factors, such as Von Willebrand factor, factor VII, factor VIII, factor X and fibrinogen enhance thrombin production in pregnancy.[7] In addition, an acquired resistance to the anticoagulant protein C and a reduction in protein S further contribute to the increased coagulability. Impaired fibrinolysis, resulting in slower breakdown of clots, also occurs.[7,8] Dehydration, subsequent to hyperemesis or infection, will increase the risk of VTE.

Venous stasis

Sluggish venous return from the lower limbs occurs when the pregnant uterus compresses the inferior vena cava, compounded by the reduction in the muscle tone of veins during pregnancy caused by progesterone.[7,9] Blood flow in the veins depends on the action of the voluntary muscles and periods of inactivity due to bed rest, air travel and or that associated with symphysis pubis dysfunction further slow blood flow. Blood remains in contact with the vessel wall for a longer time, and this may be an important factor in the development of a DVT. Incompetent venous valves are a common source of morbidity in women of reproductive age and may also contribute to venous stasis. The anatomy of the venous drainage from the lower limbs, where the left iliac vein is crossed by the right iliac artery, means that DVTs are more common in the left leg, although this is not unique to pregnancy.[10,11]

Vascular damage

The epithelial lining of veins is normally an intact, smooth, single layer of cells containing various substances to prevent platelet adhesion and clot formation.

Surgery, including caesarean section or perineal trauma, damages the vessel walls, setting off a series of chemical reactions that cause the platelets to clump together and fibrin formation that results in clot formation and increases the risk of VTE.[7,10]

PRE-CONCEPTION CARE

Ideally, those women with a high risk of VTE, including those with previous VTE, should be offered pre-pregnancy counselling with a clinician who has expertise in thrombosis in pregnancy.[12,13] 'Booking' often does not occur until near the end of the first trimester, after the stage when thromboprophylaxis should have begun. General practitioners, physicians, other health professionals and the general public need to recognise the need for pre-conception planning for women at high risk of VTE.

The MBRRACE report[12] highlighted the number of extremely obese young women who died of VTE. With over 50% of women noted to be overweight or obese at the time of their booking appointment,[14] wide-ranging public health measures to reduce obesity before pregnancy are needed.

RISK ASSESSMENT

Risk assessment and preventive measures for women found to be at higher risk of VTE are essential in improving outcomes. An assessment for risk factors for VTE should be made at booking, repeated if admitted to hospital or if factors change, and again immediately postpartum.[13,15] The midwife at the booking interview already gathers the required information (such as smoking, body mass index [BMI], previous medical or family history of VTE) required for risk assessment of VTE. Timely and efficient referral to an obstetrician/physician/haematologist as appropriate for those women found to be at increased risk is needed so that a plan of management can be determined, especially if that has not been identified in the pre-conception period.

The risk assessment tools devised by the Royal College of Obstetricians and Gynaecologists (RCOG) have been reproduced with permission.[13] (See Figures 6.2, 6.3.)

A scoring system should not replace but rather complement a common-sense approach to individual assessment. Gathering information for risk assessment requires good communication and relevant questioning. Midwives need to involve women fully in both the risk assessment and discussion regarding the need for thromboprophylaxis. Women at increased risk of VTE should be given information about the signs and symptoms of DVT and PE along with details on how to self-refer so they can quickly contact medical advice if they are concerned. Verbal discussion should be followed up with written information.

However, it has been identified that risk assessments are not always carried out at crucial times, such as admission to hospital, can be calculated incorrectly or are not followed up with the appropriate preventive treatment measures such as a weight-related regime of low molecular heparin.[3,12,16] MBRRACE have called for a consistent, easy to use, risk assessment tool that follows national guidelines.[12]

Risk factors

Inherited or acquired thrombophilia, prior VTE, co-existing medical complications, multiple gestation, immobility, infection, PPH and stillbirth are all considered significant risk factors for VTE in pregnancy[1] (see Figures 6.2 and 6.3 for a full list). Risks can also have an additive and multiplying effect, such as the combination of immobilisation and raised BMI.[15]

Previous thrombosis is the most important risk factor for developing VTE in pregnancy.[1] Women with recurrent VTE and those whose previous VTE was oestrogen-related (while on combined oral contraceptive pill) or during a previous pregnancy are unsurprisingly more likely to have another pregnancy-related VTE.

The other significant risk factor for pregnancy-related VTE is thrombophilia. An alteration in the balance between the coagulation and fibrinolytic systems caused by inherited or acquired disorders predisposes a woman to clot formation, although many women with thrombophilia do not develop thrombosis complications, indicating that the development of VTE is multicausal. Examples of thrombophilia disorders are listed in Box 6.2.

Women with high-risk thrombophilia are likely to be on long-term oral anticoagulant medication such as warfarin. As this medication is associated with damage to the fetus during development, the woman is advised to change over to LMWH when the pregnancy is confirmed, ideally within two weeks of her missed period and before the sixth week of pregnancy.[17] When planning pregnancy, she is advised to take regular pregnancy tests. The woman will require information, support and access to expert advice to facilitate this transition in her medication.

Obesity remains an important risk factor for venous thromboembolism, with women with a BMI of 30kg/m2 or greater being four times more likely to have a VTE.[12] Factors that may contribute to the increased risk include reduced mobility and reduced venous return, increased hospitalisation for other complications such as pre-eclampsia and gestational diabetes, increased rates of caesarean birth, use of the combined oral contraceptive pill

---

BOX 6.2: Thrombophilia conditions

INHERITED

- Factor V Leiden
- Antithrombin deficiency
- Protein C and protein S deficiency
- Prothrombin gene mutation G 20210A

ACQUIRED

- Antiphospholipid syndrome (APS)

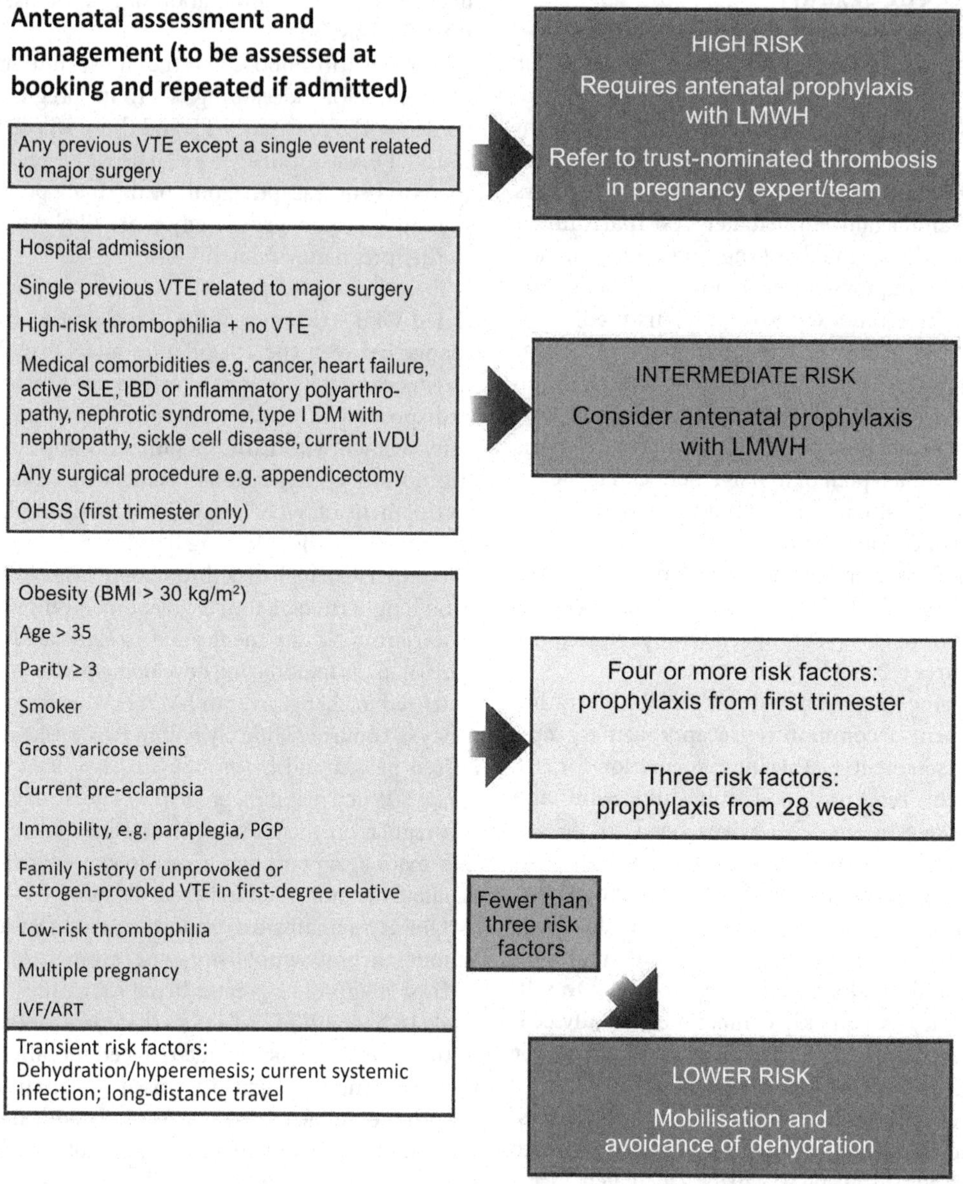

Antenatal assessment and management (to be assessed at booking and repeated if admitted)

Any previous VTE except a single event related to major surgery

→ **HIGH RISK**

Requires antenatal prophylaxis with LMWH

Refer to trust-nominated thrombosis in pregnancy expert/team

Hospital admission

Single previous VTE related to major surgery

High-risk thrombophilia + no VTE

Medical comorbidities e.g. cancer, heart failure, active SLE, IBD or inflammatory polyarthropathy, nephrotic syndrome, type I DM with nephropathy, sickle cell disease, current IVDU

Any surgical procedure e.g. appendicectomy

OHSS (first trimester only)

→ **INTERMEDIATE RISK**

Consider antenatal prophylaxis with LMWH

Obesity (BMI > 30 kg/m²)

Age > 35

Parity ≥ 3

Smoker

Gross varicose veins

Current pre-eclampsia

Immobility, e.g. paraplegia, PGP

Family history of unprovoked or estrogen-provoked VTE in first-degree relative

Low-risk thrombophilia

Multiple pregnancy

IVF/ART

→ Four or more risk factors: prophylaxis from first trimester

Three risk factors: prophylaxis from 28 weeks

Transient risk factors:
Dehydration/hyperemesis; current systemic infection; long-distance travel

Fewer than three risk factors

→ **LOWER RISK**

Mobilisation and avoidance of dehydration

APL = antiphospholipid antibodies (lupus anticoagulant, anticardiolipin antibodies, ß₂-glycoprotein 1 antibodies); ART = assisted reproductive technology; BMI based on booking weight; DM = diabetes mellitus; FHx = family history; gross varicose veins = symptomatic, above knee or associated with phlebitis/oedema/skin changes; high-risk thrombophilia = antithrombin deficiency, protein C or S deficiency, compound or homozygous for low-risk thrombophilias; IBD = inflammatory bowel disease; immobility = ≥ 3 days; IVDU = intravenous drug user; IVF = in vitro fer tilisation; LMWH = low-molecular-weight heparin; long-distance travel => 4 hours; low-risk thrombophilia = heterozygous for factor V Leiden or prothrombin G20210A mutations; OHSS = ovarian hypers timulation syndrome; PGP = pelvic girdle pain with reduced mobility; PPH = pos tpartum haemorrhage; thrombophilia = inherited or acquired; VTE = venous thromboembolism.

Figure 6.2 Obstetric thromboprophylaxis risk assessment and management: antenatal (reproduced from the Royal College of Obstetricians and Gynaecologists. 2015. *Thrombosis and Embolism during Pregnancy and the Puerperium, Reducing the Risk. Green-Top Guideline No. 37a.* London: RCOG, with kind permission of the Royal College of Obstetricians and Gynaecologists.)

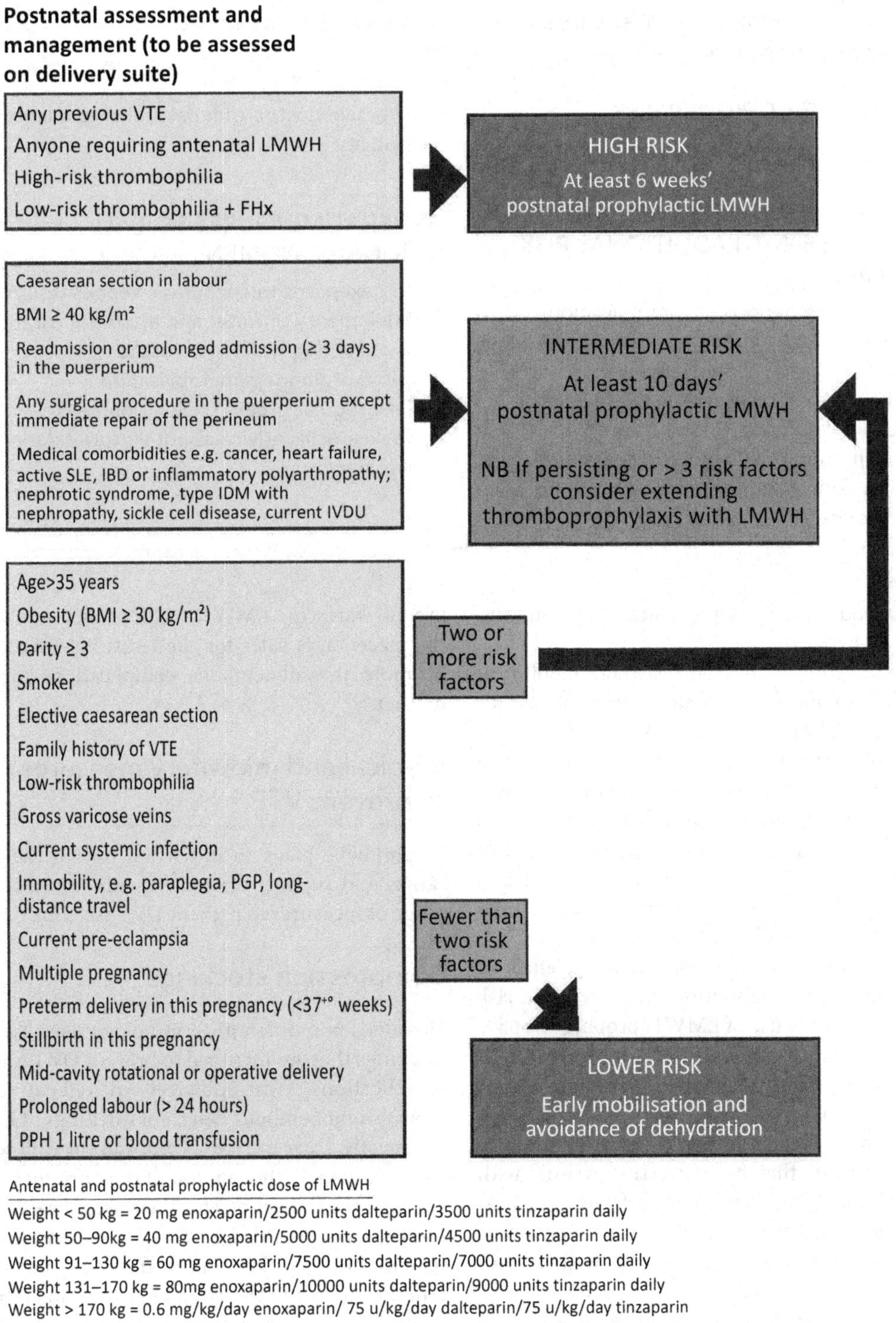

Postnatal assessment and management (to be assessed on delivery suite)

Any previous VTE
Anyone requiring antenatal LMWH
High-risk thrombophilia
Low-risk thrombophilia + FHx

HIGH RISK
At least 6 weeks' postnatal prophylactic LMWH

Caesarean section in labour
BMI ≥ 40 kg/m²
Readmission or prolonged admission (≥ 3 days) in the puerperium
Any surgical procedure in the puerperium except immediate repair of the perineum
Medical comorbidities e.g. cancer, heart failure, active SLE, IBD or inflammatory polyarthropathy; nephrotic syndrome, type IDM with nephropathy, sickle cell disease, current IVDU

INTERMEDIATE RISK
At least 10 days' postnatal prophylactic LMWH

NB If persisting or > 3 risk factors consider extending thromboprophylaxis with LMWH

Age>35 years
Obesity (BMI ≥ 30 kg/m²)
Parity ≥ 3
Smoker
Elective caesarean section
Family history of VTE
Low-risk thrombophilia
Gross varicose veins
Current systemic infection
Immobility, e.g. paraplegia, PGP, long-distance travel
Current pre-eclampsia
Multiple pregnancy
Preterm delivery in this pregnancy (<37+0 weeks)
Stillbirth in this pregnancy
Mid-cavity rotational or operative delivery
Prolonged labour (> 24 hours)
PPH 1 litre or blood transfusion

Two or more risk factors

Fewer than two risk factors

LOWER RISK
Early mobilisation and avoidance of dehydration

Antenatal and postnatal prophylactic dose of LMWH

Weight < 50 kg = 20 mg enoxaparin/2500 units dalteparin/3500 units tinzaparin daily
Weight 50–90kg = 40 mg enoxaparin/5000 units dalteparin/4500 units tinzaparin daily
Weight 91–130 kg = 60 mg enoxaparin/7500 units dalteparin/7000 units tinzaparin daily
Weight 131–170 kg = 80mg enoxaparin/10000 units dalteparin/9000 units tinzaparin daily
Weight > 170 kg = 0.6 mg/kg/day enoxaparin/ 75 u/kg/day dalteparin/75 u/kg/day tinzaparin

Figure 6.3 Obstetric thromboprophylaxis risk assessment and management: postnatal (reproduced from the Royal College of Obstetricians and Gynaecologists. 2015. *Thrombosis and Embolism during Pregnancy and the Puerperium, Reducing the Risk. Green-Top Guideline No. 37a.* London: RCOG, with kind permission of the Royal College of Obstetricians and Gynaecologists.)

BOX 6.3: Prophylactic measures that may be used to prevent thromboembolism

FOR THOSE AT HIGHER RISK

- Thromboprophylaxis with prescribed LMWH

GENERALLY AS INDICATED, AND FOR THOSE WITH ADDITIONAL RISK FACTORS

- Avoid long periods of immobilisation
- Wear correctly fitting anti-embolic stockings (AES)
- Deep-breathing exercises to encourage venous return
- Intermittent pneumatic compression devices used during operative procedures and while immobile

- Effective postpartum pain relief to enable mobility

GENERAL MEASURES FOR ALL PREGNANT WOMEN

- Leg exercises to encourage venous return
- Drink plenty of water and avoid dehydration
- Avoid sitting with legs crossed
- Avoid prolonged immobilisation
- Take regular breaks on long journeys
- Seek specific advice about air travel during pregnancy

---

and inadequate doses of preventative low molecular weight heparin.

Any travel or circumstances where mobility is restricted for more than four hours (not just air travel) should be considered a risk factor for venous thromboembolism in pregnancy.[12,13] Admission to hospital with hyperemesis combines the risk effects of immobilisation and dehydration.

Elective caesarean section doubles the risk of developing a VTE in the postnatal period, and an emergency caesarean section further doubles that risk.[6,18] Clinical practice that promotes the use of pneumatic compression devices, effective pain relief, early mobilisation, hydration and risk assessment for the use of LMWH prophylaxis have been successful in reducing mortality and morbidity, although midwives should not be complacent.

Pre-eclampsia is associated with vascular injury, which in turn is related to a disturbance in coagulation, thereby suggesting a link with thromboembolism. Confounding factors, such as bed rest and caesarean section, may also contribute to the risk of thromboembolism in women with pre-eclampsia.

Women with mechanical heart valves are likely to be taking long-term oral anticoagulation medication. They require a plan of care from the cardiologist to adjust their medication for pregnancy, balancing the risks of changing medication with the risks to fetal development associated with the use of warfarin. LMWH, which does not cross the placenta, is safer for the fetus, but there may be more thromboembolic complications for the mother.[6,19]

Medical and midwifery measures to prevent VTE

The midwife plays an important role in the education and support of women with regard to the range of measures to prevent DVT (see Box 6.3).

Compression stockings

There is some different terminology used for the stockings that are intended to prevent DVT and its complications. Most midwives will refer to them all as thromboembolic deterrent stockings (TEDS), but strictly, there are two types, and the difference between them is the amount of pressure they provide and the indications for their use. The external compression provided by stockings increases the velocity of blood flow within the veins, improves venous return and therefore reduces venous stasis. Box 6.4 outlines guidance for the correct use of compression stockings.

Anti-embolic stockings (AES) are synonymous with TEDS and provide 14–15 mm Hg pressure around the ankle. They aim to improve venous return, particularly in immobile women following

---

BOX 6.4: Guidance for correct use of compression stockings[22]

- Use manufacturer's instructions for measuring, selecting correct size and fitting stockings.
- Apply carefully, ensuring the toe hole lies under toes, the heel patch is in the correct position and the thigh gusset is over the inner thigh.
- Stockings should be smooth when fitted. Ensure they do not roll down, which gives a tourniquet effect.

- Remove daily for no more than 30 minutes.
- Check fitting daily to detect changes in leg circumference.
- Explain to women how the stockings work and why they can help reduce DVT and give advice about how to wear them.

---

surgery and/or those with significant risk factors. AES may be used in conjunction with LMWH, for women where LMWH is contraindicated (i.e., those with a high risk of bleeding) and for women travelling by air.

There is a lack of data with regard to pregnancy about which length AES (knee or thigh) offers greater benefit. Reviews on the non-pregnant population have been inconclusive,[20] although there appear to be benefits to knee-length stockings, in that they are cheaper, more likely to fit correctly and are better tolerated by the people wearing them.[21]

Accurate fitting of stockings may be difficult in pregnancy due to changing levels of oedema. Correct fitting, however, is essential – too tight can result in tissue damage and will be uncomfortable; too large and there will be no therapeutic benefit. The RCOG[23] recommends the use of properly applied thigh-length AES with knee length being considered if full-length stockings are ill-fitting or when compliance is poor.

Graduated compression stockings (GCS) are different from AES in that they provide greater ankle compression (20–40 mm Hg) and are used in the treatment of DVT on the affected leg. They are helpful in reducing oedema and pain as well as aiming to prevent the long-term problems of post-thrombotic syndrome (PTS).[24]

Intermittent pneumatic compression devices

These devices wrap around the leg and deliver pressurised air in a sequential manner up the leg. This produces a wave-like milking effect to promote venous return. They should not be used in women with a DVT or where a DVT is suspected, as there is an increased risk of pushing emboli towards the lungs. They are often put in place prior to surgery and are useful in preventing VTE when anticoagulation treatment is temporarily stopped in women at risk of bleeding.[13,25]

ANTENATAL CARE

Those women considered high risk should receive, or be considered for, antenatal thromboprophylaxis with low molecular weight heparin (LMWH) (see section on *anticoagulation treatment and prevention of DVT and PE*). Where identified, this should commence as early in pregnancy as practically possible (in view of the increased first-trimester risk). The midwife needs to complete the risk assessment tool, identify those women and make a timely and efficient referral to an obstetrician/physician/haematologist as appropriate so that a plan of management can be determined.

Box 6.5 lists some of the factors that would indicate the need for prompt referral in the early antenatal period. High risk would indicate the need for antenatal prophylaxis with LMWH from the first trimester. Intermediate risk indicates the use of LMWH prophylaxis from 28 weeks' gestation (see Figure 6.2).

Inadequate anticoagulation caused by maternal weight not being taken into account when heparin was prescribed has been implicated in deaths. There should be clear local guidelines for weight-related thromboprophylaxis and treatment doses of LMWH adjusted against the woman's booking weight.[23] The MBRRACE-UK report[12] has recommended that guidance be developed regarding the need to re-weigh women at 28 weeks' gestation and postnatally. Weight gain will influence risk assessment as well as the required dose of LMWH.

BOX 6.5: Women who will be considered for antenatal prophylaxis with LMWH[13]

- Those with previous VTE – This may have been while taking oestrogen-containing contraception, in a previous pregnancy or as an unprovoked event (a single previous VTE related to major surgery with no other risk factors is considered intermediate risk).
- Those with four or more risk factors (Figure 6.2).
- Those admitted to hospital.
- Those with a diagnosis of a high-risk inherited or acquired thrombophilia.

- Those with a medical condition such as cancer, heart disease, SLE, complications of type 1 diabetes, IV drug users and those on regular anticoagulant medication (for example, women with mechanical heart valves).
- Hyperemesis
- Surgical procedures in pregnancy

CLINICAL FEATURES

Signs and symptoms

BOX 6.6: Symptoms and Signs of DVT[26,27]

- Pain in calf, thigh, groin, buttocks (especially unilateral pain)
- Swelling (at least 2 cm difference between the two legs)
- Redness or discoloration of the affected leg
- Change in limb colour or temperature
- Limb symptoms on the left side (>80%)
- Homan's sign (pain on dorsiflexion of the foot) (unreliable)
- Low-grade pyrexia (37.5°C)
- Tachycardia
- Lower abdominal pain
- Chest pain and shortness of breath (symptoms of PE)

Deep vein thrombosis

The diagnosis of DVT in pregnancy can be difficult. Signs and symptoms (see Box 6.6) will raise suspicion of a DVT, but only a small percentage of women will have the diagnosis confirmed. During antenatal and postnatal assessments, midwives will examine the woman's legs, noting pain or any size, colour and/or temperature difference between the limbs. Midwives are likely to be the first to whom women report their symptoms. It is important for the midwife to listen carefully to the woman when she is describing symptoms and put these in context. The general discomfort and swelling of a woman's legs in pregnancy can confuse the diagnosis, and an assessment should be made in the context of additional risk factors.

DVTs in pregnancy may not be in the calf vein but higher up in the ileo-femoral region.[6] The higher the location of the clot, the more likely it is to cause a PE and the more difficult it is to be seen on ultrasound. Abdominal pain or back pain is associated with clots in higher-level veins, and there can be swelling of the entire leg.[26] Ovarian vein thrombosis, which is more likely on the right side, presents with flank, back or groin pain. Cerebral venous thrombosis (rare) may present as a severe headache.[5] Although DVT alone is not life-threatening, almost all pulmonary emboli arise from clots in the lower extremities[27] and, therefore, any signs and symptoms of DVT or possible minor or major PE should be referred immediately to medical staff and diagnosis actively pursued.

CARE

Diagnosis of DVT

Accurate diagnosis is essential, not only to prevent PE but also to protect women from unnecessary treatment with anticoagulants. *Ultrasonography* is the primary diagnostic test for detecting DVT in pregnancy. However, when results are equivocal or when iliac vein or higher-level thrombosis is suspected, MRI may be used.[26,28] Measuring blood levels of fibrin degradation products (using the D-dimer test) is a common test for DVT outside pregnancy. However, these are known to be unreliable in pregnancy and the postnatal period and, therefore, are not recommended.[28]

Treatment of DVT

Women with features of a DVT or PE should be treated with LMWH while objective tests are carried out.[29] In addition to anticoagulation, other interventions that will aid recovery are aimed at promoting good venous return, thereby preventing further clot formation. Leg elevation is recommended when sitting, but in pregnancy, inguinal congestion may occur, so the leg should not be raised at too acute an angle and pressure behind the knee should be avoided. Knee-length GCS stockings (ankle pressure greater than 23 mm Hg) need to be fitted and correctly applied to the affected leg to help reduce oedema (see section entitled 'Compression stockings'). Once LMWH treatment has begun and stockings are fitted, mobilisation should be encouraged.[5]

General measures to prevent DVT (see Box 6.3) should be emphasised. Midwives should provide women and their families with information about DVT and how to prevent further clot formation, as well as inform them about signs and symptoms of PE and when to seek further medical aid.

Pulmonary embolism

The clinical signs of pulmonary embolism (PE) (see Box 6.7) are related to the size of the clot obstructing the pulmonary circulation. Large or multiple emboli will prevent adequate oxygenation of the blood. A woman with a major PE will collapse with severe breathlessness, cyanosis, hypotension and chest pain. Sudden respiratory or cardiac arrest may occur. Warning signs and symptoms indicative of smaller emboli include unexplained pyrexia, cough, chest pain and breathlessness, which may be incorrectly diagnosed as a chest infection or be explained away as normal breathlessness of pregnancy.

Diagnosis of PE

Midwives need to identify all possible pulmonary embolism symptoms so that prompt referral, the pursuit of an accurate diagnosis and initiation of

> ### BOX 6.7: Clinical manifestations of PE[5,27]
>
> #### MOST FREQUENT SIGNS AND SYMPTOMS
> - Sudden or unexpected difficulty in breathing
> - Increased respiratory rate (tachypnoea)
> - Feeling faint
> - Tightness in chest or pleuritic chest pain
> - Increased pulse (tachycardia)
> - Cough
> - Crackles on lung auscultation
>
> #### ASSOCIATED SIGNS AND SYMPTOMS
> - Coughing up blood (haemoptysis)
> - Distended neck veins
> - Cyanosis and collapse
> - Hypotension
> - Anxiety
> - Low-grade fever
>
> These are assessed in combination with signs and symptoms of DVT.

effective treatment can be made.[29] Failure to identify the more subtle symptoms of a PE, especially in the presence of additional risk factors, has been identified as a contributing factor in some maternal deaths.[16] See Box 6.8 for the range of investigations that may be used to aid diagnosis. MBRRACE-UK has recommended the development of guidelines for imaging to ensure conclusive diagnosis.[3]

The woman's presenting symptoms and her clinical condition will determine the priority in which diagnostic testing will be done. *Compression duplex ultrasound* of both limbs will normally be the initial investigation in women suspected of having a PE and who also have leg symptoms.[18,30] The diagnosis of DVT will indirectly confirm the diagnosis of PE and treatment (which is the same for both conditions) can be maintained.[23]

Treatment of PE

Early diagnosis and treatment are vital when PE is suspected, as deaths caused by PE can occur very quickly following an embolic event. As in any emergency, if a woman collapses with a major PE, the midwife must summon senior medical staff

---

BOX 6.8: Investigations for diagnosis of PE[18,23]

- Compression duplex ultrasound: the diagnosis of DVT will indirectly confirm the diagnosis of PE.
- Chest x-ray to identify other causes for chest symptoms such as pneumonia as well as show changes that may be indicative of PE.
- Ventilation/perfusion (V/Q) scan
- Computed tomography pulmonary angiogram (CTPA)
- Electrocardiogram (ECG) and echocardiogram (ECHO) to identify if cardiac disorders are the cause of the symptoms.

BOX 6.9: Midwife's responsibilities in suspected pulmonary embolism emergency

For women presenting with cardiovascular collapse:

- Assess airway, breathing and circulation (ABC assessment).
- Summon the emergency response team.
- Administer cardiopulmonary resuscitation (CPR) as required.
- Assist with endotracheal intubation as necessary.

And for all women suspected of having PE:

- Admit to hospital and urgently refer to senior obstetrician, anaesthetist or physician as appropriate.
- Initiate IV access.
- Take blood for FBC, coagulation screen, urea, electrolytes and liver function tests.
- Assess and record cardiovascular and respiratory vital signs.
- Monitor oxygen saturations with pulse oximeter.
- Give oxygen via face mask if O_2 saturations are below 95% in air. If appropriate, sit the woman up to maximise the respiratory effort.
- Maintain accurate fluid balance including hourly urine measurement.
- Give heparin and other drugs according to medical orders.
- Record ECG.
- Assess for bleeding.
- Monitor fetal well-being as appropriate.
- Support the woman and her family.

---

and implement appropriate resuscitation procedures immediately. Box 6.9 summarises the key responsibilities of the midwife when a woman is suspected of having a PE.

Where PE is suspected, anticoagulation treatment should be started immediately and without waiting for a confirmed diagnosis. The pharmacological treatment of choice for non-life-threatening PE is LMWH, whereas in life-threatening PE, a bolus weight-related dose of intravenous (IV) unfractionated heparin (UH) is recommended Systemic thrombolytic therapy and surgical embolectomy should also be considered in life-threatening situations.[12,31] (See section 'Anticoagulation treatment and prevention of DVT and PE').

The woman, if conscious, will be extremely apprehensive and agitated. A calm, confident, sympathetic approach by the midwife may help to minimise this apprehension. Members of the woman's family will also require support, guidance and information at the time and following this event. Midwifery staff may also need to take responsibility for the care of the newborn.

Treatment with therapeutic (as opposed to prophylactic) doses of LMWH should be continued for the remainder of the pregnancy and until at least six weeks postnatally.[18,23,29] At least three months of treatment is required in total.[23] Induction of labour or CS may be planned to enable a transition to UH so that the level of anticoagulation can be adjusted to safe levels for the birth.[29]

Midwives will be involved in teaching women to give their daily injections, advise about side effects such as bleeding from gums and bruising and generally provide on-going support following what may have been a very frightening experience.

Anticoagulation treatment and prevention of DVT and PE

Anticoagulation treatment aims to prevent extension of the clot, restore venous patency and limit the risk or recurrence of a PE. *Low molecular weight heparin* (LMWH) has largely replaced *unfractionated (standard) heparin* (UH) in the prevention and treatment of VTE in pregnancy. *Unfractionated (standard) heparin* (UH) can be administered via the IV or subcutaneous route. It is now mostly used only in acute treatment of major PE, for those at high risk of bleeding, those with a cardiac and/or renal compromise and around the time of birth in those women at high risk of thrombosis.[19,23,30] Midwives should familiarise themselves with local guidelines for intravenous heparin use in acute events.

Heparin (both LMWH and UH) doesn't break down a clot but prevents further clot formation by enhancing the action of antithrombin, allowing time for the normal process of fibrinolysis to break down the clot. This stabilises the clot, preventing fragmentation and clot formation in other locations. Heparin is a large molecule that does not cross the placenta, so the risk of teratogenesis or bleeding in the fetus is minimal. It is, therefore, considered safe for use during pregnancy and lactation.[32]

Anticoagulation therapy can be influenced by renal and liver function. As conditions such as pre-eclampsia may affect renal and liver function, blood should be tested for full blood count, coagulation screen, urea, electrolytes and liver function tests. The risk of bleeding should be assessed before giving anticoagulants. The presence of active bleeding, liver disorders, low platelets and inherited bleeding disorders such as Von Willebrand's disease warrant individualised assessment by senior medical staff.

Low molecular weight heparin (LMWH)

There are several LMWHs, and examples used in pregnancy include enoxaparin (Clexane®) and dalteparin (Fragmin®).[32] LMWH is administered by subcutaneous injection. LMWH is commonly used for prophylaxis or in the longer-term phase of treatment, but studies have confirmed that LMWH is also safe and effective for the treatment of acute thromboembolism in pregnancy.[32] Both the prophylactic and therapeutic doses of LMWH are maternal weight-dependent. The RCOG guidelines[13,23] provide weight-related LMWH dose recommendations based on booking or early pregnancy weight. LMWH generally has minimal side effects, although bleeding may be a problem in around 2% of pregnancies.[6] LMWH is considered safe in breastfeeding.[13]

Other anticoagulants

Warfarin is an oral anticoagulant and, unlike heparin, is able to cross the placenta. There is a risk of damage to the embryo if taken between six- and 12-weeks' gestation. It is not generally recommended for use in pregnancy but may be an alternative to LMWH in the postpartum period. Regular assessment of blood for the international normalised ratio (INR) is necessary, particularly in the first ten days of treatment, which can prove inconvenient in the immediate days after birth. New anticoagulants that work as direct thrombin or factor Xa inhibitors (for example, dabigatran, rivaroxaban) are not recommended for use in pregnancy or breastfeeding due to lack of evidence of safety.[28,33,34]

Labour care

Women who are prescribed low molecular weight heparin in the antenatal period are at risk of bleeding at the time of birth. A plan of care regarding the dose and duration of treatment and plans for halting the regime for labour and restarting in the postnatal period needs to be documented.[3,6,12]

The woman taking prophylactic dose LMWH should be advised to omit the dose once labour begins as an epidural cannot be given within 12 hours of the last dose.[19] They are advised to attend the hospital for assessment by the medical, obstetric and anaesthetic team. Therapeutic dose low molecular weight heparin should be stopped 24 hours before procedures, including epidural insertion, and this will require specific planning of the time of birth to achieve this.[19] Planned induction of labour or a caesarean section may be required. Intravenous unfractionated heparin around the time of planned birth allows more flexibility in timings. Other measures, such as flowtron boots and antiembolic stockings, will aid prevention of VTE in this period but not as effectively as LMWH.[3]

Box 6.10 provides a checklist for midwives regarding thromboprophylaxis and the use of LMWH around the time of birth.

Postnatal Care

The first three weeks postpartum is the period of greatest risk for VTE, and triggers for risk will now be lower than they were in the antepartum period.

> ## BOX 6.10: Checklist for midwives regarding the use of LMWH around the time of birth
>
> - The woman should have a clear plan documented in both handheld and hospital-based notes by the obstetric and medical team who have seen the woman in the antenatal period.[3,12]
> - The midwife should advise women who are experiencing signs of labour and are taking LMWH to omit any scheduled dose and come to hospital for assessment by the medical, obstetric and anaesthetic team.
> - Laboratory assessment on admission to hospital will include platelet count and a coagulation screen.
> - As there will be a need to balance the risk of VTE against the risk of bleeding at the time of delivery, mechanical and non-pharmacological methods of preventing VTE will now be very important. Hydration, mobilisation, use of AES, use of intermittent pneumatic compression devices, leg exercises, deep breathing exercises and effective pain relief are all relevant interventions the midwife can promote to prevent VTE.
> - The midwife should liaise directly with the anaesthetist regarding the insertion and removal of the epidural catheter and the timing of the next LMWH dose.

The risk assessment at this time will indicate who requires thromboprophylaxis and for how long. Women at high risk of VTE will be recommended to have six weeks of prophylaxis, and those at intermediate risk will be advised to have at least ten days of prophylactic LMWH.[13] Some women may change to the oral anticoagulant warfarin about a week after the birth, especially those who were taking maintenance doses of warfarin before pregnancy.

Midwives should ensure all women, regardless of risk, mobilise and avoid dehydration during and following delivery. (See section on *medical and midwifery measures to prevent VTE.*)

Women need information about choosing between LMWH and oral anticoagulants for postnatal prevention of VTE. The need for regular blood tests for warfarin should be considered, and discussion with the woman should seek to find the most acceptable medication that will improve her motivation to continue the treatment.[3] Both warfarin and LMWH are safe for breastfeeding.[3] There are new oral anticoagulants (such as Apixoban) that are more stable and don't require frequent blood test monitoring; however, they are contraindicated in pregnancy and breastfeeding.[31] It is key that women are supported to breastfeed and alternative medication is offered if necessary.

It has been noted that many women will stop their course of LMWH when their supply runs out,[3] so it is helpful if women are provided with the required medication for the course of their treatment prior to discharge from hospital. At each point of contact with health professionals in the postnatal period, women should be asked if they are giving the LMWH injections and if they are having any side effects they are concerned about.[12] The demands of having a new baby and the unpleasant aspects of giving the injections and developing side effects such as bruising, pain and gum bleeding make it a challenge for women to stay motivated. Information about the medication and encouragement are required to aid adherence. Liaison with the GP about the course of treatment is essential.

Education, advice and support for women taking anticoagulant treatment

Women may show initial reluctance to give themselves heparin injections, and the midwife should work through the requirements with the woman to develop her confidence. LMWH involves only small volumes, which are pre-loaded and given with a fine gauge needle. The site of subcutaneous injection should rotate between the thighs and abdominal wall. Grasping some flesh, the injection is made at right angles to the skin surface. Women should be advised not to rub the injection site. Bruising inevitably occurs at the site of injection, although rubbing the site will make that worse. The woman should take precautions in situations that may cause bleeding or injury; for example, a soft bristle toothbrush will protect from bleeding gums. Arrangements for safe disposal of needles should be made.

A phone call or visit from the midwife within days of discharge from hospital may be timely to offer support to the woman as she comes to terms with what may be prolonged treatment. Women should be given information about modification of any existing risk factors such as smoking cessation, weight management and avoiding periods of immobility as relevant. If appropriate, a discussion regarding the management of any future pregnancies should be made at a suitable time. The woman's risk of recurrent DVT, if this has occurred, and the use of the combined contraceptive pill should be discussed. Verbal discussion should be backed up with written information that includes the signs and symptoms of PE with instructions on accessing further help.

Follow-up/long-term issues

For a woman that has a VTE in pregnancy, a joint postnatal review with obstetrics and haematology will enable a plan for suitable contraception and plans for the early start of prophylaxis in a future pregnancy.[3]

Women who have a DVT in pregnancy are at higher risk of post-thrombotic syndrome (PTS), which causes pain, swelling, eczema and venous ulcers and was found to impact quality of life.[4] It occurs in around 42% of women following a DVT in pregnancy.[35] It has been recommended that GCS should be worn for up to two years to prevent PTS, although the strength of evidence supporting this recommendation is not clear.[36]

Summary of midwifery responsibilities

- Provide detailed booking assessment and complete risk assessment tool that uncovers the range of risk factors for VTE, including a previous history of a VTE.
- Repeat the risk assessment tool on admission to hospital when any change occurs and immediately postnatally.
- Ensure appropriate and prompt referral in the early antenatal period of those women at high risk.

- Ensure women do not become dehydrated post-delivery, particularly after CS. The midwife can assess the concentration of the urine as an easy evaluation of hydration.
- Provide effective pain relief, especially after CS, to ensure women can take deep breaths (promote venous return) and can mobilise.
- Provide instruction to the woman regarding self-administration of LMWH.
- Ensure the correct fitting and use of compression stockings.
- Educate all women regarding general measures such as mobilisation and hydration to prevent VTE and for women to recognise when and how to seek help.
- Midwives need to be able to recognise features of DVT and/or a PE and seek a prompt referral for diagnosis and treatment.
- Administer appropriate life support in situations of life-threatening PE.

FURTHER READING AND RESOURCES

Royal College of Obstetricians and Gynaecologists (RCOG). Green-top guideline no. 37a: reducing the risk of venous thrombembolism during pregnancy and the puerperium. London: RCOG; 2015.

Royal College of Obstetricians and Gynaecologists (RCOG). Green-top guideline no. 37b: thrombembolic disease in pregnancy and the puerperium: acute management. London: RCOG; 2015.

RCOG. Information for you: reducing the risk of venous thrombosis in pregnancy and after birth. 2015. [Accessed 7 July 2023]. Available from: www.rcog.org.uk/media/q4cneyel/pi-reducing-the-risk-of-vt-in-pregnancy.pdf
Evidence-based guidance for women on preventing VTE and recognising features of DVT and PE.

REFERENCES

1. Edebiri O, Ní Áinle F. Risk factors, diagnosis and management of venous thromboembolic disease in pregnancy. Breathe (Sheff). 2022 Jun;18(2):220018. Available from: <doi:10.1183/20734735.0018-2022>.

Epub 2022 Jul 12. PMID: 36337136; PMCID: PMC9584596.

2. Knight M, Bunch K, Patel R, Shakespeare J, Kotnis R, Kenyon S, Kurinczuk JJ, On behalf of MBRRACE-UK, editors. Saving Lives, Improving Mothers' Care Core Report. Lessons learned to inform maternity care from the UK and Ireland confidential enquiries into maternal deaths and morbidity 2018–20. Oxford: National Perinatal Epidemiology Unit, University of Oxford; 2022.

3. Knight M, Kelly T, Magee L, Russell R, Nelson-Piercy C on behalf of the MBRRACE-UK VTE morbidity chapter-writing group. Messages for the prevention and treatment of thromboembolism. In Knight M, Bunch K, Tuffnell D, Shakespeare J, Kotnis R, Kenyon S, Kurinczuk JJ, On behalf of MBRRACE-UK, editors. Saving Lives, Improving Mothers' Care – Lessons learned to inform maternity care from the UK and Ireland Confidential Enquiries into Maternal Deaths and Morbidity 2016–18. Oxford: National Perinatal Epidemiology Unit, University of Oxford 2020: p36–42.

4. Kourlaba G, Relakis J, Kontodimas S, Holm MV, Maniadakis N. A systematic review and meta-analysis of the epidemiology and burden of venous thromboembolism among pregnant women. International Journal of Gynecology & Obstetrics. 2016;132:4–10. Available from: <doi:10.1016/j.ijgo.2015.06.054>

5. Nelson-Piercy, C 2020, Handbook of Obstetric Medicine, Taylor & Francis Group, Milton. Available from: ProQuest Ebook Central. [29 May 2023].

6. Mc Lintock C. Thromboembolism in pregnancy: challenges and controversies in the prevention of pregnancy-associated venous thromboembolisation and management of anticoagulation in women with prosthetic heart valves. Best Practice & Research Clinical Obstetrics and Gynaecology. 2014;28:519–536.

7. Blackburn ST. Maternal, fetal, & neonatal physiology: a clinical perspective. 5th ed. Philadelphia: Saunders; 2018; Bourjeily G, Paidas M, Khalil H et al. Pulmonary embolism in pregnancy. The Lancet. 2010 Feb 6;375:500–512.

8. Unger HW, Bhaskar S, Mahmood T. 'Venous thromboembolism in pregnancy', Obstetrics, Gynaecology & Reproductive Medicine. 2018;28(11–12):360–365. Available from: <doi:10.1016/j.ogrm.2018.11.002>

9. Taylor J, Hicks CW, Heller JA. The hemodynamic effects of pregnancy on the lower extremity venous system. Journal of Vascular Surgery: Venous and Lymphatic Disorders, 2018;6(2):246–255. Available from: <doi:10.1016/j.jvsv.2017.08.001>

10. Chan W, Spencer FA, Ginsbergm JS. Anatomic distribution of deep vein thrombosis in pregnancy CMAJ. 2010;182(7):657–666.

11. Lamont MC, McDermott C, Thomson AJ, Greer IA. United Kingdom recommendations for obstetric venous thromboembolism prophylaxis: evidence and rationale. Seminars in perinatology, 2019;43(4):222–228. Available from: <doi:10.1053/j.semperi.2019.03.008>

12. Knight M, Bellis A, Wise A, Lucas S, Nelson-Piercy C, On Behalf of the MBRRACE-UK Thromboembolism Chapter-Writing Group. Messages for the prevention and treatment of thromboembolism In Knight M, Bunch K, Tuffnell D, Patel R, Shakespeare J, Kotnis R, Kenyon S, Kurinczuk JJ, On behalf of MBRRACE-UK, editors. Saving lives, improving mothers' care – lessons learned to inform maternity care from the UK and Ireland confidential enquiries into maternal deaths and morbidity 2017–19. Oxford: National Perinatal Epidemiology Unit, University of Oxford; 2021. p. 34–51.

13. Royal College of Obstetricians and Gynaecologists (RCOG) (RISK). Green-top Guideline No. 37a: Reducing the Risk of Venous Thrombembolism during Pregnancy and the Puerperium. London: RCOG; 2015.

14. NMPA Project Team. National Maternity and Perinatal Audit: Clinical Report 2022. Based on births in NHS maternity services in England and Wales between 1 April 2018 and 31 March 2019. London: RCOG; 2022.

15. Ewins, K, Ní Ainle F. VTE risk assessment in pregnancy. Res Pract Thromb Haemost. 2020;4:183–192. Available from: <doi:10.1002/rth2.12290>

16. Tuffnell D, Knight M and Mackillop L on behalf of the MBRRACE-UK VTE chapter-writing group. Lessons for prevention and treatment of thrombosis and thromboembolism. In Knight M, Bunch K, Tuffnell D, Jayakody H, Shakespeare J, Kotnis R, Kenyon S, Kurinczuk JJ, On behalf of MBRRACE-UK, editors. Saving Lives, Improving Mothers' Care – Lessons learned to inform maternity care from the UK and Ireland Confidential Enquiries into Maternal Deaths and Morbidity 2014–16. Oxford: National Perinatal Epidemiology Unit, University of Oxford 2018: p34–41.

17. Galambosi PJ, Ulander V, Kaaja RJ. The incidence and risk factors of recurrent venous thromboembolism during pregnancy. Thrombosis Research. 2014;134:240–245.

18. Donnelly JC, D'Alton ME. Pulmonary embolus in pregnancy. Seminars in Perinatology. 2013;37:225–233.

19. National Institute for Health and Care Excellence (NICE). Intrapartum care for women with existing medical conditions or obstetric complications and their babies. NG.121. 2019. [Accessed 7 July 2023]. Available from: www.nice.org.uk/guidance/ng121

20. Wade R, Paton F, Rice S, Stansby G, Millner P, Flavell H, Fox D, Woolacott N. Thigh length versus knee length antiembolism stockings for the prevention of deep vein thrombosis in postoperative surgical patients; a systematic review and network meta-analysis. BMJ Open. 2016;6(2):e009456. Available from: <doi:10.1136/bmjopen-2015-009456>

21. Wade R, Paton F, Woolacott N. Systematic review of patient preference and adherence to the correct use of graduated compression stockings to prevent deep vein thrombosis in surgical patients. Journal of Advanced Nursing. 2017;73(2):336–348. Available from: <doi:10.1111/jan.13148>

22. Gee E. How to apply antiembolism stockings to prevent venous thromboembolism. Nursing Times [online] 2019;115(4): 24–26.

23. Royal College of Obstetricians and Gynaecologists (RCOG) (MANAGE). Green-top Guideline No. 37b: thrombembolic disease in pregnancy and the puerperium: acute management. London: RCOG; 2015.

24. Calderwood CJ Thanoon OI. Venous thromboembolism in pregnancy. Obstetrics, Gynaecology and Reproductive Medicine. 2013;22(8):227–230.

25. Kurtoglu M Sivrikoz E. Venous thrombemolism prophylaxis: Intermittent pneumatic compression. Reviews in Vascular Medicine. 2013;1:71–75.

26. Devis P, Knuttinen MG. Deep venous thrombosis in pregnancy: incidence, pathogenesis and endovascular management. Cardiovascular Diagnosis and Therapy. 2017;7(Suppl 3):S309–S319. Available from: <doi:10.21037/cdt.2017.10.08>

27. Heuser CC, Ware Branch D. Disorders of coagulation in pregnancy. Chapter 38 in: James DK, Steer PJ, Weiner, CP, Gonik B, Robson SC, editors. High-risk pregnancy: management options. 5th ed. Cambridge: Cambridge University Press; 2017. p. 1085–1107.

28. Khan F, Vaillancourt C, Bourjeily G. Clinical update: diagnosis and management of deep vein thrombosis in pregnancy. BMJ. 2017:357. Available from: <doi:10.1136/bmj.j2344>

29. McLintock C, Brighton T, Chunilal S, Dekker G, McDonell N. et al. Recommendations for the diagnosis and treatment of deep venous thrombosis and pulmonary embolism in pregnancy and the postpartum period. Australian and New Zealand Journal of Obstetrics and Gynaecology. 2012;52:14–22.

30. Leung AN, Bull TM, Jaeschke R, Lockwood CJ, Boiselle PM, Hurwitz LM, et al. American Thoracic Society documents: an official American Thoracic Society/Society of Thoracic Radiology clinical practice guideline – evaluation of suspected pulmonary embolism in pregnancy. Radiology. 2012;262(2):635–646.

31. Regitz-Zagrosek V, Roos-Hesselink JW, Bauersachs J, Blomstrom-Lundqvist C, Cifkova R, De Bonis M, et al. 2018 ESC Guidelines for the management of cardiovascular diseases during pregnancy. European Heart Journal. 2018 Sep 7;39(34):3165–3241. Available from: <doi:10.1093/eurheartj/ehy340>

32. Greer IA, Nelson-Piercy C. Low molecular-weight heparins for thromboprophylaxis and treatment of venous thromboembolism in pregnancy: a systematic review of safety and efficacy. Blood. 2005;106(2):401–407.

33. Lameijer H, Aalberts JJJ, van Veldhuisen DJ, Meijer K, Pieper PG. Efficacy and safety of direct oral anticoagulants during pregnancy; a systematic literature review. Thrombosis Research. 2018;169:123–127. Available from: <doi:10.1016/j.thromres.2018.07.022>

34. Myers B, Neal R, Myers O, Ruparelia M. Unplanned pregnancy on a direct oral anticoagulant (Rivaroxaban): a warning. Obstetric Medicine. 2016;9(1):40–42.

Available from: <doi:10.1177/1753495X15621814>

35. Wik HS, Jacobsen AF, Sandvik L, Sandset PM. Prevalence and predictors for post-thrombotic syndrome 3 to 16 years after pregnancy-related venous thrombosis: a population-based, cross-sectional, case-control study. J Thromb Haemost. 2012 May;10(5):840–847.

36. Mol GC, Dronkers CEA, van de Ree MA, van der Pas SL, Tegelberg-Stassen MJAM, Sanders FBM, et al. Elastic compression stockings one year after DVT diagnosis: who might discontinue? Thrombosis Research. 2019;173:35–41. Available from: <doi:10.1016/j.thromres.2018.11.002>

7

Pre-eclampsia and associated conditions

MAUREEN BOYLE

PRE-ECLAMPSIA   104
Introduction   104
Pathophysiology   104
Risk/pre-disposing factors   105
Clinical features   106
ECLAMPSIA   113
Introduction   113
Pathophysiology   113
Care   113
HELLP SYNDROME   115
Introduction   115

Pathophysiology   115
Clinical features   115
ACUTE FATTY LIVER OF PREGNANCY (AFLP) 117
Introduction   117
Pathophysiology   117
Clinical features   118
FOLLOW-UP/LONG-TERM ISSUES FOR
    HYPERTENSIVE DISORDERS   119
Summary of midwifery responsibilities 119
References   120

BOX 7.1: Definitions

PRE-ECLAMPSIA (PET) is defined[1] as new-onset hypertension (>140mmHg systolic or >90mmHg diastolic) after 20 weeks of pregnancy and the coexistence of one or more of the following new-onset conditions:

- *proteinuria*: urine protein:creatinine ratio ≥30 mg/mmol or albumin:creatinine ratio ≥ 8 mg/mmol, or ≥1 g/L (2+) on dipstick testing
- *other maternal organ dysfunction*, including features such as renal or liver involvement, neurological or haematological complications or uteroplacental dysfunction (such as fetal growth restriction (FGR), abnormal umbilical artery Doppler waveform analysis, or stillbirth)

Severe pre-eclampsia is considered to be pre-eclampsia with severe hypertension (≥160/110) that does not respond to treatment or is associated with on-going or recurring severe headaches, visual scotomata, nausea or vomiting, epigastric pain and/or oliguria as well as progressive deterioration in laboratory blood tests such as rising creatinine or liver transaminases or falling platelet count, or failure of fetal growth or abnormal Doppler findings.

Fulminating pre-eclampsia is likewise severe but is often used to describe the very rapid progression of the disease.

Chronic hypertension is hypertension that is present at booking or before 20 weeks of

DOI: 10.4324/9781003382195-7

pregnancy or if the woman is already taking antihypertensive medication when referred to maternity services.

- *essential hypertension* (primary) – no underlying cause
- *secondary hypertension* – associated with underlying disease, including obesity

Gestational hypertension is new hypertension present after 20 weeks without significant proteinuria or other signs of pre-eclampsia and resolution within three months after birth. It is sometimes called *'pregnancy induced hypertension'* (PIH).

INTRODUCTION

Pre-eclampsia may be described as an unpredictable and progressive condition with the potential to cause multi-organ dysfunction and failure that can be detrimental to the health of both the woman and her baby. In fact, although the definition (see Box 7.1) appears clear, there are many varied presentations of pre-eclampsia, and presenting signs and symptoms may not always fit the classical definitions.

In resource-rich countries, pre-eclampsia is considered a major cause of maternal morbidity and mortality, but in other parts of the world with limited antenatal care, the numbers are much higher. Worldwide, pre-eclampsia is reported to occur in 2–8% of pregnancies[2] and accounts for more than 50,000 maternal deaths each year.[3] Pre-eclampsia also contributes significantly to the number of preterm births, stillbirths and neonatal deaths.[4,5]

APEC[6] (Action on Pre-eclampsia) suggests that in the UK, about 10% of first pregnancies are complicated by mild pre-eclampsia and 1–2% by a more serious form of the disease. Other estimates vary, which underlines the challenge of defining pre-eclampsia; however, as currently there are increasing numbers of pregnancies at high risk for pre-eclampsia, it is clear that large numbers of women will present with this condition.

In a recent Confidential Enquiry report from MBRACCE-UK,[7] maternal deaths from pre-eclampsia and associated conditions were reported at the lowest rate since these records began. However, the latest report[8] cites a number four times higher. It must also be remembered that the maternal mortality figures do not take into account the level of morbidity, both for mother and baby, making these figures only part of the picture.

Although even though overall the number of women dying from hypertensive complications in the UK remains low, there is no place for complacency – every fetal death causes anguish, and a maternal death is an unimaginable tragedy for the family concerned and is possibly an indicator of failure in the care system. It is sobering to note that the most recent Confidential Enquires[8] noted that for 75% of the women who died of hypertensive disease, improvements to their care may have made a difference to the outcome.

Midwives at the forefront of maternity care delivery are ideally placed for primary surveillance and early detection of pre-eclampsia. It is acknowledged that pre-eclampsia is a complex and frustrating condition, especially with regard to the prediction of progression. Changes associated with the condition worsening do not necessarily follow a logical, sequential or linear progression. However, it is likely that effective monitoring and care during the early stages of the condition will reduce the need for an 'emergency' response and improve the outcomes for the woman and baby. Nevertheless, pre-eclampsia is a particularly difficult disease, and all experienced midwives will recall women with severe symptoms who made an uncomplicated recovery, as well as women with relatively mild symptoms who suffered a tragic outcome, all emphasising that pre-eclampsia is a particular challenge for health professionals.

PATHOPHYSIOLOGY

The precise aetiology of pre-eclampsia remains unknown, although recent scientific studies have improved understanding. The changes seen in pre-eclampsia appear to be caused by a complex interplay of abnormal genetic, immunological and placental factors.[9]

In a healthy pregnancy uncomplicated by pre-eclampsia, trophoblastic cells invade the maternal uterine arteries at both the decidual and myometrial levels, resulting in erosion of the muscle layer and enlargement of the lumen. Additionally, there is increased synthesis of prostacyclin, nitric oxide and thromboxane A2, which creates a change in homeostatic balance and tendency to vasodilatation of the uterine arteries. This alteration in function results in lowered resistance in the arteries, absence of maternal vasomotor control and a substantial increase in blood supply to the placenta to meet the demands of the developing fetus.

In a pregnancy complicated by pre-eclampsia, the trophoblastic invasion of the placental bed spiral arteries is confined to the decidual level. Because of this impeded trophoblastic invasion, adrenergic nerve supplies to the uterine spiral arteries are not disrupted, systemic vascular resistance remains high and a relatively ischaemic (under-perfused) placenta results, compromising the growth and well-being of the fetus.

This placental hypoperfusion is accompanied by an imbalance of key angiogenic factors that are important in the development of blood vessels. Concentrations of Placental Growth Factor (PlGF) increase until around 30 weeks, after which it declines. It is important in promoting blood vessel formation, and low levels of PlGF are associated with pre-eclampsia.[10,11] Measurement of PlGF, or the ratio of PlGF to sFlt (a tyrosine kinase protein with antiangiogenic properties), is the basis of a maternal blood test, which aims to identify women at greater risk of pre-eclampsia.[1,12]

The persistently under-perfused placenta causes oxidative stress, which results in the release of inflammatory cytokines and an imbalance of angiogenic factors that can cause widespread damage to the endothelial cells that line maternal blood vessels.[13] This damage to the endothelial cells underlies the varied multi-organ dysfunction seen in pre-eclampsia.

The total peripheral vascular resistance increases in pre-eclampsia (as contrasted with the reduction expected in a normal pregnancy), and this is one of the causes of raised blood pressure. In addition, enhanced contraction of damaged blood vessels facilitates aggregation of platelets at the site of endothelial injury and may pre-dispose to problems with coagulation.

In the kidneys, glomerular capillary endothelial swelling occurs accompanied by deposits of fibrinogen within and under the endothelial cells. This results in the general renal function being impaired, causing rising serum creatinine, uric acid and urea levels. In addition, increased glomerular permeability allows the protein to escape into the urine.

The hypoalbuminaemia of pre-eclampsia causes a lower colloid osmotic pressure, affecting fluid transport across the capillaries, resulting in too much fluid in the interstitial spaces (oedema) and too little in the vascular compartment (hypovolaemia). In addition to the cardiovascular and renal affects described previously, reduced organ

---

BOX 7.2: Pre-disposing/risk factors[1]

HIGH RISK

- Hypertensive disease during a previous pregnancy
- Chronic kidney disease
- Autoimmune disease such as systemic lupus erythematosus or antiphospholipid syndrome
- Type 1 or Type 2 diabetes
- Chronic hypertension

MODERATE RISK

- First pregnancy
- Age 40 years or older
- Pregnancy interval of more than ten years
- BMI of 35kg/m^2 or more at first visit
- Family history of pre-eclampsia
- Multiple pregnancy

---

perfusion in the liver, pulmonary system and the brain can contribute to the serious and potentially fatal outcomes seen in pre-eclampsia.

RISK/PRE-DISPOSING FACTORS

Although it is acknowledged that pre-eclampsia is a very unpredictable disease and may occur in those with no pre-disposing factors, it can be useful to identify those who may be at increased risk (see Box 7.2).

Other conditions apart from those identified by NICE (Box 7.2) have also been mentioned in the literature, including the genetic contribution of the father in increasing the risk of pre-eclampsia. Pre-eclampsia has been noted in a second or subsequent pregnancy with a new partner[14,15] and women with partners who previously fathered a baby resulting in a pregnancy with pre-eclampsia,[16,17] as well as a pregnancy involving donor material.[14] The presence of abnormal placental material, such as hydatidiform mole, or other anomalies, such as hydrops fetalis[18] or polyhydramnios,[19] are also considered risk factors for pre-eclampsia.

A study comparing risk factors for early onset (<34 weeks) pre-eclampsia with those for late-onset (≥ 34 weeks) pre-eclampsia found younger maternal age, nulliparity and diabetes mellitus were more strongly associated with late-onset pre-eclampsia.[20]

CLINICAL FEATURES

Pre-conception care

Women who have a pre-existing condition, especially those who are taking medication, should access pre-conception care to ensure they are in optimum health as well as to have their medication assessed to ensure safety in pregnancy. Those women with chronic hypertension taking ACE (angiotensin-converting enzyme) inhibitors and ARBs (angiotensin II receptor blockers) will be advised to change their drugs as there is an increased risk of congenital abnormalities if these are taken during pregnancy.[1] If a woman is booking without accessing this care and is taking these drugs, the midwife must ensure the woman is referred urgently to medical colleagues for medication assessment.

Salt restriction is not generally recommended, but women with chronic hypertension should be encouraged to keep their dietary sodium intake low.[1]

Antenatal screening and specific care

PREDICTION

Many suggestions have been made regarding methods to specifically identify those women who are at high risk of pre-eclampsia and would benefit from increased monitoring. These include early blood tests, Doppler assessment of uterine blood flow, ultrasound studies[21] and other procedures.[22] Although many assessments look promising, at present, NICE has not recommended any of these tests for routine use.

Higher levels of liver enzymes AST and ALT during the first 20 weeks of pregnancy are associated with a higher risk for the development of severe pre-eclampsia in the second half of the pregnancy; however, no clinical cut-off value has yet been established.[23,24]

Currently, NICE[1] recommends regular fetal assessment for women who previously suffered severe, early or complicated pre-eclampsia, commencing at 28–30 weeks gestation (or at least two weeks before the previous gestational age of onset). The assessment comprises an ultrasound to assess growth, amniotic fluid volume and umbilical artery Doppler velocimetry.

For a woman whose signs and symptoms are unclear, the placental growth factor-based (PIGF) testing of maternal blood (either using sFlt1:PIGF ratio or PIGF alone), together with standard clinical assessment, can help to underpin care for those between 20–36 + 6 weeks gestation.[25]

Prevention

Although there is some evidence to support thrombophilia treatment in those women at risk of FGR, this remains an area in need of further research[26] and is not recommended by NICE[1] at present.

However, aspirin treatment in those at risk of pre-eclampsia has become recommended care[1,27,28]. Current advice is 75–150mg aspirin daily from 12 weeks until the birth of the baby[1] for those at high risk or with more than one moderate risk factor (see Box 7.2). Although a larger dose of aspirin is available as an over-the-counter medication, pharmacists cannot currently issue low-dose aspirin without a prescription.

CLINICAL FEATURES

A low maternal death rate, as well as avoidance of any adverse outcome for all women and babies, can only be achieved with early identification and optimal management of hypertensive conditions. See Box 7.3 for signs and symptoms of pre-eclampsia.

BOX 7.3: Signs and symptoms of pre-eclampsia

- A rise in blood pressure >140/90 mm/Hg
- Proteinuria/oliguria
- Development of epigastric or right upper quadrant pain/pain below the ribs/liver tenderness
- Nausea and vomiting
- Cerebral disturbances (headache, altered consciousness)
- Visual field disturbances (including blurred vision, flashing lights)
- Progressive, or rapid onset, oedema (frequently can be easily observed on the woman's face/hands)
- Abnormal renal function tests
- Abnormal liver enzymes
- Bleeding tendency: platelet count decreasing and/or clotting factors abnormality
- Clonus (large or repetitive muscular reaction from reflex or stretching)
- Abnormalities in fetal assessment, including FGR, reduced liquor volume and/or CTG recording (in some cases, restriction of fetal growth can precede the woman's symptoms)

Antenatal care

The main aims of care of a woman with pre-eclampsia are to:

- Control blood pressure to prevent strokes
- Monitor/restrict fluids to prevent pulmonary oedema
- Consider anticonvulsant therapy with magnesium sulphate to prevent eclampsia
- Identify any fetal compromise
- Plan the birth of the baby for the optimum time

Awareness of these aims underpins the testing and observations necessary for early detection of deterioration (impending seizure, organ failure and/or pulmonary oedema). Continued assessment of vital signs, analysis of symptoms, physical examination and laboratory tests will be maintained at intervals according to the woman's condition.

While the midwife may initiate many of the early clinical investigations and is eminently able to interpret findings, the scope of midwifery clinical practice must be remembered and actions should always be in accordance with the Midwives Standards,[29] referring the woman to a registered medical practitioner when there are signs of deviation from normal.

All women, but in particular those with risk factors for pre-eclampsia, should be given information about the symptoms of pre-eclampsia (see Box 7.4) and know how and when to self-refer if necessary.

BLOOD PRESSURE

Blood pressure evaluation is such a routine part of midwifery practice it would be easy to become complacent. Accuracy of assessment as part of

BOX 7.4: Women's self-assessment of pre-eclampsia symptoms

- Severe headache
- Problems with vision, such as blurring or flashing before the eyes
- Severe pain just below the ribs
- Vomiting
- Sudden swelling of the face, hands or feet
- Reduction in fetal movements

professional midwifery practice is vital for women's well-being.[4]

It has become more common for pregnant women to monitor their own BP, a practice which has long been accepted outside of pregnancy. Two large trials have studied self-monitoring of BP in both higher-risk pregnancy[30] and in women with chronic or gestational hypertension.[31] Both studies found that self-monitoring did not lead to significantly earlier clinic-based detection of hypertension; however, the practice appeared to be safe.

NICE[1] defines hypertension in pregnancy as 140/90 to 159/109 and severe hypertension as > 160/110. Antihypertensive medication is usually offered if the BP is sustained at >140/90, but whether hospital admission is necessary at this time will depend on the individual woman's other signs and symptoms, predominately blood results. A rise in blood pressure as well as the absolute value, is also important to note. A systolic blood pressure of 30mmHg above the earliest recorded pregnancy reading or a diastolic increase of 15–25mmHg may be significant.[28] Midwives are also cautioned that any rise in blood pressure occurring after 20 weeks' gestation in a previously normotensive woman should be cause for concern, as this may be the first indicator of a progressive disorder. However, blood pressure needs to be taken and interpreted in context with other signs and symptoms.

Underpinning monitoring and treatment of pre-eclampsia are regular and frequent blood pressure measurements. These may be as often as every five minutes, for a period of time when concern is high, or less frequently. However, the 'routine' regular measurements, usually four hourly, will only be a minimum. The midwife will undertake a blood pressure measurement whenever it is felt necessary, for instance, if the woman reports new symptoms or the CTG interpretation changes. Blood pressure readings will determine the management of medication, so a recording before and at a suitable interval (depending on the drug) following antihypertensive administration will provide valuable information to ensure the optimum drug, dose and timing of the drug that is being offered.

Blood pressure is frequently taken with an automated machine, and in fact, the lack of observer error and the assured regularity of the test will give an automated machine the advantage of producing an accurate trend when frequent measurement is required. However, previous reports of

Confidential Enquiries into Maternal Deaths in the UK[32] have warned against exclusive reliance on automated blood pressure recording systems. There have been reported issues with automated machines, in particular under-reading, and some maternity units will have a protocol for undertaking regular manual blood pressure recording: for instance, once a shift, or every four hours.

The MAP (mean arterial pressure) is the average pressure responsible for driving blood forward into the capillary bed of tissues. This reading may be used as a prediction of pre-eclampsia[33] or to assess the progress of pre-eclampsia and to underpin medication. The MAP will usually show up on automated blood pressure devices or can be calculated as either:

- Systolic BP plus twice the diastolic, divided by 3
- Diastolic BP plus ⅓ (systolic BP minus diastolic BP)

In severe circumstances, an arterial line may be inserted to enable continuous monitoring of blood pressure, which will be displayed on a monitor. The arterial line will also allow easy access for arterial blood gas sampling.

PROTEINURIA

Proteinuria should never be ignored. Although proteinuria is often caused by a urinary tract infection, it is also possible that it may be the first sign of pre-eclampsia in a woman with normal blood pressure. Less commonly, proteinuria is associated with chronic renal disorders.

The midwife needs to ensure an accurate assessment of proteinuria. The reagent strips ('dipsticks') commonly used in clinical practice should be considered a guide only to the presence of protein in the urine and not be accepted as an accurate quantification of protein excretion. It should also be ensured that the manufacturer's instructions concerning the care of dipsticks (such as dating the opening of bottles and replacing lids after use) are followed to ensure accuracy is optimal, and if using visual assessment, the guideline for timings followed. However, an automated reagent-strip reading device for dipstick screening for proteinuria is recommended by NICE.[1]

When 1+ or above of protein is detected, a 'clean-catch' mid-stream sample of urine should be tested to exclude the possibility of contamination. If protein is still detectable, the sample should be sent to the laboratory for investigation of infection (usually via an M,C&S investigation), together with a urine specimen for urinary spot protein:creatinine ratio (PCR) or albumin:creatinine ratio (ACR). Results over 30mg/mmol for the PCR or over 8mg/mmol for the ACR are considered significant proteinuria. A 24-hour urinary collection to assess protein is no longer routinely recommended.

It should be remembered that the quantity of protein present in urine samples may not be indicative of renal damage but instead may be a reflection of capillary leakage and, more accurately, a projection of the development of generalised oedema. Where protein loss is significant, the possibility of pulmonary and/or cerebral oedema as complications of pre-eclampsia is considerable.

BLOOD TESTS

While worsening of any of the signs and symptoms of pre-eclampsia are acceptable as reasonable predictors of increasingly severe pre-eclampsia, it is as well to remember that women with blood pressures within the normal range, especially if taking antihypertensive drugs, or in whom proteinuria was absent have had eclamptic seizures. The obvious presence of a single finding should prompt investigations for others by measuring known biochemical markers (see Box 7.5 for an example of bloods routinely taken for pre-eclampsia screening).

When bloods are taken for a PET screening, if the results are within the normal range, they can act as a baseline for future tests. A changing level, even if still within the normal range, should act as a warning sign, and these blood results should be recorded in a way that any trend is easily identifiable.

BOX 7.5: PET screening

While many tests may be undertaken, of particular importance are:

- Full blood count
- Renal function tests
- Liver function tests
- Clotting studies may also be carried out

Full Blood Count (FBC)

A full blood count is a valuable assessment of pre-eclampsia. In a normal pregnancy, there is an increase in plasma, which 'dilutes' the red cells, and thus, physiological anaemia is commonly noted. By contrast, in pregnancies complicated by pre-eclampsia, this plasma volume expansion is not as great, and the concentration of red cells and haemoglobin may remain at higher levels (similar to those outside of pregnancy). However, with increased endothelial damage, a feature of pre-eclampsia, friction within the blood vessels may lead to an increased breakdown of red cells (haemolysis) with subsequent anaemia. Furthermore, endothelial damage can cause an increased activation of platelets, and platelet count may fall. Coagulation studies are recommended when platelets are $<100 \times 10^9/l$.

Renal function tests

Urea and creatinine clearance is high in pregnancy, but blood levels at the upper end of the range may be suggestive of impaired renal clearance. A rise in serum uric acid production is secondary to tissue ischaemia, and increasing levels may be reflective of impaired renal clearance, renal medullary ischaemia and tubular damage,[28] and these findings may be the only clinical indicators of the seriousness of pre-eclampsia. The importance of this information is that a rise in serum uric acid may be detected before proteinuria becomes evident;[34] however, NICE does not recommend its routine use.[1]

Leakage of albumin through the kidneys is a positive indication of glomerular endothelial damage, the consequences of which are lowering of serum albumin levels and leakage of fluid into the extracellular space, while a marked rise in creatinine is indicative of severe renal impairment.

Liver function tests

Development of epigastric or right upper quadrant pain may be suggestive of liver involvement. Damage to the endothelial lining of blood vessels in the liver results in leakage of plasma and causes an increase in size and overstretching of the fibrous capsule. In addition, blood vessels may rupture, and a haematoma may form in the sub-capsular region, increasing the pressure on the liver peritoneum and causing referred pain.

Raised levels of liver enzymes are indicators of a significant level of liver cell damage and the development of HELLP syndrome.

FLUID BALANCE

Fluid management is vital to the successful management of pre-eclampsia. The importance of meticulous recording and evaluation of input and output cannot be over-emphasised. In most women hospitalised with moderate to severe pre-eclampsia, an indwelling urinary catheter will be used, and the urine measured hourly (output should be 0.5 ml/kg/hr and should not fall below 30 ml/hour or 100 ml/4 hourly).

All maternity unit policies for pre-eclampsia care will contain a section regarding fluid restriction, and midwives will need to remember that IV infusions, bolus drug infusions and oral intake should be included in the 'allowed' (usually about 80ml/hour) amount of fluid.

Following the birth of her baby, if the woman has had a PPH (not an uncommon scenario for a woman with pre-eclampsia), fluid management is a particular challenge. As a very fine balance between intake and output is required, this may be best achieved by monitoring via a central venous pressure (CVP) line to underpin fluid management.

The most recent Confidential Enquiries[8] credited careful attention to fluid balance in women with pre-eclampsia to previously eliminating pulmonary oedema as a cause of maternal death in women with hypertensive disorders in the UK. Fluid overload in pre-eclampsia can lead to pulmonary oedema, which can have a direct impact on both the woman's and her baby's well-being. Fluid overload (both oral and intravenous) is also associated with hyponatraemia, which is a cause of both maternal and neonatal seizures.[8]

MULTIDISCIPLINARY TEAM

The most effective approach to the care of a woman with PET is likely to be multidisciplinary, involving an obstetrician and anaesthetist at the consultant level, haematologist, the neonatal team and appropriately experienced midwives who should all be involved in the planning and provision of care.

Maternal and fetal thresholds for planned early birth before 37 weeks in women with pre-eclampsia should be documented,[1] although these, of course, will be amended if the condition of either the woman or fetus changes. Intravenous magnesium sulphate and a course of antenatal corticosteroids to benefit the newborn may be offered if early birth is planned for women with preterm pre-eclampsia, in line with the NICE guidelines.[35]

MEDICATION

A key aspect of care in pre-eclampsia is the use of antihypertensive medication to control the level of blood pressure to prevent the development of cerebrovascular accidents. In addition, magnesium sulphate reduces the risk of seizures. However, it must be borne in mind that these are not cures as they do not arrest the disease progression, and careful monitoring is required.

The choice of which drug is used in clinical practice is dependent on individual hospitals' policies. It is also suggested[36] that the choice is based on any pre-existing treatment, side-effect profiles, risks (including fetal effects) and the woman's preference. The most widely recommended antihypertensive drugs in pregnancy are labetalol (oral or IV), nifedipine or methyldopa.[36] The aim of antihypertensive treatment is to keep the level of BP at around 135/85.[1]

Midwives need to ensure knowledge of the protocol and policies of their workplace, as these will be different from unit to unit. See Box 7.6 for a description of the most common drugs.

BOX 7.6: Medications commonly used in pre-eclampsia

Labetalol is a mixed α and β blocker administered orally or intravenously. Other examples of this group of drugs the midwife may see, usually in the postnatal period, are Metoprolol and Atenolol. These drugs act on blood vessels by altering the baroreceptor sympathetic reflex response of nerves, resulting in vascular relaxation, lowered peripheral resistance and reduced cardiac output, thus lowering the blood pressure. Oral Labetalol is the recommended first line of treatment for hypertension in pregnancy[1] and can also be given in severe pre-eclampsia as an intravenous infusion. Labetalol is contraindicated in those with asthma. It has been suggested that labetalol can cause an increased risk of hypoglycaemia and bradycardia for breastfeeding infants,[37] and, therefore, routine surveillance should be undertaken by the midwife.

Nifedipine (Adalat®) is an oral calcium channel blocker and has increasingly been used in pre-eclampsia as the second line in hypertensive management where early treatment with Labetalol or Methyldopa has failed to keep maternal blood pressure below the danger level or when these drugs are contraindicated, or when a rapid response is needed.

It works by preventing the transfer of calcium ions from extracellular space and inhibits uptake by smooth muscle cells. Vascular muscle response and reflex excitation contractility are reduced, relaxation is achieved, peripheral resistance is lowered, blood vessels dilate and blood pressure falls.

The sublingual route is not normally used in pregnancy because mucosal absorption is unpredictable.[38] Nifedipine may also be used as a tocolytic drug, with no apparent drop in the blood pressure for a woman who is normotensive.[38]

Methyldopa is a central alpha-II agonist, often used in pregnancy. It acts directly on the brainstem to create vasodilation and lower blood pressure without adverse changes in heart rate, cardiac output, renal perfusion or uteroplacental blood flow. Lowering the blood pressure is slow; thus, where rapid onset of blood pressure reduction is desired, an alternative drug is preferable. Methyldopa should be stopped within two days of birth to avoid possible side effects, and another antihypertensive should be used if necessary in the puerperium.

Hydralazine, an arteriolar dilator, is usually reserved for use in cases of very high blood pressure. Given intravenously, it acts directly on the smooth muscles of the arterial wall to bring about rapid vasodilation, with the hypotensive effect lasting six to eight hours. Side effects are headaches, nausea and vomiting (signs which mimic impending eclampsia) and a possible link to thrombocytopenia in the neonate has been reported. Doses are usually titrated to the woman's blood pressure, and care needs to be taken to avoid a very rapid drop in a pregnant woman's blood pressure, which could lead to reduced placental perfusion and fetal distress. One-to-one care by the midwife is usual when the woman is receiving an IV infusion of hydralazine, as very frequent vital signs recording and continuous observation of the mother and fetus are necessary.

Magnesium sulphate is recommended as a first-line treatment of eclampsia and to prevent eclampsia in those at high risk. It is usually given as a bolus IV injection, followed by an IV infusion. (See later in this chapter for midwifery care when a woman is receiving a magnesium sulphate infusion.) Although its primary function is as an anti-convulsive, there is also a strong hypotensive effect, and further antihypertensive medication may not be necessary for the pre-eclamptic woman. Calcium gluconate can be given to treat magnesium toxicity and should be readily available.

Magnesium sulphate can also be used in labour or if birth is planned within 24 hours for neuroprotection of the preterm fetus.[39,40]

FETAL ASSESSMENT

At each antenatal visit after 24 weeks gestation,[1] the midwife will measure the symphysis-fundal height and record growth measurement on an appropriate chart. The midwife should advise the woman with regard to monitoring fetal movements, encouraging her to become familiar with her baby's normal pattern of movement and advising her to contact the maternity unit if she has concerns about the pattern or frequency of movements.

Due to vascular changes to uterine blood flow to the placenta, the fetuses of women with chronic hypertension are more at risk of fetal growth restriction, intrauterine death, placental abruption and preterm birth.[1,41] For this woman, ultrasound scans, including growth measurement, amniotic fluid assessment and umbilical artery Doppler studies, are suggested to be carried out.[1] For women with pre-eclampsia, these tests will be undertaken when pre-eclampsia is first suspected or diagnosed and then repeated every two to four weeks as clinically indicated.

When severe/fulminating pre-eclampsia is present, continuous or very frequent CTG assessments are made, as any deterioration of this may indicate a change in the woman's condition, as well as a compromised fetus.

If the woman is preterm, when it is anticipated that birth could take place imminently, a course of intravenous magnesium sulphate and a course of antenatal corticosteroids are offered[35] to aid in the maturation of the baby's lungs and help prevent complications after birth.

BOX 7.7: Summary of midwifery care in the antenatal period for the woman with pre-eclampsia

- Monitoring vital signs, with frequency dependent on the woman's condition, and attention paid to fluid balance
- Blood/urine testing dependent on the woman's condition
- Administering antihypertensive medication as prescribed, with an assessment of its effectiveness
- Administering a course of corticosteroids and/or magnesium sulphate if prescribed
- Appropriate fetal surveillance, usually involving regular CTGs, US growth scans, amniotic fluid volume assessment and umbilical artery Doppler velocimetry
- Regular discussion with the woman to assess symptoms, including fetal movements
- Regular discussion with the woman and her family to ensure all questions are answered and there is full knowledge of actions and plans

See Box 7.7 for a summary of midwifery care women admitted to an antenatal ward with pre-eclampsia should receive.

Care in Labour

If the woman's condition stabilises sufficiently to enable labour to be induced, epidural anaesthesia is often selected if the clotting studies are satisfactory. This method of pain relief offers the additional benefits of lowering blood pressure, eliminating painful stimuli that may trigger seizures and avoiding the possibility of complications which may accompany general anaesthesia and exacerbate pulmonary oedema. Spinal/epidural anaesthesia is, therefore, the preference for caesarean section but requires particular caution with regards to the fluid load in order not to alter the stable balance previously attained.

During labour, whether induced or spontaneous, the woman with any level of pre-eclampsia will need a continuation of the monitoring that she was receiving antenatally (see Box 7.8 for a summary of care that may be provided). It is salutary to remember that one in five cases of eclampsia occurs in labour, so vigilance should not be relaxed. Syntometrine should not be given for management of the third stage of labour as the ergometrine component is associated with increases in blood pressure.

Complications

An awareness of potential complications (see Box 7.9) will ensure the midwife's assessment addresses these issues, and escalation is prompt if suspicions arise.

Postnatal care

Postnatal care needs to continue with the knowledge that, although the birth of the baby is deemed to be the 'cure' for pre-eclampsia, symptoms can continue or even escalate in the initial period after the birth. Therefore, the intensity of assessment and monitoring of medications needs to be maintained or even increased.

Non-steroidal anti-inflammatory drugs should be avoided in women with pre-eclampsia as they may potentially cause pulmonary oedema if the woman is volume-depleted.[28] Methyldopa should also be avoided postpartum as it is associated with depression.[28]

NICE[1] suggests all women with pre-eclampsia have regular assessments while in hospital, appropriate antihypertensive medication as required and a plan for follow-up care in the community before discharge. All women should be counselled regarding the risk of pre-eclampsia in a future pregnancy and more long-term effects regarding cardiovascular disease.

BOX 7.8: Summary of midwifery care in labour for the woman with pre-eclampsia

- Monitor vital signs at a frequency relevant to the woman's condition: blood pressure, pulse, respirations and oxygen saturation
- Administer antihypertensive drugs as prescribed and assess the effect on blood pressure
- Monitor and record total fluid input (maintaining prescribed fluid restriction) and urinary output to achieve clear records of fluid balance
- Monitor fetal condition
- Obtain blood samples as necessary and monitor results for changes reflecting deterioration.
- Assess symptoms (see Box 7.3) to identify worsening condition
- Any significant changes in the woman's condition must be notified to the obstetrician and/or anaesthetist
- Maintain a quiet, calm atmosphere
- Provide psychological support for the woman and her family

BOX 7.9: Potential maternal complications

- Abruption
- Pulmonary oedema/aspiration
- Acute renal failure
- Liver failure or haemorrhage
- Stroke
- Visual compromise/blindness

ECLAMPSIA

BOX 7.10: Eclampsia

Eclampsia is the occurrence of convulsions that are associated with the signs and symptoms of pre-eclampsia. It is a Greek word meaning 'lightning' and often strikes with the same random ferocity and has similarly devastating effects. The randomness is illustrated by the fact that seizures may occur before proteinuria and hypertension have been documented.[42]

INTRODUCTION

The occurrence of eclampsia has declined over recent years. Knight et al.[43] for UKOSS found that rates of eclampsia were down to 26.8 per 100,000 maternities from 46 per 100,000 maternities previously. This may directly result from the increasingly common use of magnesium sulphate as a treatment to prevent those with moderate/severe pre-eclampsia from developing eclampsia.

PATHOPHYSIOLOGY

The seizure that is the key feature of eclampsia is thought to be due to intense vasospasm of the cerebral arteries, oedema secondary to ischaemic damage of the vascular endothelium and/or intravascular clot formation.

An eclamptic seizure usually includes three defined phases:

- *Prodromal phase*, in which the imminent seizure is heralded by possible reports of visual disturbances, muscular twitching, facial congestion, foaming at the mouth and/or deepening loss of consciousness.
- *Tonic-clonic phase*, where initially generalised muscular contractions are present, and respiration is absent. This is followed by repeated strong, jerky, irregular muscular activity.
- *Abatement phase*, which occurs within 60–90 seconds of onset, during which time respiration is re-established and there is a gradual return to consciousness, but perhaps with a confused and agitated state.

CARE

Immediate care

Eclampsia can occur in the antenatal, intrapartum or postnatal period, and the care will be fundamentally the same.

It is futile to attempt any action within the short interval of the tonic-clonic phase apart from calling for urgent help and protecting the woman from injury. However, immediate subsequent care should be aimed at damage limitation by placing the woman in the recovery position as soon as possible. Suction should be used to clear secretions from the mouth and nasal passage to maintain a clear airway, and oxygen should be administered. These measures help to boost the maternal oxygen saturation and improve delivery to the fetus, which would have been deprived of oxygen during the tonic-clonic phase of the seizure. Further urgent measures are imperative to prevent the recurrence of further seizures and optimise maternal and fetal well-being (see Box 7.11).

There is an association of eclampsia with cardiac arrest and intracerebral haemorrhage.[44] However, it is more usual for the seizure to last about 90 seconds,[42] for the woman to be successfully stabilised and then receive close monitoring by the midwife, both before and after the birth. It must be remembered that despite birth being the 'cure' for pre-eclampsia, 44% of eclamptic episodes have been reported as occurring in the postnatal period.[42] Therefore, care and careful assessment need to continue into the postpartum period as appropriate.

On-going care

Care of the woman will be by the multidisciplinary team and includes close monitoring of the following:

- Frequent monitoring of vital signs: O_2 saturations, BP, pulse, respirations
- Observe for signs of toxicity if receiving a magnesium sulphate infusion (see Box 7.12)
- Continuous ECG

BOX 7.11: Immediate care of a seizure

- Summon assistance (anaesthetist, obstetrician and additional midwifery help) via the emergency call bell if in hospital. If not in hospital, call for emergency paramedic help (dial 999 in the UK) to arrange immediate transfer to hospital.
- Protect the woman from injury during the tonic-clonic phase
- Maintain airway (clear by suctioning if necessary)
- Provide supplementary oxygenation if possible
- Place the woman in the left lateral (recovery) position as soon as possible
- *As help arrives, the following actions will probably happen concurrently:*
- Obtain intravenous access, take appropriate blood specimens and monitor fluid balance
- Treat the seizure (magnesium sulphate is usual)
- Monitor vital signs and beware of bleeding (abruption or PPH)
- If pregnant, assess fetal well-being (risk of fetal distress from hypoxia or abruption)
- If pregnant, once the woman's condition is stabilised, a plan for the birth of the baby needs to be made urgently and carried out without delay

---

BOX 7.12: Care for women receiving a magnesium sulphate (MgSO$_4$) infusion

- Close monitoring of respirations and O$_2$ saturations, as respiratory depression is a sign of magnesium toxicity
- Assessment of the woman's overall responses: drowsiness, slurring of speech, flushing, double vision and weakness can all be signs of magnesium toxicity
- Close monitoring of BP, as magnesium sulphate is a powerful depressant of neuromuscular transmission; therefore, care must be taken to avoid sudden hypotension, particularly if the woman is concurrently receiving large doses (especially if administered intravenously) of antihypertensives
- Assessment of deep tendon reflexes, usually hourly, as loss of reflexes is a sign of magnesium toxicity
- Cardiac monitoring with on-going three-lead ECG is common because of the potential effect on the cardiac system by magnesium sulphate
- Careful fluid balance (with maintenance of fluid restriction if necessary) as part of renal function assessment, as well as to identify any fluid overload
- Blood tests: regular renal function tests (as MgSO$_4$ is excreted via the kidneys, impaired renal clearance could result in toxic levels being quickly reached) and other tests such as PET bloods, coagulation studies, as necessary
- On-going psychological care for the woman and her family

Magnesium sulphate toxicity can be treated with calcium gluconate IV, and the midwife should ensure this is easily available.

- Urine output/fluid balance
- Blood tests as required, ABG if necessary, bedside blood glucose testing
- If pregnant: fetal assessment (continuous CTG) and preparation for birth

In rare situations where seizures are recurrent or prolonged, the woman may need to be medically paralysed and ventilated.

Once the woman's condition has stabilised and the baby has been born, the aggressive approach to management needs to be maintained as the risk of eclamptic seizures occurring during the postpartum period remains.

HELLP SYNDROME

BOX 7.13: HELLP

HELLP syndrome is a serious complication of pre-eclampsia in which many women do not develop significant hypertension or proteinuria:

> Haemolysis
> Elevated Liver enzymes
> Low Platelets

INTRODUCTION

HELLP is the most common cause of severe liver disease in pregnancy. On admission, it can be difficult to differentiate between several conditions, especially when there is liver involvement: HELLP and AFLP symptoms can also be caused by hepatitis, thrombotic microangiopathy, thrombotic thrombocytopenic purpura, SLE, antiphospholipid syndrome and severe sepsis.[45] Women are likely to present with quite vague symptoms. The midwife is well placed to observe signs and symptoms, as well as trends in blood results and vital signs, to aid diagnosis.

For some women, the condition may develop rapidly, while for others, the progression of the disease may be more gradual and/or occur late in the pregnancy or the postnatal period. The suggestion of HELLP is a clear indication for close surveillance. Monitoring of the condition is similar to that of pre-eclampsia with an added emphasis on the assessment of liver enzymes. Treatment is also similar to that of pre-eclampsia and the 'cure' is the same: birth of the baby. Following birth, as in pre-eclampsia, there is an initial period of continued risk, followed by stabilisation, and there is a possibility of recurrence in the next pregnancy.

PATHOPHYSIOLOGY

The multisystem failure in HELLP can be associated with changes in renal and hepatic function. Evidence of anaemia may indicate excessive breakdown of red cells, one of the early features of HELLP. It must be remembered that irrespective of the cause of anaemia (haemolysis or iron deficiency), its presence will increase the cardiac workload and thus worsen hypertension.

As in pre-eclampsia, thrombocytopenia develops from the reduction of the life span of platelets and utilisation at sites of endothelial damage. In addition, reduced circulatory volume, ischaemia, renal tubular necrosis and reduced renal clearance lead to a rise in the serum levels of urea, creatinine and urates, which are indicators of marked maternal and fetal compromise.

Infarctions and oedema occurring in the liver will impair its capacity to maintain adequate metabolic activities, such as the synthesis of clotting factors, while an increase in liver size may lead to capsular rupture triggering a combined medical, surgical and obstetric emergency.

CLINICAL FEATURES

Diagnosis

Diagnosis is based on a combination of laboratory findings and clinical signs and symptoms (see Box 7.14), even though these may vary significantly. HELLP is usually considered to be a third-trimester condition; however, it has been suggested that 30% of cases are first expressed or progress in the postpartum period.[46]

The most common presenting signs for women with HELLP include epigastric or abdominal pain, nausea or vomiting, headache or visual changes. Although new-onset hypertension and/or new-onset proteinuria may be present, up to 15% of women lack either symptom.[46] It is suggested that a diagnosis of HELLP syndrome should be considered in any pregnant woman presenting in the second half of gestation or immediately postnatal, with significant new-onset epigastric/RUQ pain until proven otherwise. See Box 7.14 for further possible signs and symptoms.

Antenatal care

Hospitalisation is usually required to enable more intense monitoring of the maternal and fetal condition (see Box 7.15) with the aim of stabilisation and expediting the birth at the optimum time. The

BOX 7.14: HELLP syndrome: signs, symptoms and possible laboratory findings

Possible signs and symptoms

- Right upper quadrant pain (frequently with a positive liver recoil test)
- Epigastric pain
- Nausea and vomiting
- Malaise
- Fatigue
- Generalised oedema
- Headache
- Gastro-intestinal bleed
- Hypertension
- Proteinuria
- Reduced urine output

Possible laboratory findings

- Haemolysis
- Anaemia
- Low platelet count (<100 x 10^9/L)
- Elevated liver enzymes

BOX 7.15: Optimal care for women with HELLP syndrome

- Timely diagnosis and on-going accurate assessment of the severity
- Control of blood pressure if necessary
- Prevention of seizure
- Management of fluid and strict fluid balance
- Assessment and monitoring of fetal condition
- Administration of magnesium sulphate and steroids for the benefit of the neonate if appropriate
- Plan for time and mode of birth
- Judicious care to manage the potential for haemorrhage
- High dependency or intensive care for the woman postpartum, with awareness of the continued risk of multiple organ failure
- Good psychological care to be provided for the woman and her family throughout

Although birth is the only cure, serious manifestations can continue into the immediate postpartum period, so on-going observations for the woman should not be stepped down until it is clear the woman has recovered.

time available for measures to be initiated is dictated by the woman's condition.

If immediate delivery is not indicated, on-going fetal assessment by ultrasound and CTG and, if preterm, administration of corticosteroids and magnesium sulphate for the benefit of the neonatal condition may be undertaken. The woman's condition must be closely observed for signs of disease progression, indicated by deterioration in her blood results or increasing severity of physical signs and symptoms.

Due to the potential rapid progress of the disease, in particular thrombocytopenia, a FBC and usually clotting studies are necessary within two hours of planned epidural or spinal siting for induction of labour or caesarean section.

It has been suggested that regular maternal doses of corticosteroid administration for women with HELLP may improve the platelet count and prevent severe morbidity. However, this is currently controversial, and corticosteroids are not recommended for routine care at present.[47] More research is needed to determine if corticosteroids can improve outcomes for women affected by HELLP syndrome in pregnancy.

Potential complications of HELLP

Morbidity is common among women with HELLP syndrome and includes reactions to the blood products administered, admissions to an intensive/critical care ward, eclampsia, renal impairment or failure, pulmonary oedema, subarachnoid hemorrhage, sepsis, hepatic encephalopathy and subcapsular liver haematoma.

Approximately 1% of women with HELLP syndrome have a subcapsular hepatic haematoma.[48] Common signs and symptoms to be evaluated are in Box 7.16, but for an accurate diagnosis of subcapsular liver haematomas, CT (computed tomography) scanning, ultrasound or MRI will be used. If the haematoma ruptures, this is an emergency, and the woman will probably present with acute shock symptoms.[48,49]

BOX 7.16: Potential signs and symptoms for hepatic haematoma

- Right upper quadrant, epigastric or right shoulder pain
- Pyrexia
- Hypotension
- Hepatomegaly
- Hepatic tenderness and rebound tenderness with peritonitis
- Shock, renal or respiratory failure
- Leukocytosis
- Anaemia
- Highly elevated serum aminotransferase

Risks to the fetus/neonate include fetal demise, FGR, stillbirth and prematurity.[50]

ACUTE FATTY LIVER OF PREGNANCY (AFLP)

BOX 7.17: Acute Fatty Liver of Pregnancy (AFLP)

AFLP is a rare but potentially fatal obstetric complication described as acute liver failure secondary to fatty infiltration. Effects of this can include coagulopathy, electrolyte abnormalities and multisystem organ dysfunction.

There has previously been controversy about whether AFLP and pre-eclampsia are the same disease; however, most authorities now accept AFLP as a variant of pre-eclampsia.

INTRODUCTION

The most widely quoted incidence for AFLP in the UK is 1:7,000 to 20,000 pregnancies.[28] In the UK, increased knowledge, early intervention and aggressive management of complications have led to recent improvements in maternal and fetal/infant mortality and morbidity.[51] Previous (1980s) estimates of maternal mortality were over 70%, but currently around 2% is suggested.[51]

The USA recently reported similar incidences[52] and maternal mortality rates,[53] with perinatal mortality estimated to be 10 to 20%.[53] The US Acute Liver Failure Study Group reported AFLP to be the most common cause of acute liver failure during pregnancy, more common than drug-induced causes and hepatitis.[54]

The initial presenting symptoms can make diagnosis challenging. AFLP can be confused initially with HELLP syndrome, fulminant hepatitis of pregnancy, other liver diseases or pancreatitis, but blood tests will contribute to the correct diagnosis. Hepatic imaging is also usually undertaken to exclude other disorders or detect hepatic haemorrhage.[28]

PATHOPHYSIOLOGY

The exact pathogenesis of AFLP is not known, however the aetiology, in at least some cases, is suggested to involve abnormalities in fetal hepatic mitochondrial fatty acid oxidation,[55] related to an autosomal recessive mutation that causes deficiency of the long-chain 3-hydroxyacyl coenzyme A dehydrogenase (LCHAD). This results in the fetus being unable to metabolise some fatty acids, which can build up, transfer across the placenta to the woman and affect the maternal liver. However, not all babies who are later found to have LCHAD deficiency had mothers who developed AFLP.

Women with AFLP have multi-organ fatty infiltration, and this can cause severe effects on the kidneys, pancreas, endothelial cells and placenta.

Most women with AFLP have no known risk factors[53] (see Box 7.18 for some risk factors that have been suggested).

Pre-conception care

Women who have had previous pregnancies affected by AFLP should access carrier screening for fatty acid oxidation defects for both partners.

BOX 7.18: Pre-disposing/risk factors for AFLP

- Primigravidae
- BMI <20
- Association with male fetuses (3:1)
- Multi-fetal pregnancy
- Non-steroidal anti-inflammatory drugs

CLINICAL FEATURES

Signs and symptoms

AFLP may start antenatally (usually in the third trimester),[28] but it may not become apparent until after the birth. Signs and symptoms usually present gradually and may be fairly non-specific initially, with women complaining of anorexia, nausea, emesis (severe vomiting in 60%), malaise, fatigue and headache. About half of women may have epigastric or RUQ pain, and about half will demonstrate signs of pre-eclampsia, although usually mild.[28] There may also be hepatic tenderness (this may be accidentally identified when the midwife does her normal palpation before starting a CTG), but there is usually no hepatomegaly. Jaundice is a late sign, usually appearing after about two weeks of symptoms.

As many of these are initially mild symptoms, a woman may not immediately seek advice from a midwife or doctor. Therefore, the first contact the woman may have can be in response to worsening of symptoms or a severe symptom such as unexpected bleeding (it is suggested 90% have DIC), which is often the presenting symptom.[9,28] Other serious signs and symptoms may involve various systems:

- Hepatic: ascites with abnormal LFTs, fulminant liver failure, hepatic encephalopathy
- Renal: associated kidney injury, including lactic acidosis and raised ammonia, acute renal failure, polyuria
- Pancreas: pancreatitis, hypoglycaemia (up to 70%), which may be severe
- Sepsis[51]
- There may also be polydipsia and features of DIC[28]

Diagnosis

Diagnosis is made by identifying signs and symptoms on a criteria list (see Box 7.19). The Swansea Criteria for diagnosis of acute fatty liver of pregnancy list is accepted at present for a clear diagnosis, but other markers may also be taken into consideration.[56,57] A liver biopsy is the gold standard diagnostic test but is rarely done due to coagulopathy.

BOX 7.19: Swansea Criteria for diagnosis of AFLP

Six or more criteria are required in the absence of another cause:

- Vomiting
- Abdominal pain
- Polydipsia/polyuria
- Encephalopathy
- Elevated bilirubin > 14 µmol/L
- Hypoglycaemia < 4 mmol/L
- Elevated urea > 340 µmol/L
- Leukocytosis > 11 x 10^9/L
- Ascites or bright liver on ultrasound scan
- Elevated transaminases (AAT or ALT) 42 > IU/L
- Elevated ammonia > 47 µmol/L
- Renal impairment; creatinine > 150 µmol/L
- Coagulopathy; prothrombin time > 14 seconds or APPT > 34 seconds
- Microvesicular steatosis on liver biopsy

Antenatal care

A woman with acute AFLP will be cared for in a critical care unit, and if necessary, transfer to a liver unit may occur. However, the midwife may be the first professional to see the woman on initial presentation, and her assessments and speedy referral may be critical in reaching a diagnosis as quickly as possible, as delay may lead to poor outcomes for the woman and baby.[58]

Due to the uncertain diagnosis, a full range of vital signs should be undertaken and repeated frequently in order to obtain a trend. Close monitoring of oxygen saturation and respirations may indicate early deterioration of the woman's condition. As with vital signs, a full range of blood tests is necessary, with particular attention to blood sugar (70% of women have profound hypoglycaemia),[28] liver function tests, renal function tests and clotting factors. A woman presenting with signs of AFLP will usually have a history of vomiting and will need appropriate IV fluid replacement. However, as she may also have signs of polyuria and/or compromised renal function, close fluid balance is necessary in order to evaluate her condition. An indwelling urinary catheter with urometer for hourly measurement is usual.

BOX 7.20: Potential complications of AFLP[28,59]

- Renal failure
- Hypoglycaemia
- Infection
- Severe PPH
- Gastrointestinal haemorrhage
- Coagulopathy
- Fulminant hepatic failure
- Stillbirth

Care in labour

Following stabilisation of the woman's condition, the birth of the baby will be initiated as soon as possible.

Postnatal care

As the woman with AFLP is usually very ill, she will be cared for initially in a critical care unit. In acute cases, a temporary or permanent liver transplant may be considered. Other potential complications are included in Box 7.20.

Although there is controversy about the cause of AFLP, the association with LCHAD deficiency in the baby means the babies of women with AFLP need to be screened for fatty acid oxidation disorders and also monitored for complications of hypoglycaemia and metabolic derangements.[53]

FOLLOW-UP/LONG-TERM ISSUES FOR HYPERTENSIVE DISORDERS

Although the birth of the baby is necessary to 'cure' all the conditions discussed, care needs to continue into the puerperium, with the knowledge that many women become more ill before starting to improve, and the largest number of seizures occur in the postnatal period.

Maintaining regular vital sign observations at a frequency depending on the woman's condition is vital. NICE[1] suggests that women with pre-eclampsia who have given birth need to be asked about severe headache and epigastric pain each time the blood pressure is measured. Attention needs to continue to be paid to fluid balance, at least until creatinine levels are within the normal range.[1]

Pre-eclampsia, HELLP syndrome and AFLP are all conditions which can recur in a future pregnancy, and women should be aware of this risk and may choose to access pre-conception counselling before becoming pregnant again. In particular, if a woman persists in requiring anti-hypertension medication, it is important to access pre-conception care when planning a further pregnancy so medications can be assessed and changed if necessary.

Women who have had gestational hypertension or pre-eclampsia should be informed that these conditions are associated with an increased risk of developing high blood pressure and its complications in later life[60,61] and, therefore, long-term monitoring is needed. One study[60] identified that those with hypertensive disorders of pregnancy had an increased risk of developing new chronic hypertension, heart failure, cardiovascular disease and cardiomyopathy within 24 months after birth.

In addition to the physical care the woman requires, there is the need for psychological support as there may be many questions the woman wishes to have answered. The skills of the midwife as a communicator will be essential in providing information that is timely, appropriate, accurate and as comprehensive as possible to assist with the process of adjustment to what may have been a life-threatening event. The midwife might also consider informing the woman and her partner about APEC (Action on Pre-eclampsia), an organisation where continued support and information can be obtained (www.apec.org.uk).

SUMMARY OF MIDWIFERY RESPONSIBILITIES

It is vital to maintain up-to-date knowledge of all aspects of related conditions, as this is an area where treatments, including drugs, change frequently.

All women should be screened for PET at every encounter and should be informed of relevant signs and symptoms that they should report.

Midwives must ensure skills of assessment, including BP monitoring, are always optimum and develop further areas of expertise, such as the care of women with CVP and arterial lines, as these are frequently used for women with PET and associated conditions.

Many situations around PET can be true emergencies, requiring a prompt response. All midwives should have a detailed knowledge of local policies, be able to access rarely used drugs and operate specialised monitoring equipment with speed and competence while continuing to engender a feeling of safety in the woman.

When dealing with women with highly complex conditions, meticulous record keeping is vital to ensure subtle changes in the woman's signs and symptoms are observed, and communication between the MDT and midwives changing shifts is optimum.

Pre-eclampsia and associated conditions are unpredictable and yet have the potential to be life-threatening – women will need high levels of psychosocial support to cope both during the time of diagnosis, during treatment and following. A referral for long-term support should be made if appropriate.

FURTHER READING AND RESOURCES

Fox R, Kitt J, Leeson P, Aye C, Lewandowski A. Preeclampsia: risk factors, diagnosis, management, and the cardiovascular impact on the offspring. Journal of Clinical Medicine. 2019;8:1625. Available from: <doi:10.3390/jcm8101625>

An up-to-date comprehensive article focusing on pre-eclampsia and the fetus/infant.

Action on Pre-eclampsia (APEC)

www.apec.org.uk

A charity which aims to raise public and professional awareness of pre-eclampsia, improve care and ease or prevent physical and emotional suffering caused by the disease. They offer information and support to members of the public who are affected by pre-eclampsia, as well as providing online accredited courses for professionals.

NICE. Hypertension in pregnancy: diagnosis and management. 2019 – updated 2023. Available from: www.nice.org.uk/guidance/ng133

REFERENCES

1. NICE (National Institute for Health and Care Excellence). Guideline NG133: hypertension in pregnancy: diagnosis and management. 2019 updated 2023. Available from: www.nice.org.uk/guidance/ng133

2. Buschman AR, Rep A. Pre-eclampsia: understanding clinical complexity. Evol Med Public Health. 2018 Sep 12;2018(1):211–212. Available from: <doi:10.1093/emph/eoy028>. PMID: 30323930; PMCID:PMC6177543.

3. Wang W, Xie X, Yuan T et al. Epidemiological trends of maternal hypertensive disorders of pregnancy at the global, regional and national levels: a population-based study. BMC Pregnancy and Childbirth 2021;21:364. Available from: <doi:10.1186/s12884-021-0389-2>

4. Nathan H, Duhig K, Hezelgrave N, Chappell L, Shennan A. Blood pressure measurement in pregnancy. The Obstetrican & Gynaecologist. 2015;17:91–98.

5. Hodgins S. Pre-eclampsia as underlying cause for perinatal deaths: time for action. Glob Health Sci Pract. 2015;3(4):525–527. Available from: <doi:10.9745/GHSP-D-15-00350>

6. Action on Pre-eclampsia (APEC). [Accessed 30 December 2022]. Available from: www.apec.org.uk

7. Harding K, Redmond P and Tuffnell D on behalf of the MBRRACE-UK Hypertensive disorders of pregnancy chapter writing group. Caring for women with hypertensive disorders of pregnancy. In: Knight M, Nour M, Tuffnell D, Kenyon S, Shakespear J, Brocklehurst P, Kurinczuk JJ, on behalf of MBRRACE-UK, editors. Saving Lives, Improving Mothers' Care – Surveillance of maternal deaths in the UK 2012–14 and lessons learned to inform maternity care from the UK and Ireland Confidential Enquiries into Maternal Deaths and Morbidity 2009–14. Oxford: National Perinatal Epidemiology Unit, University of Oxford; 2016. p. 69–75.

8. Marian Knight, Kate Harding, Louise Page, Nicki Pusey and Samantha Holden on behalf of the MBRRACE-UK hypertensive disorders chapter-writing group. Chapter 6: lessons on prevention and treatment of hypertensive disorders. In: Knight M, Bunch K, Patel R, Shakespeare J, Kotnis R, Kenyon S, Kurinczuk JJ, On behalf of MBRRACE-UK,

editors. Saving Lives, Improving Mothers' Care Core Report – Lessons learned to inform maternity care from the UK and Ireland Confidential Enquiries into Maternal Deaths and Morbidity 2018–20. Oxford: National Perinatal Epidemiology Unit, University of Oxford 2022: p63–73. © 2022 Healthcare Quality Improvement Partnership and National Perinatal Epidemiology Unit, University of Oxford; 2022.

9. Bothamley J, Boyle M. Medical conditions affecting pregnancy and childbirth. 2nd ed. London: Routledge; 2021.

10. Armaly Z, Jadaon JE, Jabbour A, Abassi ZA. Preeclampsia: novel mechanisms and potential therapeutic approaches. Frontiers in Physiology, 2018;9:973. Available from: <doi:10.3389/fphys.2018.00973>

11. Sharp A, Chappell LC, Dekker G, Pelletier S, Garnier Y, Zeren O, et al. Placental growth factor informed management of suspected pre-eclampsia or fetal growth restriction: the MAPPLE cohort study. Pregnancy Hypertension: An International Journal of Women's Cardiovascular Health. 2018;14:228–233. Available from: <doi:10.1016/j.preghy.2018.03.013>

12. Duhig KE, Myers J, Seed PT, Sparkes J, Lowe J, Hunter RM, et al. Placental growth factor testing to assess women with suspected pre-eclampsia: a multicentre, pragmatic, stepped-wedge cluster-randomised controlled trial. The Lancet. 2019;393(10183):1807–1818. Available from: <doi:10.1016/S0140-6736(18)33212-4>

13. Calimag-Loyola APP, Lerma EV. Renal complications during pregnancy: in the hypertension spectrum. Disease-a-Month. 2019;65(2):25–44. Available from: <doi:10.1016/j.disamonth.2018.03.001>

14. Higgins L, Haezell A. Severe preeclampsia and eclampsia. Chapter 4 in: Chandraharan E, Arulkumaran S, editors. Obstetric and intrapartum emergencies. Cambridge: Cambridge University Press; 2012.

15. Galaviz-Hernandez C, Sosa-Macias M, Teran E, Garcia-Ortiz JE, Lazalde-Ramos BP. Paternal Determinants in Preeclampsia. Front Physiol. 2019 Jan 7;9:1870. Available from: <doi:10.3389/fphys.2018.01870>

16. Jaatinen, N, Jääskeläinen, T, Ekholm, E, Laivuori, H, for FINNPEC. Searching for a paternal phenotype for preeclampsia. Acta Obstet Gynecol Scand. 2022;101:862–870. Available from: <doi:10.1111/aogs.14388>

17. Skjaerven R, Vatten L, Wilcox A, Rønning T, IrgensL and Lie R. Recurrence of pre-eclampsia across generations: exploring fetal and maternal genetic components in a population based cohort. BMJ. 2005;331(7521):877–885.

18. Burwick R, Pilliod R & Caughey A. Fetal hydrops and the risk of severe preeclampsia. 2015;212(Suppl 1):S412-S413 Available from: <doi:10.1016/j.ajog.2014.10.1067>

19. Burwick R, Pilliiod R & Caughey A. Polyhydramnios as a risk factor for pre-eclampsia. American Journal of Obstetrics & Gynecology 2015;212(Suppl 1):S412. Available from: <doi:10.1016/j.ajog.2014.10.1066>

20. Lisonkova S & Joseph K. Incidence of preeclampsia: risk factors and outcomes associated with early- versus late-onset disease. Am J Obstet Gynecol 2013;209(6):544–546.

21. Lai J, Syngetaki, Nicolaides K, Dadelszen P & Magee L. Using ultrasound and angiogenic markers from a 19-to-23-week assessment to inform the subsequent diagnosis of preeclampsia. American Journal of Obstetrics & Gynecology 2022;2227:294. e1.-11. Available from: <doi:10.1016/J.ajoh.2022.03.007>

22. MacDonald T, Walker S, Hannan N, Tong S & Kaitu'u-Lino T. Clinical tools and biomarkers to predict preecclampsia. EBioMedicine 2021;75:103780. Available from: <doi:10.1016/j.ebiom.2021/103780>

23. Mei-Dan E, Wiznitzer A, Sergienko R et al. Prediction of preeclampsia: liver function tests during the first 20 gestational weeks. The Journal of Maternal-Fetal and Neonatal Medicine 2009;26(3):250–253.

24. Lee SM, Park JS, Han YJ, Kim W, Bang SH, Kim BJ, Park CW, Kim MY. Elevated Alanine Aminotransferase in Early Pregnancy and Subsequent Development of Gestational Diabetes and Preeclampsia. J Korean Med Sci. 2020 Jul 6;35(26):e198. Available from: <doi:10.3346/jkms.2020.35.e198>

25. NICE. DG49:PLGF-based testing to help diagnose suspected preterm pre-eclampsia. 2022. Available from: www.nice.org.uk/guidance/dg49

26. Gibson P, Nerenberg KA. TIPPing practice away from anticoagulation in pregnancy. Lancet. 2014;384:1648–1649.

27. Jin J. Use of aspirin during pregnancy to prevent preeclampsia. JAMA. 2021;326(12):1222. Available from: <doi:10.1001/jama.2021.15900>

28. Nelson-Piercy C. Handbook of obstetric medicine. 6th ed. Abington: CRC Press; 2020. ISBN:9781000173710.

29. Nursing and Midwifery Council (NMC). Standards for midwives. 2023. Available from: www.nmc.org.uk/Standardsformidwives-TheNursingandMidwiferyCouncil

30. Tucker K, Mort S, Yu L et al. Effect of self-monitoring of blood pressure on diagnosis or hypertension during higher-risk pregnancy The BUMP 1 Randomized Clinical Trial. JAMA 2022;327(17):1656–1665 doi:10.1001/jama.2022.4712.

31. Chappell L, Tucker K, Galal U et al. Effect of self-monitoring of blood pressure control in pregnant individuals with chronic or gestational hypertension: the BUMP 2 Randomized Clinical Trial JAMA 2022;327(17):1666–1678 doi:10.1001/jama.2022.4726.

32. Lewis G, editor. The confidential enquiry into maternal and child health (CEMACH). saving mothers' lives: reviewing maternal deaths to make motherhood safer – 2003–2005. The Seventh Report on Confidential Enquiries into Maternal Deaths in the United Kingdom. London: CEMACH; 2007.

33. Mayrink J, Souza RT, Feitosa FE, et al. Mean arterial blood pressure: potential predictive tool for preeclampsia in a cohort of healthy nulliparous pregnant women. BMC Pregnancy Childbirth. 2019;19:460. Available from: <doi:10.1186/s12884-019-2580-4>

34. Bellos I, Pergialiotis V, Loutradis D, Daskalakis G. The prognostic role of serum uric acid levels in pre-eclampsia: a meta-analysis. J Clin Hypertens. 2020;22:826–834. Available from: <doi:10.1111/jch.13865>

35. NICE (National Institute for Health and Care Excellence). Guideline NG25: preterm labour and birth. 2015 updated 2022. Available from: www.nice.org.uk/guidance/ng25

36. Ashworth D, Battersby C, Green M, Hardy P, McManus R, Cluver C & Chappell L. Which antihypertensive treatment is better for mild to moderate hypertension in pregnancy? British Medical Journal 2022;376:e066333. doi.10.1136/bmj-2021–066333.

37. Bateman B, Patorno E, Desai R et al. Late pregnancy β-blocker exposure and risks of neonatal hypoglycaemia and bradycardia. Pediatrics. 2016;138(3):e20160731. Available from: <doi:10.1542/peds.2016-0731>

38. Royal College of Obstetricians and Gynaecologists (RCOG). Nifedipine in pregnancy. British Journal of Obstetrics and Gynaecology 2000;107:299–307.

39. RCOG (Royal College of Obstetrics & Gynaecology). Magnesium Sulphate to Prevent Cerebral Palsy following Preterm Birth. Scientific Impact Paper No. 29;2011.

40. De Silva DA, Synnes AR, von Dadelszen P, Lee T, Bone JN, MAG-Cp CPN, et al. MAGnesium sulphate for fetal neuroprotection to prevent Cerebral Palsy (MAG-CP)-implementation of a national guideline in Canada. Implementation Science: IS. 2018;13(1), 8. Available from: <doi:10.1186/s13012-017-0702-9>

41. Webster S, Waugh J. Hypertension in pregnancy. Chapter 32 in: James DK, Steer PJ, Weiner CP, Gonik B, Robson SC, editors. High-risk pregnancy: management options. 5th ed. Cambridge: Cambridge University Press; 2017. p. 847–899.

42. Burns R, Dent K. MOET (managing obstetric emergencies and trauma). 4th ed. Chapter 27: pre-eclampsia and eclampsia. Cambridge: Wiley Blackwell; 2022. p. 231–242.

43. Knight M on behalf of UKOSS. Eclampsia in the United Kingdom. BJOG. 2007;114(9):1072–1078. Available from: <doi:10.1111/j.1471–0528.2007.01423.x>

44. Leslie D, Collis M. Hypertension in pregnancy. BJA Education. 2016;16(1):33–37. Available from: <doi:10.1093/bjaceaccp/mkv020>

45. Pourrat O, Coudroy R, Pierre F. Differentiation between severe HELLP syndrome and thrombotic microangiopathy, thrombotic thrombocytopenic purpura and other imitators. European Journal of Obstetrics and Gynecology and Reproductive Biology. 2015;189:55–58.

46. American College of Obstetricians and Gynecologists. Gestational Hypertension and Preeclampsia: ACOG Practice Bulletin No.222.Obstetrics & Gynecology. 2020;135(6):e237–e260.

47. Magee L, Nicohaides K, von Dadelszen P. Preeclampsia. The New England Journal of Medicine 2022;386:1817–1832. Available from: <doi:10.1056.NEJMre210952>

48. Dekker G. Hypertension. Chapter 35 in: James D, Steer P, Weiner C, Gonik B, et al., editors, High risk pregnancy. 4th ed. St Louis, USA: Elsevier; 2011.

49. Bradke D, Tran A, Ambarus T, Nazir M, Markowski M, Juusela A. Grade III subcapsular liver hematoma secondary to HELLP syndrome: a case report of conservative management. Case Rep Womens Health. 2019 Dec 24;25:e00169. Available from: <doi:10.1016/j.crwh.2019.e00169>. PMID: 31908974; PMCID: PMC6940712.

50. Fitzpatrick K, Kim Hinshaw K, Kurinczuk J, Knight M. Risk factors, management, and outcomes of hemolysis, elevated liver enzymes, and low platelets syndrome and elevated liver enzymes, low platelets syndrome. Obstet Gynecol. 2014;123(3):618–627.

51. Knight M, Nelson-Piercy C, Kurinczuk J, Spark P & Brocklehurst P. A prospective national study of acute fatty liver of pregnancy in the UK. Gut 2008;57:951–956. Available from: <doi:10.1136/gut.2008.148676>

52. Nelson D & Schell R. Acute Fatty Liver of Pregnancy. Contemporary OB/GYN Journal 2021;66:6 Available from: www.contemporaryobgyn.net/view/acute-fatty-liver-of-pregnancy

53. Naoum E, Leffert L, Chitilan H, Gray K, Bateman B. Acute Fatty Liver of Pregnancy. Anesthesiology 2019;130(3):446–461. Available from: <doi:10.1097/ALN.0000000000002597>

54. Lee W. Acute liver failure study group: adult acute liver failure study (V2) [Dataset]. NIDDK Central Repository; 2023. Available from: <doi:10.58020/9n48-q075>

55. Perera I et al. A case of fatal acute fatty liver of pregnancy and literature review. International Journal of Reproduction, Contraception, Obstetrics and Gynecology. 2018;7(5):2026–2030. Available from: <doi:10.18203/2320-1770.ijrcog20181950>; www.ijrcog.org/index.php/ijrcog/article/view/4589

56. Morton A, Laurie J. Physiological changes of pregnancy and the Swansea criteria in diagnosing acute fatty liver of pregnancy. Obstetric Medicine. 2018;11(3):126–131. Available from: <doi:10.1177/1753495X18759353>

57. Minakami H, Morikawa M, Yamada T et al. Differentiation of acute fatty liver of pregnancy from syndrome of hemolysis, elevated liver enzymes and low platelet counts. Journal of Medical Ethics 2014;40(3):641–649.

58. Ziki E, Bopoto S, Madziyire M et al. Acute fatty liver of pregnancy: a case report. BMC Pregnancy and Childbirth. 2019. Available from: <doi:10.1186/s12884-019-2405-5>

59. Yucesoy G, Ozkan S, Bodur et al. Acute fatty liver of pregnancy complicated with disseminated intravascular coagulation and haemorrhage: a case report. International Journal of Clinical Practice 2005;147(Suppl):82–84.

60. Ackerman-Banks C, Lipkind H, Palmsten K et al. Association between hypertensive disorders of pregnancy and cardiovascular diseases within 24 months after delivery. Am J Obstet Gynecol 7th April 2023 online.

61. Hilden K, Magnuson A, Montgomery S et al. Previous pre-eclampsia, gestational diabetes mellitus and the risk of cardiovascular disease: a nested case-control study in Sweden. BJOB [online]. 2023 March 27.

8

Malpresentations

MAUREEN BOYLE

BREECH	124	Pathophysiology	136
Introduction	125	Clinical features	136
Pathophysiology	126	FACE PRESENTATION	137
Risks/predisposing factors	126	Introduction	137
Clinical features	126	Pathophysiology	137
Care	127	Clinical features	137
TRANSVERSE OR OBLIQUE LIE	133	Care	138
Introduction	133	Postnatal	138
Clinical features	134	Complications associated with	
Compound presentation	135	malpresentations	139
Clinical features	135	Summary of midwifery responsibilities	139
Care	135	Further reading and resources	139
BROW PRESENTATION	136	References	139
Introduction	136		

BOX 8.1: Malpresentation

A malpresentation is when the fetus has a body part other than the vertex presenting into the pelvic outlet. This is commonly a breech presentation but could also involve an abnormal lie, such as oblique or transverse, when the presenting part may be an arm or shoulder. Other non-vertex presentations include face and brow.

BREECH

BOX 8.2: Breech presentation

A breech presentation is a longitudinal lie, with the fetal buttocks or feet presenting in the lower pole of the uterus and the head in the upper pole. There are three classifications of breech (see also Figure 8.1).

Extended breech (Frank): The extended breech presents with flexion at the hips and extension at the knees so that the feet are lying near the fetal head (Figure 8.1a), which results in a

DOI: 10.4324/9781003382195-8

well-fitting presenting part. This presentation is most common in primiparous women who have firm abdominal muscles.

Flexed breech (Complete): The flexed breech presents with flexion at the hips and the knees, with the feet beside the buttocks (Figure 8.1b), which results in a poor fitting presenting part and increases the risks of early rupture of membranes and cord prolapse.

Footling breech (Incomplete): The footling breech presents with extension at both the hips and the knees, leading to one or both feet or knees presenting (Figure 8.1c). This is the rarest of the breech presentations and has a high risk of cord prolapse, given the ill-fitting nature of the presenting part.

INTRODUCTION

Where the lie is longitudinal with the breech presenting, experienced care is vital, and current UK guidelines generally recommend a prelabour external cephalic version (ECV) where appropriate, followed by a discussion concerning the mode of birth if this is unsuccessful.[1] Worldwide, in resource-rich areas, most breech-presenting births are managed by caesarean sections (CS); however, there is a slow increase in the trend towards considering planned vaginal births in carefully selected cases in many countries, such as Canada,[2] Australia and New Zealand.[3] The Royal College of Obstetricians and Gynaecologists[1] in the UK have published guidelines concerning vaginal birth with breech presentation. However, regardless of antenatal planning, a breech presentation may be identified for the first time in labour; therefore, it is important that all midwives are competent to support women with unanticipated breech presentations during birth, regardless of location or ability to refer to other practitioners.

The incidence of breech presentation at 28 weeks has been found to be around 20% of fetuses. However, by 37 weeks, the number of breech presentations will decrease to between 3–4% due to spontaneous version.[1,4] It has been suggested that up to 30% of breech presentations are not diagnosed until labour[5] as it has, repeatedly, been found that clinical examination by abdominal palpation is not always reliable, with one recent study suggesting it may be only approximately 57–70% accurate.[6]

Historical Context

While there have been reports of the increased risks associated with breech births for centuries,[7] vaginal breech births remained the norm throughout much of the last century. However, as early as 1959, it was proposed that all breech presentations should be delivered abdominally to reduce perinatal morbidity and mortality.[8] From around this time onwards, throughout most resource-rich areas of the world, the number of breech vaginal births has steadily

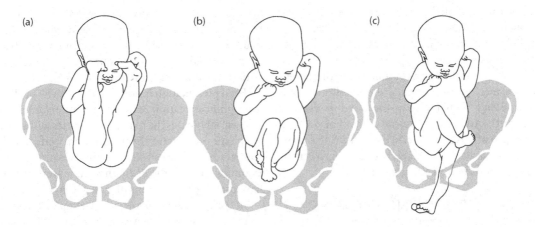

Figure 8.1 Classifications of breech presentation (a) Extended breech, (b) Flexed breech (c) footling breech

declined,[9] with the publication of the Term Breech Trial (also known as the Hannah Trial) in 2000[10] leading to the almost universal recommendation for breech presenting births to be carried out as planned caesarean sections. While the validity of their research findings has been much questioned and critiqued,[9,11,12,13] the fact remains that currently, in the UK, very few practitioners have extensive clinical experience of vaginal breech births.

As planned vaginal breech births are not common in the UK, most midwives working within the NHS will only experience them through skills drills and the occasional undiagnosed breech when women present in advanced labour. It is, therefore, valid to consider breech births within the context of 'birth emergencies', as both the risks and anxiety of those providing care are significantly increased. Although the finding of a breech presentation in labour would usually necessitate immediate referral to senior obstetricians, midwives at the point of qualification are expected to be able to support the safe birth of an undiagnosed breech.[14] This underpins the importance of skills drills and practice being on-going.

PATHOPHYSIOLOGY

In some cases, a breech presentation can be caused where there is too much amniotic fluid (polyhydramnios), allowing the fetus greater ability to continuously change its position, or where there is too little amniotic fluid (oligohydramnios), where the fetus does not have the room to turn to a vertex presentation easily. Uterine shape, including bicornuate or septate uterus, or the presence of fibroids may influence a fetus to stay in a breech presentation and can explain why, for some women, all their babies are breech. Placental location may also influence how the fetus can comfortably position itself. There is also some evidence that breech presentation may be a symptom of a problem in fetal morphogenesis or function.[15] This potentially higher risk of congenital abnormalities means these babies should receive increased assessment after birth. Additionally, research has shown that if either parent was born breech, their offspring is more than twice as likely to be breech, suggesting a genetic predisposition to a breech position.[16]

RISKS/PREDISPOSING FACTORS

Often, there is no identifiable reason for a breech presentation. However, there are features which make it more likely (see Box 8.3).

BOX 8.3: Predisposing and risk factors to a breech presentation[15,16,17,18]

- Low gestational age/premature labour
- Primiparity (tight abdominal muscles)
- Grand multiparity (lax abdominal muscles)
- Older maternal age
- Female infant
- Polyhydramnios
- Congenital fetal abnormalities
- Smoking/intake of substances, which may cause reduced fetal movements, such as anticonvulsive medications or alcohol
- Septum or partial septum (bicornuate uterus)
- Fibroids or uterine tumours
- Placenta praevia
- Previous uterine surgery

Consideration should also be given to the fact that for some women, all their babies adopt a breech presentation, suggesting that perhaps their pelvic shape is better suited to breech position. Although pelvic classification is rarely practiced, obstetric texts frequently refer to an increased risk of breech with some pelvic shapes, making cephalic pelvic entry more challenging. The possibility of a genetic predisposition to breech position also needs to be noted.[16]

CLINICAL FEATURES

Abdominal palpation is used to determine the lie, presentation and position of the fetus during routine antenatal examinations and where there is uncertainty, it needs to be confirmed by ultrasound. On admission in labour, a vaginal examination can aid in diagnosis (see Box 8.6).

Fetal presentation is not considered to be of clinical significance until 36 weeks gestation (unless in preterm labour), as the majority of fetuses will adopt a cephalic presentation by term. Often, women with complex pregnancies will have multiple ultrasound examinations, so it is likely that these women will have breech presentations diagnosed early.

In the UK, women at low risk of complications are primarily seen by midwives, where current practice does not recommend routine ultrasound scans after 20 weeks gestation,[19,20] so the midwife's skill in performing abdominal palpation is vital to diagnosis.

While approximately 25–30% of breech presentations remain undiagnosed at term[1,5] and there is some evidence that those with less experience are more likely to mistake a breech for a cephalic presentation,[21] so vigilance and practice in abdominal palpation are vital. It is also suggested that a senior opinion is sought whenever there is any uncertainty.

Abdominal examination

Prior to undertaking an abdominal palpation, it is important for the midwife to complete a thorough history, as any risk factors (see Box 8.3) may alert the midwife to the possibility of a breech presentation. Additionally, women with a breech presentation often complain of increased discomfort under the ribs and heartburn, which is caused by the proximity of the fetal head. Therefore, a discussion with the woman regarding her pregnancy symptoms and comfort can also provide the midwife with useful clues to the fetal position before she has even begun to palpate. However, as any woman may present with a breech presentation, a midwife should always be open to the possibility.

On inspection, there is likely to be little difference; the lie is longitudinal, although on palpation, the size may palpate larger than expected, particularly if the presenting part has not yet descended into the pelvis. Using a Pawlik's grip, the head is located in the fundus and palpated as a round, hard mass, which may move independently of the back by gently balloting it between both hands. However, in a frank breech (see Figure 8.1), if the feet are 'splinting' the head, then the diagnosis may be more difficult.

On auscultation, the fetal heart sounds are often best heard at or above the level of the umbilicus and laterally on the side of the fetal back. The use of a pinard stethoscope can be helpful, as they require more specific placement in terms of location. It is generally recommended that if there is any suspicion of breech presentation by 36 weeks gestation, then an ultrasound scan should be performed to confirm and assist in care planning.

Antenatal diagnosis

When midwives diagnose a breech presentation after 36 weeks (or according to local policy), a referral is usual, depending on individual hospital guidelines, to obstetric colleagues, a 'breech team' or a birth options clinic. The woman can then be given full and in-depth information on the risks and benefits of ECV (see Box 8.4), elective CS or a planned vaginal breech birth.

BOX 8.4: Possible contraindications for ECV[21,23]

- Prior indication for CS
- Placenta praevia
- Rh sensitisation
- Coagulation disorders
- Recent antepartum haemorrhage/placental abruption
- Major uterine anomaly
- Previous CS or other uterine surgery: individual assessment is needed
- Pre-eclampsia
- Multiple pregnancy
- Ruptured membranes
- Oligohydramnios
- Known fetal compromise
- Fetal growth restriction (FGR)
- Fetal anomaly
- Intrauterine fetal death

While it may appear that there are many contraindications, it has been found that only 4% of breech presentations have a contraindication to ECV.[24]

CARE

Turning breech to cephalic presentation

EXTERNAL CEPHALIC VERSION (ECV)

ECV (see Box 8.5) is the manipulative transabdominal conversion of the breech to cephalic presentation, and it has been an RCOG-recommended standard for many years.[1] This procedure has been carried out since the time of Hippocrates and was continued throughout the Middle Ages, but during the 1970s and 80s, the practice fell out of favour, and its availability diminished.[8,21] However, with further studies and as the option of vaginal breech birth decreased, it has since been widely reintroduced with most maternity units in the UK now offering an ECV service. The procedure has been the subject of significant scientific appraisal, and a number of studies have been carried out which demonstrate that when offered at term, there is a reduction in the rate of planned caesarean sections without increased risks to the baby.[21,22] Nevertheless, there are some contraindications to offering this procedure (see Box 8.4).

BOX 8.5: External Cephalic Version (ECV)

Following an assessment by CTG and/or ultrasound, the woman is required to either lie on her side with the fetal back uppermost or on her back with an appropriate wedge tilt to the side. Using the palmer surfaces of both hands, the practitioner will gently disengage the breech from the maternal pelvis (if needed). Once disengaged, the breech is encouraged laterally upward to encourage fetal flexion and for the fetus to 'follow its nose' around. The whole procedure should be gentle and unhurried. In a study comparing the use of gel or talc on the operator's hands, it was found gel resulted in less pain for the woman.[25]

The midwife should stay with the woman and be alert to any signs of discomfort as, although the procedure can be uncomfortable, if significant pain is experienced, this would always be an indication to stop the procedure. Women should be reassured that most find the discomfort manageable,[26] and where needed, Entonox or regional analgesia may be used.[21,27] The fetal heart should be auscultated after each attempt and a maximum of three attempts is considered appropriate.[1,21] A CTG should be repeated following the procedure and if the mother is Rhesus negative then blood for a Kleihauer test should be taken and Anti-D administered.

Following a successful ECV, it is important to discuss signs of spontaneous labour and when the woman should contact her midwife if there are any concerns, paying particular attention to fetal movements and any vaginal bleeding. If unsuccessful, plans should be made with the obstetrician to discuss the mode of birth or, if appropriate, another ECV may be attempted at a later date.

Factors that increase the likelihood of ECV success include:[21,22]

- Multiparity
- Increased/normal amniotic fluid volumes
- Posterior placenta
- Non-extended breech
- Skilled ECV practitioner
- BMI of less than 25
- Use of tocolytic drugs

Potential risks associated with ECV:[21,23,28]

- Transient fetal heart rate anomalies
- Persisting abnormal cardiotocography (CTG)
- Inadvertent ROM/cord prolapse
- Placental abruption
- Significant feto-maternal haemorrhage is possible but very rare
- Even after a successful ECV, the risk of CS in labour is increased
- Increased risk of instrumental vaginal birth

While deemed very safe, it is recommended that the procedure should always be undertaken in a place where the baby can immediately be delivered by caesarean section should this become necessary.

ALTERNATIVE AND COMPLEMENTARY THERAPIES

Moxibustion

Moxibustion is a form of Traditional Chinese Medicine (TCM) where moxa sticks (usually *Artemesia vulgaria* or a smokeless variety) are burned close to the skin of the outer aspect of the fifth toenails of both feet. This is a traditional acupuncture point. The moxa burns with a slow but intense heat, which stimulates heat receptors on the skin of the toe and, according to TCM theory, moxa has a tonifying and warming effect that promotes movement and activity. This effect is utilised to encourage the fetus to become more active and thus increase the chance of a spontaneous version to cephalic.[29]

There is, however, conflicting evidence for the use of moxibustion.[29,30,3]. A Cochrane review stated that there is some evidence that, when used in conjunction with knee/chest positioning, it may reduce the incidence of non-cephalic presentations at term and recommended further studies to evaluate its effectiveness.[32] A more recent Cochrane review[29] also suggests there may be a positive effect to using moxibustion.

Whilst the evidence of its effectiveness is conflicting, it is non-invasive, appears to be safe and is an option some women are likely to consider in their desire to avoid an operative birth. It is, therefore, important that midwives have a basic understanding of moxibustion as a treatment some women will seek out.

In some areas, midwives have developed the use of moxibustion as an extended skill which can be offered to women from 33 weeks gestation.[33] However, as with all things, midwives are reminded that they are accountable for their practice and so should only offer a service if properly trained and competent to do so.[34]

Other alternative therapies

It has been suggested that the following may also be beneficial in encouraging breech to cephalic version, although research into their effectiveness has generally been small studies which lack rigor. All would benefit from further evaluation and they should, therefore, not be routinely recommended.

- Ginger paste
- Homeopathy
- Chiropractic
- Fetal acoustic stimulation
- Hypnotherapy
- Yoga positions, swimming positions

Posture and positioning

Much has been written regarding the use of the knee-chest, all-fours position as a means of encouraging spontaneous version from breech to cephalic presentation. A Cochrane review[35] examined studies where women were encouraged to adopt this position for varying time periods in late pregnancy. The evidence was unable to demonstrate any significant benefit in breech version, so they concluded that there is no reason to recommend this intervention but suggested that further large-scale studies were warranted. However, as this is a non-invasive intervention and may be considered a safe practice, it is likely that some women will continue to make use of it. As mentioned in the previous section, if women are making use of moxibustion, then it is possible that, in conjunction with the knee-chest position, the success rate may be improved.[29]

Undiagnosed Breech in Labour

IMMEDIATE CARE/TREATMENT

It is not uncommon, even for women who have accessed regular antenatal care, to present in labour

BOX 8.6: Vaginal Examination (VE)

Prior to undertaking a vaginal examination, the midwife will gain consent and carry out an abdominal examination which, as described earlier, will hopefully alert the midwife to the possibility of a breech presentation. On vaginal examination, the smooth, hard round head with its familiar landmarks is absent. The presenting part is often high, soft and irregular, and sometimes the anal orifice or male genitalia can be felt. If landmarks can be felt, they will be in a line (e.g., the fetal ischial tuberosities and the anus), although in a very compressed breech, the cleft between the buttocks may be mistaken for the sagittal suture. After rupture of membranes, fresh meconium is often seen, especially on the examining finger after identification of the anus, and this is diagnostic. Occasionally, the midwife may also feel a foot or, rarely, a knee. However, diagnosis of a breech from a vaginal examination, particularly in early labour, can be challenging, and mistakes are sometimes made. Any doubt should result in confirmation by ultrasound.

with an unknown breech presentation, which will ideally be diagnosed on admission. It is estimated that up to 30% of all breech presentations at term will be undetected prior to labour.[1,36,37] All midwives should be alert to the possibility of previous palpations and even vaginal examinations being incorrect (or even of a late position/presentation change) and, therefore, each examination should be conducted without preconceived expectations. (See Box 8.6 for characteristics of a breech presentation during VE).

The first action when a breech is diagnosed in labour is to explain the finding to the woman calmly and to refer or otherwise obtain assistance. In a hospital setting, this would initially be senior midwifery and obstetric colleagues and, prior to birth, anesthetic and neonatal team members should be on standby. If available, it would also be appropriate to call a specialist breech midwife or midwife with breech experience. In the community, emergency services (dial 999 in the UK) should be called to enable swift transfer to an obstetric unit and/or assistance if the birth is imminent.

When the diagnosis is made in labour, particularly advanced labour, it is much harder to ensure the woman is both given adequate information and is able to understand this in order to give informed consent to either a vaginal birth or, where available, an emergency CS. However, every effort should be made to ensure the woman is making a choice that is right for them. The individual discussion will probably be underpinned by the specific situation, for example, parity, previous obstetric history and medical history. Any contra-indications that would have applied to a planned vaginal birth (see Box 8.7) may also be relevant to the decision-making. There is some evidence that there is a difference in risk when the breech is identified in early or late labour[37] and, therefore, this should be reflected in the information given. The RCOG[1] does not recommend that women near or in the active second stage of labour be routinely offered caesarean section.

Care during labour

While it is anticipated that senior obstetric assistance will usually be available in a hospital, it is imperative that every midwife is familiar with and able to support a woman birthing in the breech position. Many babies will need resuscitation, so it is vital that this is prepared for prior to the birth, regardless of location.

Careful assessment of the fetal condition is necessary, and the current RCOG guidelines,[1] as well as other authorities,[2] recommend continuous electronic fetal monitoring. But if the woman is upright, this may be a challenge, and meticulous intermittent monitoring may need to be carried out. Once the baby has descended through the pelvis and the fetal heart cannot be heard, assessment of the tone and colour of the visible legs and torso is important.

If the birth is taking place on labour ward, the RCOG[1] suggests it is not necessary to be in theatre. The position the woman adopts should be her choice, and if the decision for a vaginal breech birth was identified in the antenatal period, information and discussion to enable the woman to make an informed choice would have been possible. However, in the case of an unexpected breech birth, it is suggested that, with the woman's consent, whichever position the midwife feels most capable of supporting the woman in is likely to be the safest. But the midwife should be able to support instinctive actions by the woman, so ideally both positions – upright/all-fours or semi-recumbent/lithotomy – are prepared for.[1,38] One study[39] identified that 70% of successful breech births in the upright/all-fours position occurred spontaneously. However, 10% of women had to change position to semi-recumbent/lithotomy to enable assistance to be given – this underpins the importance that midwives should be able to offer care in whichever position is chosen.

It is vital that the temperature of the birthing room is warm and without draughts, as the baby's body will be exposed before drying/wrapping is possible and cold air can stimulate respiration before the head is born.

Prior to the birth, it is important to ensure the woman's bladder is empty.

A vaginal examination (VE) is advisable to clearly identify the second stage, as the fetal body could potentially slip through a cervix which is not fully dilated, leading to head entrapment. If this occurs, a retractor or finger should be used to gently push aside the cervix in front of the baby's face, urgent medical aid should be sought and delivery must be expedited. Active pushing should be avoided prior to the breech distending the introitus, and anal dilation should be visualised[1] to potentially prevent head entrapment.

Amniotomy should only be used for specific clinical indications, and an immediate VE following spontaneous membrane rupture to ensure there is no cord prolapse is advised.[2]

In any position, the recommendation is, wherever possible, minimal handling is the best approach. This traditional principle of '**hands off the breech**' is valid as long as there is good progress and clear signs of fetal well-being. Any handling of the baby is liable to stimulate premature respiration, as well as activate the 'startle reflex' causing the baby to extend its arms and, therefore, touching should only be done if necessary. However, it is vital that when there is a delay, the midwife is able to understand what may cause this and assist as necessary to reduce the risk of cord compression or oxygen deprivation.

It is important to keep an awareness of the time throughout the birth, as avoiding prolonged lack of oxygen to the fetus is crucial to good outcomes. There is a need to expedite the birth if the fetal heart rate becomes abnormal or compromised tone/colour is observed in the exposed baby. Delay in the birth process should be avoided: it is recommended < 5 minutes from the birth of the buttocks to the head or < 3 minutes from umbilicus to head,[1] but, of course, the condition of the baby will depend on the resources the fetus had when the second stage began.

Avoidance of traction is crucial to a safe birth; however, assistance without traction is required if there is delay or evidence of poor fetal condition.[1] It is imperative that the baby's back should always remain uppermost in relation to the anterior maternal pelvis. To avoid confusion when caring for a woman who changes position, consideration should be made of the reminder that during the birth, 'only one back' should be seen by the caregiver – the maternal back if the woman is in upright/all-fours position, or the baby's back if the woman is in semi-recumbent/lithotomy position.[40]

The baby's legs should deliver spontaneously, but if necessary, they can be assisted by placing two fingers in the popliteal fossa to bend the leg. The leg is then flexed towards the abdomen and then down. Traction or additional handling of the baby should be avoided. The second leg often delivers spontaneously, but this manoeuvre can be repeated if necessary.

Following the birth of the legs and trunk, the cord should be visualised – there is no evidence that pulling a loop of the cord is beneficial as it could cause arterial spasms and should, therefore, be avoided.

Manoeuvres to aid the birth of the baby's arms

With further expulsion, well-flexed arms may deliver spontaneously. If they do not, or if it is necessary to expedite the birth, then it may be possible to simply hook them down from the elbow or, with two fingers passed over the shoulder, gently pull the humerus across the chest, sweeping the arms across the body and downwards. It is suggested that a sternal crease is seen when the arms are under the sacrum and not entrapped.[41] If, however, the arms are extended (nuchal), the midwife must intervene. The Løvset's manoeuvre (see Box 8.8 and Figure 8.2) can be carried out when the woman is

> ### BOX 8.8: Løvset's manoeuvre in maternal semi-recumbent/lithotomy position
>
> Once the scapulae are visible, the baby should be held carefully by the fetal pelvic girdle (avoiding any pressure on the soft tissues of the abdomen) (see Figure 8.2), and a gentle downward motion with rotation is carried out. Care must be taken to always keep the fetal back towards the mother's front (i.e., the fetal back must be uppermost if the woman is in the semi-recumbent/lithotomy position). The baby is then rotated so the shoulder that was posterior is now anterior (under the woman's symphysis) to splint the posterior arm across the baby's face and change it to an anterior position.
>
> If the arm does not deliver spontaneously during the rotation, the midwife should slide a finger over the shoulder and along the humerus, apply pressure to the antecubital fossa to flex the elbow and draw the arm gently down over the face and chest. The baby is then rotated 180 degrees back in the opposite direction so that the second arm is anterior and can be delivered using the same technique where necessary, remembering to ensure that the fetal back stays anterior (baby's back to the woman's front).

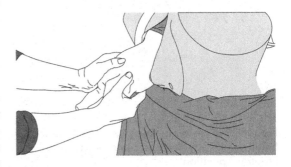

Figure 8.2 Løvset's manoeuvre in maternal semi-recumbent/lithotomy position

in a semi-recumbent/lithotomy position, or if she is upright/all-fours the rotation is done using the bony prominences of the shoulder girdle rather than the pelvis.

The head will move through the pelvis in a transverse position until it rotates spontaneously to bring the occiput under the symphysis pubis. It is important to wait for this to happen, using maternal pushing and the weight of the baby, and for the nape of the neck to be visible before manoeuvres are used to assist with the birth of the head. If the woman is in the semi-recumbent/lithotomy position and there appears to be a delay, then an assistant should apply suprapubic pressure to assist with flexion of the head.

Manoeuvres to aid the birth of the baby's head

While the fetal head may birth spontaneously and without problems, it is important to ensure the birth of the head is not too rapid and so it may be prudent to carry out a *modified Mauriceau-Smellie-Veit* (MSV) manoeuvre (Figure 8.3). This is particularly important if the head is not well flexed, as it aims to enhance flexion. When the woman is in a semi-recumbent/lithotomy position, the baby's body is laid along the midwife's dominant arm with the palm upwards supporting the chest. The index and second fingers of the midwife's hand are placed on the malar (cheek) bones of the baby's face, taking care to avoid the eyes. The midwife should then place the other hand across the baby's shoulders with the middle fingers on the occiput to increase

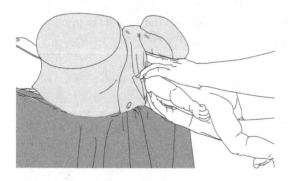

Figure 8.3 Assisted birth of the head: Mauriceau-Smellie-Veit with maternal semi-recumbent/lithotomy position

flexion. The other fingers can be placed over the baby's shoulders. An assistant can provide external support for flexion by providing suprapubic pressure throughout this manoeuvre. As the head is flexed, it is drawn out gently until the sub-occipital region appears, the face is born, and the head is rotated around the symphysis pubis. It is important to ensure this is done slowly and gently to avoid cervical nerve damage,[41] as rapid delivery of the fetal head could lead to compression and decompression of the fetal skull bones, which may cause tentorial tears and intracranial haemorrhage.[40]

The MSV is commonly used with the woman in a semi-recumbent/lithotomy position, but it is also possible to perform MSV with the woman in all-fours. This is the commonly called a *Mauriceau-Cronk manoeuvre*, which involves manually flexing the fetal head by elevating the occiput and downward pressure on the maxilla.[41] Practicing with both maternal positions during skills drills will enable midwives to be more competent in supporting women's choices.

The *Bracht manoeuvre* is when the fetal body is actively rotated over the maternal symphysis.[21] Following the birth of the arms, the baby is grasped by the hips and lifted with both hands (without any traction) towards the woman's abdomen, causing the neck to pivot around the symphysis. An assistant can apply suprapubic pressure to facilitate the birth of the aftercoming head.

Emergency breech extraction

This is rarely undertaken and is inappropriate for a singleton, term breech birth.[21] It would only be undertaken by an obstetrician as an emergency procedure to achieve immediate delivery if there is severe fetal distress and when an emergency caesarean section is not an option. It is most commonly used to assist the birth of a second twin[1] in an oblique or transverse lie after internal podalic version.[42] A hand must be placed into the uterus and both feet are grasped. The legs are then pulled down and the head is pressed upwards with the outside hand. Traction must be maintained on the delivered legs until the breech is fixed. Traction takes the place of contractions, and the breech can then be delivered using the manoeuvres previously described. As the arms will be extended due to traction, Løvset's manoeuvre (Box 8.8) will be necessary.

BOX 8.9: Vaginal breech birth checklist

- Abdominal palpation
- Vaginal examination to assess cervical full dilation
- Confirm maternal bladder is empty
- Ensure the woman is positioned appropriately or able to move spontaneously, which may not only help women to cope but also may ensure the fetus adopts and maintains an optimum position
- Make sure the room is warm and there are no draughts
- Continuous CTG/regular auscultation of the fetal heart
- 'Hands off the breech'
- Monitor the condition of the fetus through observation as well as FH, and apply appropriate manoeuvres necessary or if a delay occurs
- Prepare for probable neonatal resuscitation
- Third stage management/observation for PPH
- Clear and contemporaneous record-keeping
- Maintain the baby's temperature
- Early skin-to-skin and feeding
- Ensure there is a full neonatologist/paediatrician assessment of the baby

Possible complications of a vaginal breech delivery, which may need ongoing care

Baby:

- Fractures of the humerus, clavicle or femur
- Dislocation of the hip or shoulder
- Erb's palsy
- Internal organ damage by rough or incorrect handling (e.g., kidneys, liver, spleen)
- Dislocation of the neck
- Spinal cord damage or fracture
- Intracranial haemorrhage
- Soft-tissue damage

- Hypoxia/birth asphyxia; this may be due to cord compression, cord prolapse or premature placental separation
- Potential cold injury and/or hypoglycaemia
- Long-term neurological damage
- Congenital dislocation of the hip, especially with frank breech; this is usually a complication of the presentation and not the birth process

Mother:

- Urethral trauma
- Vaginal or perineal trauma
- Postpartum haemorrhage

The majority of these complications are rare and can be minimised by correct techniques during the birth and immediate identification and referral as appropriate.

RCOG[1] suggests that planned vaginal breech birth increases the risk of low Apgar scores and serious short-term complications in the baby but has not been shown to increase the risk of long-term morbidity. Maternal complications are least with a successful vaginal birth, but the risk is highest with emergency CS.

TRANSVERSE OR OBLIQUE LIE

BOX 8.10: Transverse Lie

A transverse lie denotes a fetus with its longitudinal axis perpendicular to the long axis of the uterus (see Figure 8.4). The transverse lie can occur with either the curvature of the fetal spine orientated upwards (dorsosuperior), or downwards (dorsoinferior). In an oblique lie, the head or the breech will be located within the iliac fossa (see Figure 8.4). Most often, these presentations form part of an unstable lie when the fetus moves between longitudinal, transverse and oblique lies after 37 weeks gestation.

INTRODUCTION

The incidence of transverse/oblique lie is difficult to estimate and varies significantly depending on

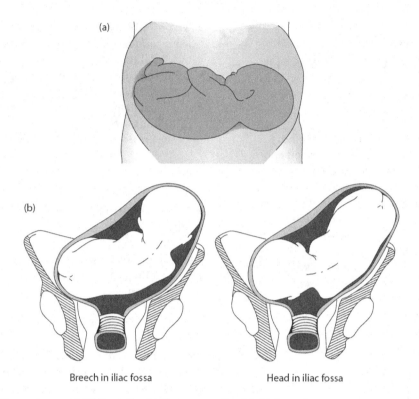

(a)

(b)

Breech in iliac fossa   Head in iliac fossa

Figure 8.4 Transverse and Oblique lie: (a) Transverse lie, (b) Oblique lie

population variables. However, where grand multiparity is uncommon, the incidence is between 1:300–1:400 pregnancies.[43]

Pathophysiology

Box 8.11 lists some of the associated conditions which may lead to transverse or oblique lie.

CLINICAL FEATURES

Diagnosis

Diagnosis is usually made antenatally. On inspection of the abdomen, the uterus appears broad and on palpation, the fetal poles will not be felt in either the pelvis or the fundus. Additionally, the woman may experience discomfort when the lower uterine segment is touched. Referral to the obstetrician should be made as appropriate, and an ultrasound examination and review would be recommended to rule out any relevant causes/associations (see Box 8.11) and to plan care.

On vaginal examination (VE), very little is likely to be felt as the presenting part remains high. It may

> **BOX 8.11: Suggested causes and associations with transverse or oblique lie**
>
> - Grand multiparity
> - Contracted maternal pelvis
> - Placenta previa
> - Prematurity
> - Polyhydramnios
> - Uterine abnormalities such as transverse septum or leiomyomas (fibroids).
> - Fetal macrosomia
> - Fetal abnormalities
> - Multiple pregnancy (second twin)

be possible to feel the shoulder, ribs or, on occasion, the fetal arm may prolapse through the cervix. A cord prolapse is a very real risk in these situations, and this, too, may be felt. It would be prudent to avoid VE until after ultrasound confirmation if an oblique or transverse lie is suspected from palpation due to the potential presence of a placenta praevia or the risk of cord prolapse following accidental ROM.

Care

ANTENATAL

Antenatally, prior to term, there is little clinical significance; however, the woman should be informed to attend immediately if premature labour is suspected or if there is prelabour rupture of membranes as the risk of cord prolapse (see Chapter 9) is significant. Inpatient care from 37+ weeks to reduce these risks is often recommended. Additionally, ECV may be attempted, but in an unstable lie, the fetus may revert back. Where the fetus persists in a transverse/oblique lie at term or in early labour the obstetrician may attempt ECV, possibly with a controlled ARM; however, in most cases, CS is required.

Labour

There is no mechanism for labour, and without version or emergency CS, the labour becomes obstructed and contractions may become tonic with no relaxation of the uterus. Uterine rupture, death of the fetus and/or possible maternal death may ensue if no action is taken.

If diagnosed in labour, it would be important to explain the situation to the woman and her birth partner clearly, while making an immediate referral to an obstetrician. If not in hospital, arrangements for urgent transfer to a labour ward must be made.

Postnatal

If emergency ECV is done at term or when the woman is in labour, there is the potential for injury to maternal organs, such as the bladder, or to the baby. Careful examination and monitoring after the birth is necessary.

COMPOUND PRESENTATION

> **BOX 8.12: Compound presentation**
>
> A compound presentation is when a fetal extremity presents alongside the presenting part. The majority of compound presentations involve the fetal hand or arm presenting with the vertex.

> **BOX 8.13: Causes, risks and associations with compound presentation**
>
> - Premature rupture of membranes
> - Premature labour, low gestational weight
> - Pelvic mass displacing the fetal pole
> - Induction of labour with a high presenting part
> - Cord prolapse
> - Multiple pregnancy

Introduction

The incidence of compound presentation is rare and usually described anywhere from 1 in 250 to 1 in 1500 births.[44]

PATHOPHYSIOLOGY

Any situation which gives the fetus the space to move an extremity to lie next to the presenting part can give rise to a compound presentation. Some suggested causes, risks and associations with compound presentation are included in Box 8.13.

CLINICAL FEATURES

DIAGNOSIS

Compound presentation is a finding that may be diagnosed on vaginal examination when the extremity is felt alongside the presenting part. Most often, a hand or fingers are felt alongside the vertex, although, rarely, a foot may be felt beside the vertex or an arm may be present together with the breech. Even less commonly, more than one extremity may be involved.[44]

CARE

Mechanism/immediate care

Many cases resolve spontaneously. If the hand is presenting, it may retract as labour progresses and care can continue as normal. Additionally, as the fetus already has the reflexes which are associated with newborns, it is possible to encourage retraction with gentle stimulation to the fingers. So long as labour is progressing normally, a compound presentation can usually be safely ignored, and the fetus is likely to self-correct the situation.

Referral

However, if the hand or arm has prolapsed below the presenting part, it is likely the increased presenting diameter will necessitate a caesarean birth, and therefore, timely obstetric referral and transfer (if required) is necessary. It has been suggested that up to 25% of cases require CS due to a non-reassuring fetal status.[44]

Similarly, a foot presenting by the fetal head is more complicated as the size of the leg makes retraction less likely and significantly increases the diameter of the presenting part. Occasionally vaginal birth may still occur, but augmentation is to be avoided, and instrumental delivery is contraindicated with a compound presentation.

Postnatal

Any specific care will depend on the outcome of the compound presentation and how the birth took place. There is a possibility of injury to the fetus, and ongoing, careful checks of the baby are necessary. If manipulation is needed, there is potential for damage to the woman's bladder, and therefore, urine output/renal function should be observed postnatally to ensure this is normal. If a vaginal birth, there is an increased risk of perineal damage, and this should be assessed and treated in the usual way.

BROW PRESENTATION

BOX 8.14: Brow presentation

In a brow presentation, the fetal head is halfway between full flexion (vertex) and hyperextension (face presentation: see next section). The presenting part of the fetal head is between the orbital ridge and the anterior fontanelle. The frontal bones are the point of designation and can present (as with the occiput in a vertex presentation) in any position relative to the maternal pelvis.

INTRODUCTION

The reported incidence of brow presentations varies significantly and has been stated to be between 1:177–1:1,500 births.[45]

PATHOPHYSIOLOGY

Conditions which prevent the fetus from flexing the head have the potential to become a brow presentation. These can include impediments to flexion such as a fetal goitre or a thick cord several times around the neck. Fetal conditions such as hydrocephalus or anencephaly can also cause a brow presentation.

A fetus can also extend to a brow position when having difficulty fitting through the pelvis; for example, an OP (occipital posterior) position may result in the fetus becoming held up at the pelvic brim and contractions promoting the extension of the fetal head.

Some suggested causes, risks and associations with brow presentation are included in Box 8.15.

CLINICAL FEATURES

Diagnosis

Diagnosis prior to labour is difficult, although a brow presentation may be suspected with a post-dates pregnancy where a larger head is palpable abdominally. Confirmation may be sought from ultrasound scan; however, at this stage, the fetus may manage to manoeuvre and descend into the pelvis. Since more than 50% of brow presentations convert to vertex or face presentation before labour,[46] no intervention is usually undertaken, apart from careful assessment and observation when labour begins.

BOX 8.15: Suggested risks and associations with brow presentation

- Post-dates
- Prematurity
- Cephalopelvic disproportion
- Fetal malformations
- Polyhydramnios
- Associated with OP positions

On vaginal examination, the pelvis may feel empty, although it may be possible to reach the presenting part, which will usually remain high. The anterior fontanelle may be felt on one side of the pelvis and the orbital ridges on the other. However, if descent had taken place, the landmarks may be obscured by oedema.

Labour

IMMEDIATE CARE

When a brow is suspected in early labour, it may flex (to vertex presentation) or extend (to face presentation), possibly allowing labour to continue and, therefore, conservative management and a watch and wait for approach[45] with appropriate multi-professional collaboration is recommended.

Where a brow presentation persists, the large mentovertical (13.5cm) diameter is considered too large to fit through the pelvis unless the fetus is very small or preterm, and labour will become obstructed, necessitating a CS.

Where a brow presentation is suspected, it is worth early discussion with the woman and obstetric team to reduce the risk of an emergency transfer of care or unanticipated CS.

Postnatal

A late diagnosis, when the woman has been in labour for some time, has the potential for injury to maternal organs, such as the bladder, or to the baby. Following the birth of a baby in a brow position, referral to the neonatologist/paediatrician should be made for assessment of possible causative fetal issues. Careful examination and monitoring of both the woman and baby should be undertaken after the birth.

FACE PRESENTATION

> ### BOX 8.16: Face presentation
>
> A face presentation is the result of a complete extension of the fetal head, where the area from the glabella (the flat area of bone between the eyebrows) to the underside of the mentum (chin) lies over the cervical os and the occiput is flexed against the upper back.

INTRODUCTION

The incidence of face presentation is reported to be between 1:500–1:1,000 births.[45]

PATHOPHYSIOLOGY

Occasionally, the face may be the primary presenting part at the start of labour. See Box 8.17 for associations with a primary face presentation.

However, more often, a deflexed posterior presentation develops into a face presentation as labour progresses. This is called a secondary face presentation and is caused when the deflexed posterior position (OP) gets held up at the pelvic brim, and contractions promote the extension of the fetal head.

CLINICAL FEATURES

Diagnosis

Although almost impossible to diagnose from abdominal examination, palpation may suggest a high head with a sharp angulation noted between the fetal occiput and back. However, it is expected that most face presentations will not be diagnosed until labour.

On vaginal examination, the presenting part is often high and will feel soft and irregular, with

> ### BOX 8.17: Suggested risks and associations with face presentation
>
> - Tumours of the fetal neck, e.g., goitre or cystic hygroma (which are usually diagnosed during antenatal ultrasound)
> - Anencephaly (which is usually diagnosed during antenatal ultrasound)
> - Prematurity
> - Low birth weight
> - Birth weight > 4kg
> - Polyhydramnios
> - Uterine abnormalities
> - Loops of cord around the neck (preventing flexion)
> - Cephalopelvic disproportion
> - Fetal musculoskeletal abnormalities
> - Multi-fetal pregnancy
> - Multiparity

the orbital ridges, nose, mouth and malar bones palpable. It is even possible that the fetal mouth may suck the examiner's finger. Initially, it can be hard to distinguish between a face presentation and a breech, especially if oedema is present, as this can distort the landmarks. However, the distinguishing feature is that the mouth and two malar prominences will be felt as a triangle (whereas with a breech presentation, the two ischial tuberosities and anus will be in a straight line). When examining the mouth, gums will be felt. Care must be taken during examination so as not to damage the eyes.

CARE

BOX 8.18: Mechanism of face presentation birth

The mentum (chin) is the denominator, which is used to define the position, with the submentobregmatic diameter (9.5 cm) being the largest diameter to pass through the pelvis. This is very similar to the biparietal diameter, and so a vaginal birth is often achievable; however, it must be remembered that face bones do not mould. Most often, the face enters the brim of the pelvis in the transverse position and, with descent, progresses into the mento-anterior (chin anterior) position, in which case it is possible to expect a vaginal birth 60–90% of the time[45] with the fetal head being born by hyperflexion of the neck.

After anterior rotation and descent, the chin and mouth appear at the vulva. The nose, eyes, brow and occiput sweep the perineum, and the head is born by flexion. Restitution then takes place where the chin rotates back towards the side in which it entered the brim and the shoulders are born as usual. However, it is important to note that the occiput can cause significant perineal distension, so perineal trauma may be increased.

A mento-posterior position at the beginning of labour may rotate to mento-anterior; however, if the face persists in the mento-posterior position, vaginal birth is not possible as the fetal skull is unable to pass under the symphysis pubis, and therefore, a CS will be necessary.

Immediate care

It has been suggested that over 50% of face presentations are not diagnosed until the second stage of labour.[47] However, a more recent study found an approximately 70% diagnosis rate on admission in labour,[48] and while in that study, all proceeded to CS, it is generally agreed that intervention is only warranted when there is fetal distress or arrest of dilation/descent. A French study[49] identified that spontaneous vaginal birth, with mento-anterior presentation, occurred in 73%.

REFERRAL

If a face presentation is suspected, the midwife should discuss with obstetric colleagues, and if at home or in a Birth Centre, transfer into an obstetric labour ward is necessary. If birth is imminent in the community, paramedic help should be called in case resuscitation is necessary and for subsequent transfer for a neonatologist/paediatrician examination.

It is vital that the midwife inform the woman and her birth partners immediately and sensitively of her findings so that they can be prepared, as most face presentation babies have significant bruising and facial swelling, which, while it will generally resolve within a few days, can be distressing to parents. On rare occasions, the neonate may need temporary admission to the neonatal unit for support if excessive oedema compromises respiration.

While fetal heart rate abnormalities during labour may be more common, it is important that fetal blood sampling, fetal scalp electrodes and ventouse delivery are avoided with a face presentation. Additionally, if required, it is safer to perform a CS in the first stage of labour with careful delivery of the fetal head as there is an increased risk of extension to the uterine incision and CS birth becomes more challenging in the second stage.

POSTNATAL

Because oedema and bruising for the baby with a face presentation are common, support to establish feeding may be challenging and will include exploring different feeding positions and teaching the woman to hand express to provide colostrum and support regular breast stimulation if the baby is initially unable to feed. If the baby is admitted to the neonatal unit, the usual care for a woman separated from her baby will be necessary.

COMPLICATIONS ASSOCIATED WITH MALPRESENTATIONS

There are many possible complications which are commonly associated with all malpresentations listed in Box 8.19.

SUMMARY OF MIDWIFERY RESPONSIBILITIES

- Attend all relevant skills and drills and revision sessions, to ensure skills and knowledge are kept current.
- Identify malpresentations antenatally whenever possible to enable forward planning and non-urgent, informed decision-making by the woman

- Monitor the progress of labour and refer as appropriate
- Monitor well-being and position of the fetus
- Refer to obstetric colleagues and transfer to an obstetric labour ward when necessary
- Prepare for neonatal resuscitation and potential PPH as appropriate
- Keep the baby warm
- Early skin-to-skin and feeding
- Neonatologist/paediatrician assessment
- Observe for any maternal complications following births associated with malpresentations and refer as appropriate
- Psychological and emotional support for the woman and her family throughout the birth
- Ongoing psychological support as necessary (See Chapter 16)

BOX 8.19: Possible complications which are commonly associated with all malpresentations

Woman:

- Prolonged latent phase
- Primary dysfunctional labour/slow progress
- Prolonged second stage of labour
- Exhaustion, dehydration and ketosis
- Obstructed labour
- Instrumental/operative interventions
- Perineal lacerations and trauma
- Trauma from operative or instrumental delivery
- Risk of infection associated with prolonged rupture of membranes
- Psychological trauma

Fetus/baby:

- Hypoxia resulting from prolonged labour
- Cord prolapse (predisposed to by a high presenting part)
- Risk of infection if there is prolonged rupture of membranes
- Cerebral haemorrhage from unfavourable upward moulding
- Injury to the baby from presentation or interventions
- Hypothermia or hypoglycaemia if hypoxic or if resuscitation has been required

---

FURTHER READING AND RESOURCES

Bogner G, Strobl M, Schausberger C, Fischer T, Reisenberger K, Jacobs VR. Breech delivery in the all fours position: a prospective observational comparative study with classic assistance. J Perinat Med. 2015 Nov;43(6):707–713. Available from: <doi:10.1515/jpm-2014-0048>. PMID: 25204214.

One of the first modern studies of women with breech positions undertaking vaginal birth in the 'all fours' position.

Impey LWM, Murphy DJ, Griffiths M, Penna LK, On Behalf of the Royal College of Obstetricians and Gynaecologists. Management of breech presentation. BJOG. 2017;124:e151–e177. Available from: <doi:10.1111/1471-0528.14465>

Current UK guidelines for care when there is a breech presentation.

REFERENCES

1. Impey, LWM, Murphy, DJ, Griffiths, M, Penna, LK on behalf of the Royal College of Obstetricians and Gynaecologists. RCOG greentop guideline no 20b: management of breech presentation. BJOG. 2017;124:e151–e177. Available from: <doi:10.1111/1471-0528.14465>

2. Kotaska A & Menticoglou S. SOGC Clinical Practice Guideline No. 384: management of Breech Presentation at Term. Journal of Obstetrics and Gynaecology Canada 2019;41(8):1193–1205. Available from: <doi:/10.1016/j.jogc.2018.12.018>

3. The Royal Australian and New Zealand College of Obstetricians and Gynaecologists (RANZCOG). Management of breech presentation. 2021. Available from: https://ranzcog.edu.au/wp-content/uploads/2022/05/Management-of-breech-presentation.pdf

4. Nassar N, Roberts C, Morris J. Breech presentation. BMJ Best Practice. 2023. Available from: https://bestpractice.bmj.com/topics/en-gb/668

5. Hemelaar J, Lim L, Impey L. The impact of an ECV service is limited by antenatal breech detection: a retrospective cohort study. Birth 2015;42(2):165–172. Available from: <doi:10.1111/birt.12162>

6. Wastlund D, Moraitis A, Dacey A, Sovio U, Wilson E, Smith G. Screening for breech presentation using universal late-pregnancy. PLoS Med. 2019;16(4):e1002778. Available from: <doi:10.1371/journal.pmed.1002778>

7. Hobby EAE, editor. The midwives book, or the whole art of midwifry discovered. Oxford: Oxford University Press; 1999. ISBN:0195086538.

8. Wright RC. Reduction of perinatal mortality and morbidity in breech delivery through routine use of cesarean section. Obstet Gynecol. 1959;14:758–763.

9. Steen M. Vaginal or caesarean delivery? How research has turned breech birth around. Evidence Based Midwifery. 2008;6(3):95–99.

10. Hannah ME, Hannah WJ, Hewson SA, Hodnett ED, Saigal S, Willan AR. Planned caesarean section versus planned vaginal birth for breech presentation at term: a randomised multicentre trial: term breech trial collaborative group. Lancet. 2000;21:1375–1383.

11. Glezerman M. Five years to the term breech trial: the rise and fall of a randomized controlled trial. American Journal of Obstetrics & Gynecology. 2006;194(1):20–25.

12. Deans CL, Penn Z. The case for and against vaginal breech delivery. The Obstetrician & Gynaecologist. 2008;10:139–144.

13. Lawson GW. The term breech trial ten years on: primum non nocere? Birth. 2012 39: 3–9.

14. Nursing and Midwifery Council (NMC). Standards of proficiency for midwives. London: NMC; 2019 Nov 18.

15. Macharey G, Gissler M, Toijonen A, Heinonen S & Seikku L. Congential anomalies in breech presentation: a nationwide record linkage study. Congenit Anom (Kyoto) 2021;61(4):112–117. Available from: <doi:10.1111/cga.12411>. Epub 2021 Feb 18. PMID:33559256.

16. Nordtveit TI, Melve KK, Albrechtsen S, Skjaerven R. Maternal and paternal contribution to intergenerational recurrence of breech delivery: population based cohort study. BMJ. 2008 Apr 19;336(7649):872–6. Available from: <doi:10.1136/bmj.39505.436539.BE>. Epub 2008 Mar 27. PMID: 18369204; PMCID: PMC2323052.

17. Cammu H, Dony N, Martens G, et al. Common determinants of breech presentation at birth in singletons: a population-based study. European Journal of Obstetrics and Gynecology and Reproductive Biology. 2014;177:106–109.

18. Vendittelli F, Rivière O, Crenn-Hébert C, et al. Is a breech presentation at term more frequent in women with a history of cesarean delivery? Am J Obstet Gynecol. 2008;198:521.e1–521.e6.

19. Bricker L, Medley N, Pratt JJ. Routine ultrasound in late pregnancy (after 24 weeks' gestation). Cochrane Database of Systematic Reviews. 2015;6. Art. No.: CD001451. Available from: <doi:10.1002/14651858.CD001451.pub4>

20. National Institute for Health and Care Excellence (NICE). Antenatal care NG201. 2021. Available from: www.nice.org.ukk/guidance/ng201

21. Burns R, Dent K. Chapter 37: breech delivery and ECV in managing obstetric emergencies and trauma. 4th ed. Cambridge: Cambridge University Press; 2022. P. 205–317.

22. Leung VKT, Suen SSH, Sahota DS, et al. External cephalic version does not increase the risk of intra-uterine death: a 17-year

experience and literature review. The Journal of Maternal-Fetal and Neonatal Medicine. 2012;25(9):1774–1778.

23. Impey LWM, Murphy DJ, Griffiths M, Penna LK on behalf of the Royal College of Obstetricians and Gynaecologists. External cephalic version and reducing the incidence of term breech presentation: green-top guideline no. 20a. BJOG 2017; 124:e178–e192. Available from: <doi:10.1111/1471–0528.14466>

24. Burgos J, Melchor JC, Pijoan JI, et al. A prospective study of the factors associated with the success rate of external cephalic version for breech presentation at term. International Journal of Gynecology and Obstetrics. 2011;112(1):48–51.

25. Vallikkannu N, Nadzratulaiman W, Omar S, Si Lay K & Tan P. Talcum powder or aqueous gel to aid external cephalic version: a randomised controlled trial. BMC Pregnancy Childbirth 2014;14:49. Available from: <doi:10.1186/1472-2393-14-49>

26. Vlemmix F, Kuitert M, Bais J, et al. Patient's willingness to opt for external cephalic version. Journal of Psychosomatic Obstetrics and Gynecology. 2013;34(1):15–21.

27. Burgos J, Cobos P, Osuna C, et al. Nitrous oxide for analgesia in external cephalic version at term: prospective comparative study. Journal of Perinatal Medicine. 2013;41(6):719–723.

28. Salzer L; Nagar R; Melamed N; et al. Predictors of successful external cephalic version and assessment of success for vaginal delivery. The Journal of Maternal-Fetal and Neonatal Medicine. 2015;28(1):49–54.

29. Coyle ME, Smith C, Peat B. Cephalic version by moxibustion for breech presentation. Cochrane Database of Systematic Reviews 2023, Issue 5. Art. No.: CD003928. Available from: <doi:10.1002/14651858.CD003928.pub4>

30. Coulon C, Poleszczuk M, Paty-Montaigne M-H, Gascard C, Gay C, Houfflin-Debarge V, Subtil D. Version of breech fetuses by moxibustion with acupuncture: a randomized controlled trial. Obstetrics & Gynecology. July 2014;124(1):32–39. Available from: <doi:10.1097/AOG.0000000000000303>

31. Zanchin C. Breech presentation and moxibustion: should it be offered to improve maternal outcomes? British Journal of Midwifery 2021;29:12 Available from: <doi:10.12968/bjom.2021.29.12.692>

32. Coyle ME, Smith CA, Peat B. Cephalic version by moxibustion for breech presentation. Cochrane Database of Systematic Reviews. 2012;5. Art. No.: CD003928. Available from: <doi:10.1002/14651858.CD003928.pub3>

33. Weston M1, Grabowska C. Moxibustion to turn the breech. Pract Midwife. 2012 Sep;15(8):S3–S4.

34. Nursing and Midwifery Council (NMC). The code: professional standards of practice and behaviour for nurses, midwives and nursing associates. 2015 updated 2018. Available from: https://www.nmc.org.uk/standards/code/

35. Hofmeyr GJ, Kulier R. Cephalic version by postural management for breech presentation. Cochrane Database of Systematic Reviews. 2012;10. Art. No.: CD000051. Available from: <doi:10.1002/14651858.CD000051.pub2>

36. Ressi B & O'Beirne 2015 Detecting breech presentation before labour: lessons from a low-risk maternity clinical J Obstet Gynaecol Can 37:702–706. Available from: <doi:10.1016/S1701–2163(15)30174–2>

37. National Institute for Health and Care Excellence (NICE). Intrapartum care for women with existing medical conditions or obstetric complications and their babies [O] evidence review for breech presenting in labour NICE guideline NG121. 2019. Available from: www.nice.org.uk/guidance/ng121

38. Mattiolo S, Spillane E & Walker S. Physiological breech birth training: an evaluation of clinical practice changes after a one-day training program. Birth. 2021;48:558–565. Available from: <doi:10.1111/birt.12562>

39. Bogner G, Strobl M, Schausberger C, Fischer T, Reisenberger K, Jacobs VR. Breech delivery in the all fours position: a prospective observational comparative study with classic assistance. J Perinat Med. 2015 Nov;43(6):707–13. Available

from: <doi:10.1515/jpm-2014-0048>. PMID: 25204214.

40. Mirza E, Chandraharan E. Chapter 9: breech delivery in obstetric and intrapartum emergencies. 2nd ed. Editor. Chandraharan E, Arulkumaran SS. Cambridge: Cambridge University Press; 2021. P. 56–65.

41. Reitter A, Halliday A, Walker S. Practical insight into upright breech birth from birth videos: a structured analysis. Birth. 2020;47:211–219. Available from: <doi:10.1111/birt.12480>

42. Burns R, Dent K. Chapter 38: twin pregnancy in managing obstetric emergencies and trauma. 4th ed. Cambridge: Cambridge University Press; 2022. P. 319–322.

43. Simm A. Fetal malpresentation. Obstetrics, Gynaecology and Reproductive Medicine. 2007;17(10):283–288. Available from: <doi:10.1016/j.ogrm.2007.07.007>

44. Devin K & Chambliss L. A compound presentation resulting in compartment syndrome in a newborn. Journal of Pediatric Surgery Case Reports. 2022;78. Available from: <doi:10.1016/j.epsc.2022.102199>

45. Talaulikar VS, Arulkumaran S. Malpositions and malpresentationd of the fetal head. Obstetrics, Gynaecology and Reproductive Medicine. 2012;22(6):155–161.

46. Olsen M. Malpresentation. Chapter 20 in Obstetric Care edited by M Olsen pp. 188–196. Cambridge University Press; 2017. Available from: <doi:10.1017/9781316662571.021>

47. Sinha S, Talaulikar V & Arulkumaran S. Malpositions and malpresentations of the fetal head. Obstetrics, Gynaecology and Reproductive Medicine 2018;28(3):83–91.

48. Tapisiz OL, Aytan H, Altinbas SK et al, Face presentation at term: a forgotten issue. The Journal of Obstetrics and Gynaecology Research. 2014;40(6):1573–1577.

49. Ducarme G, Ceccaldi PF, Chesnoy V, Robinet G, Gabriel R. Face presentation: retrospective study of 32 cases at term. Gynecol Obstet Fertil. 2006;34(5):393–396. French. Available from: <doi:10.1016/j.gyobfe.2005.07.042>

Cord prolapse

CLARE GORDON

Introduction   143
Pathophysiology   144
Risk/pre-disposing features   144
Clinical Features   144
Care   145
Management   145

Outcomes/follow-up/long term   148
Professional considerations   149
Summary of midwifery responsibilities 149
Further resources   149
References   150

BOX 9.1: Definitions

Cord prolapse is a well-documented obstetric complication, but the definitions are not always consistent in the literature. However, it is recognized that there are two types of cord prolapse.[1]

Overt cord prolapse is where the umbilical cord lies in front of the presenting part when the membranes have ruptured and may be visible at the vulva.

Occult cord prolapse is defined as the descent of the umbilical cord through the cervix, lying alongside the presenting part but not in front of the fetal presenting part.

Cord presentation is when any part of the umbilical cord is between the presenting part and the cervix with or without membrane rupture.[1,2]

INTRODUCTION

The incidence of cord prolapse has declined since the 1940s from 6.4 per 1,000 live births to 1.7 per 1,000 live births in the 2000s.[3] This can largely be attributed to less grand multiparity and a significant increase in caesarean sections. With this, there is clear evidence of a decrease in mortality rates.[3] This can also be related to the changes in obstetric practices around breech birth. A significant study found that cord prolapse occurred in around 19.4% of twin pregnancies, 41.9% in breech presentation, 66.7% in multigravidas and 34.4% were <37/40 gestation.[4]

Better access to antenatal care hopefully leads to greater detection of an abnormal lie, and women who are known to have a non-cephalic presentation in the later stages of pregnancy are more likely to have this confirmed on ultrasound scans as well as by palpation. Practices around obstetric advice for women whose babies are breech have changed dramatically in the last few decades. RCOG guidelines now recommend external cephalic version, and if this is unsuccessful, an elective caesarian section for all breech presentations at term.[5] See Chapter 8 for a further discussion concerning breech presentation.

Current expectations are that babies of lower gestations are expected to have better outcomes than in previous years, and in addition, those babies who formerly would not have survived now do; therefore, care must reflect this, with antenatal admission a

DOI: 10.4324/9781003382195-9

common response when any risk is identified.[6] If an unstable lie is detected, women are advised to remain an inpatient or have greater access to outpatient services and be managed expectantly at home,[7] which will optimise care if a cord prolapse does occur.

PATHOPHYSIOLOGY

Once the position of the cord becomes compromised, especially when out of the vagina, the fetal blood supply is obstructed. This is either because of the drop in temperature and spasm of the vessels or compression between the bony pelvis and the presenting part; therefore, the amount of time from prolapse to birth determines the level of injury to the baby. This starts as fetal hypoxia in varying degrees, and if delivery is not imminent, it may be followed by fetal or neonatal death. However, less than 3% of babies suffering from a prolapsed cord will die if birth is expedited.[8] The condition of the baby at the moment of prolapse and subsequent asphyxia is predicative of outcome. Therefore, low birthweight, premature babies and those suffering anomalies are likely to have less good outcomes.[9]

RISK/PRE-DISPOSING FEATURES

There are recognised risk factors for cord presentation and cord prolapse – most associated with malpresentation, smaller babies and multiparous women. If there is room for the cord to slip in front of the presenting part, there is the risk of a cord presentation or prolapse (Table 9.1). Women who present with transverse/oblique or unstable lie or a footling breech presentation after 37 + 0 weeks of pregnancy are usually offered admission to an antenatal ward within an obstetric-led unit that can accommodate an emergency caesarean section should the need arise. Any labour or SROM when the baby is an abnormal lie is an indication for urgent referral and probably emergency caesarean section.[7]

Around half of all reported cases of cord prolapse have occurred after an intervention.[10] Women who opt for external cephalic version of a breech presentation should be informed of all associated risks (see Chapter 8), and the midwife should be prepared for a cord prolapse, providing the appropriate environment accordingly.[9,10] Induction of labour itself is cited as a possible risk factor; however, whether this is related to artificial rupture of membranes specifically is disputed.[6,9,10,11]

CLINICAL FEATURES

Diagnosis

In almost all cases, overt cord prolapse is diagnosed by vaginal examination. The cord may be visible at the introitus or a pulsating mass may be felt on vaginal examination.[10] It is important to note that occult cord prolapse is less easily diagnosed as the

Table 9.1 Associations with cord prolapse and cord presentation[7]

General	Procedure related
Multiparity	Artificial rupture of membranes with high presenting part
Low birthweight (<2.5kg)	Vaginal manipulation of the fetus with ruptured membranes
Preterm labour (less than 37 weeks)	External cephalic version (during procedure)
Fetal congenital abnormalities	Internal podalic version
Breech presentation	Stabilising induction of labour
Transverse, oblique and unstable lie*	Insertion of intrauterine pressure transducer
Second twin	Large balloon catheter induction of labour (if filled >180 mls)
Polyhydramnios	
Unengaged presenting part	
Low-lying placenta	

* Unstable lie is when the longitudinal axis of the fetus (lie) is changing repeatedly after 37[+0] weeks.
Reproduced from: Royal College of Obstetricians and Gynaecologists. 'Umbilical Cord Prolapse. Green-top Guideline No. 50, London: RCOG; November 2014, with the permission of the College.

cord will not be felt on vaginal examination. Fetal bradycardia or variable decelerations may be seen on a CTG or heard during auscultation. Whilst this is not definitive, it should be considered a differential diagnosis as having an origin in malpresentation of the cord.

CARE

When discussing the place of birth with women and providing them with information with which to make a decision, the position of her baby is one area of discussion during a risk assessment. If the woman is considering or requesting support to birth at home or in a midwife-led birth centre, she should be informed that the position of her baby will be an issue for further discussion should the lie of her baby become unstable, transverse and/or oblique, or a breech presentation (see Chapter 8 for further discussion of breech presentation).

Before performing a vaginal examination, if, during the preliminary abdominal palpation, the midwife finds any mobility of the presenting part, she should consider whether a VE could initiate a cord prolapse. Any high head should alert the midwife to inform other members of the team, ensuring the ability to respond in case an inadvertent ROM during the VE causes a cord prolapse during the procedure.

It is normal midwifery practice to assess fetal well-being after spontaneous rupture of membranes (SROM). It is also pertinent to consider the merits of performing a VE in all women known to have a non-engaged presenting part as, if the head remains high; there may be a cord prolapse without immediate compromise to the fetal condition.

MANAGEMENT

Regardless of location, whether in hospital or in a community setting, if a cord presentation or prolapse is suspected or diagnosed, assistance must be called and pressure from the cord relieved. In hospital, this would usually necessitate an emergency response – or crash call – in order to mobilise the necessary staff to facilitate a potential emergency caesarean delivery. In a community situation, during either a planned or unplanned homebirth, this is an emergency situation. The midwife should provide immediate support measures as detailed in what follows and instruct either the woman, her birth partner or any other person present to call emergency services (dial 999 in the UK) for an immediate transfer to hospital. The instructions to the operator must be clear and concise. Local policies and procedures may prescribe the wording for such emergencies.

Current evidence does not recommend attempting to replace the cord or wrapping warm swabs around the prolapsed cord. In fact, these procedures may delay delivery.[9,10,12] However, although evidence is insufficient to support this practice, midwives in an emergency situation outside of an obstetric unit will utilise every skill available to them and gentle replacement of the cord to within the vagina while awaiting the emergency services may help to keep it warm and viable. However, it must be remembered that handling may also cause the cord to spasm, and extreme care must be paramount.

Procedures must not inflict any time delay towards delivery – if the cord has prolapsed, the aim is delivery.

1. To alleviate cord compression, the presenting part is elevated – in the first instance, use fingers to push the head away from the cord, then, if a delay before delivery is anticipated, fill the bladder (see Box 9.2). In hospital, it would be pertinent to call for help and then digitally

---

BOX 9.2: Filling the bladder following a cord prolapse

To fill the bladder, a Foley urinary catheter is sited, 500–750mls of sterile saline solution is inserted and the tubing is then clamped. With the clamp still in place, drainage tubing and a drainage bag are attached, ready for the clamp to be removed when the caesarean section commences.[9] If available, an IV/blood-giving set can be inserted into the catheter to expedite filling.[1,10]

It is often suggested that once the bladder is filled, it is still necessary to digitally displace the presenting part; however, a study by Bord et al.[13] found no significant difference in outcome when the presenting part was supported digitally once the bladder had been filled.

Catheterisation and other necessary equipment must be available at a planned homebirth.

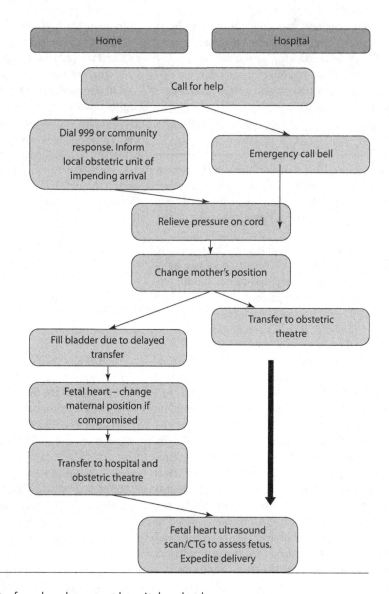

Figure 9.1 Management of cord prolapse – at hospital and at home

elevate the presenting part whilst others assist. At home, once assistance has been called, the bladder can be filled and/or digital manipulation continued.

2. Maternal position – either knee-chest position (see Figure 9.1) or exaggerated Sims (see Figures 9.2 and 9.3) until birth is imminent. If transferring from home to hospital, the knee-chest position is not safe in an ambulance; therefore, the midwife should change the woman to exaggerated Sims whilst keeping pressure off the cord, either with digital

elevation or with the bladder still full. In a hospital, the woman is usually transferred to the operating theatre on her bed – the midwife can sit on the bed, maintaining elevation of the fetal head during the transfer.

3. Ensure patent IV access.
4. Provide facial oxygen, if available, at 8 L/min.
5. Stop any oxytocin infusion.
6. A tocolytic may be considered if there is an unavoidable delay and if there is enough assistance available, provided this does not delay the procedures needed to expedite delivery.

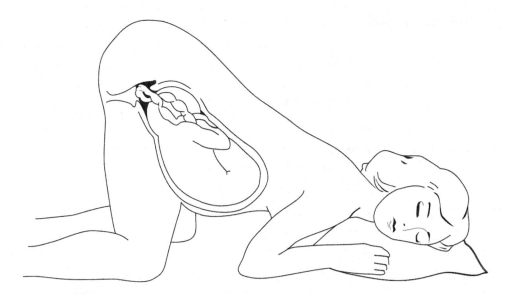

Figure 9.2 Knee-chest position

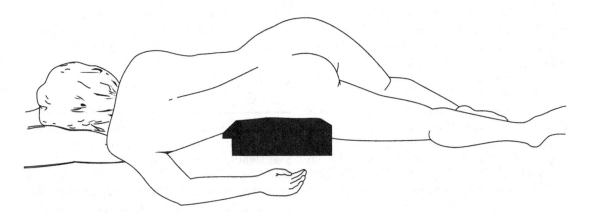

Figure 9.3 Exaggerated Sims position

In hospital, the fetal heart is not usually monitored until after the emergency call for help and transfer to labour ward/theatre, as this could delay delivery. Then, auscultation and/or continuous fetal monitoring will display if fetal bradycardia or any pathological heart rate patterns are present, which will indicate an immediate caesarean. An emergency caesarean section should be performed with the aim of delivering the baby within 30 minutes or less.[7]

However, at home, after the initial responses, while waiting for the emergency services and during the transfer from home to hospital, the midwife should endeavour to continue to monitor the fetal heart. If heart rate abnormalities occur, it may be pertinent to alter maternal position and/

or management. If digital displacement has moved the presenting part above the pelvic brim, a midwife may consider continuous suprapubic pressure upwards.[14] Midwives should always put the woman at the centre of care, and therefore, they will decide on an individual basis if they feel the extra manipulations would be of benefit in the context.

Mode of Birth

When at home or in a midwifery-led birth centre, if the woman's cervix is fully dilated, the midwife must make a judgement as to whether the baby can be delivered quickly vaginally (by maternal effort and perhaps with the aid of an episiotomy) or

Table 9.2 Checklist to manage cord prolapse

Consider	**Assess Risk:**
	Malpresentation
	High presenting part
	Every VE in labour
	At every fetal heart rate anomaly, particularly after SROM
	After SROM with risk factors
Call for help	**At home:**
	Emergency services (999 in UK)
	In hospital:
	Emergency crash call
Relieve	**Pressure from cord:**
	Maternal position
	Digital displacement
	Fill bladder
Birth	Emergency transfer by quickest means to an obstetric theatre

whether the insult to the baby would be better alleviated by undertaking the measures described previously and transfer to obstetric care. Regardless of her decision, emergency help must be called for, as even after a successful vaginal delivery, the baby will likely need resuscitation.

In hospital, an assessment of fetal viability will determine the course of action.

Once fetal viability has been confirmed, the stage of labour needs to be established. If the cervix is fully dilated, it may be possible to expedite delivery either with maternal effort (more likely if multiparous), ventouse or forceps if the head is fully engaged and the requirements for instrumental delivery are met. If vaginal delivery is not likely to be swift, then an early resort to caesarean section is necessary.

If the woman's cervix is not fully dilated and no CTG abnormalities are detected, continuous electronic fetal monitoring should be maintained and preparation for surgery instigated. The speed of this preparation will be defined by the fetal condition, with an emphasis on minimising any insult and long-term effects on the baby. Women should provide verbal consent, and the bladder must be emptied prior to incision. At all times, communication is paramount to inform the woman and her birth companions of events.

If there is any fetal heart activity, then emergency procedures must be followed to expedite

delivery. If an ultrasound scan confirms no heartbeat is present, then the sequence of events is not an emergency situation (Table 9.2).

OUTCOMES/FOLLOW-UP/ LONG TERM

Outcomes for the baby do depend on where the mother is when the prolapse takes place and the availability of an obstetric theatre and relevant staff. The prognosis for the baby is generally very good if accessibility to a fully staffed obstetric theatre is available.[15] When prolapse occurs outside of hospital or in a lower-resourced setting, outcomes for the baby are less predictable. Perinatal mortality is increased by more than ten-fold when cord prolapse occurs outside hospital when compared to inside. The length of time to delivery – with the emergency procedures described in place – appears to predict outcomes. If more than 30 minutes pass from prolapse until delivery, then the outcomes for the baby are less favourable.[10]

Cord prolapse, although potentially fatal for the baby, is not associated with increased morbidity for the mother, providing due care and attention is paid to preparing her for emergency surgery. Despite the extremely rapid delivery needed by the fetus, the maternal physical and psychological risks are that of an emergency caesarean and potential psychological disturbance.[8,12]

PROFESSIONAL CONSIDERATIONS

As with all obstetric emergencies, actions must be accompanied by communication with the woman and her birth partners. Sudden onset changes, such as necessitating emergency management techniques, need to be communicated calmly and sensitively in order to minimise distress and still keep the woman informed.

It is vital to document a clear chain of events, not only to provide evidence for peer reflection and risk management review but also to provide the family with a transparent review of the care they received. Some hospital Trusts have developed a proforma with which to document the chain of events, and if not, then usual midwifery standards apply. As discussed in Chapter 1, documentation should be clear, concise, factual and as contemporaneous as possible.[16]

In order to improve practice, it is necessary to reflect on what has worked well and what needs improvement. In a review of multidisciplinary team working in responding to obstetric emergencies, it is evident that the ability to communicate events relies not only on the documentation but on the ability of all members of the multidisciplinary team to function effectively.[17,18] Simulation training for cord prolapse is often omitted from multidisciplinary team training despite large amounts of evidence that it should be included alongside other obstetric emergencies.[19,20] It is possibly dependent on whether midwives or doctors are responsible for delivering the programme, as midwives report that training improves their practice more than doctors.[17]

Each Trust or organisation will have its own procedures to report such incidents for further investigation, either a clinical incident form or another. As a midwife involved in the case, there should be a liaison with the team to ensure this has been completed.

SUMMARY OF MIDWIFERY RESPONSIBILITIES

- **Call for help** – In hospital, use the 'crash call system' – the senior midwife, senior obstetric team, anaesthetic team and neonatologists are needed. An emergency caesarean section is the most likely outcome.

- In a home/community environment – stay with the woman and get someone else to call emergency services (dial 999 in the UK). Immediate transfer to the nearest obstetric unit will most likely be needed. If the woman is delivering, then paramedics may be helpful for neonatal resuscitation as well as subsequent transfer.

- **Management procedures** – Maternal – Reposition to relieve cord compression and relieve pressure on cord digitally. Consider filling the bladder.

- **Fetal** – Auscultate the fetal heart, ensuring maternal heart rate is differentiated when the previously mentioned actions are in place but do not delay transfer to the operating theatre.

- **Communicate** – With the woman and her birth companions.

- **Document** – Use a proforma if available. If not, ensure a concise, streamlined and factual chain of events.

- **Reflect** – With peers and MDT.

- **Risk Management** – Explore any risk factors that were present. Any multidisciplinary team training issues following emergency procedures should be identified. Complete incident reports for Trust or organisation clinical governance purposes.

- **Debrief** – Offer the woman and any birth companions who were present the opportunity to discuss and debrief.

FURTHER RESOURCES

Royal College of Obstetricians and Gynaecologists (RCOG) Chebsey CS, Bristol BS, Fox R, Draycott TJ, Siassakos D, Winter C. Royal college of obstetricians and gynaecologists umbilical cord prolapse green-top guideline no. 50.257. 2014 Nov. [Accessed 17 July 2023]. Available from: www.rcog.uk

Pagan M, Eads L, Sward L, Manning N, Hunzicker A, Magann EF. Umbilical cord prolapse: a review of the literature. Obstet Gynecol Surv. 2020;75(8):510–518 Available from: <doi:10.1097/OGX.0000000000000818>

Collins S, Hayes K, Arulkumaran S, Arambage K, Impey L, editors. Oxford textbook of obstetrics and gynaecology. Oxford: Oxford University Press; 2023.

REFERENCES

1. Wong L, Hoi Wan Kwan A, Ling Lau S, To Angla Sin W, Yeung Leung T. Umbilical cord prolapse: revisiting its definition and management. Am J Obstet Gynecol [Internet] 2021. [Accessed 10 July 2023]. Available from: <doi:10.1016/j.ajog.2021.06.077>

2. Doumouchtsis, SK. Emergencies in obstetrics and gynaecology. Oxford: Oxford University Press; 2016.

3. Gibbons C, O'Herlihy C, Murphy JF. Umbilical Cord Prolapse- changing patterns and improved outcomes: a retrospective cohort study BJOG: Int J Obstet Gynaecol.[Internet] 2014; 121 (13): 1705–1708. Available from: <doi:10.1111/1471-0528.12890>

4. Gannard-Pechin E, Ramanah R, Cossa S, et al. Umbilical cord prolapse: a case study over 23 years. J Gynecol Obstet Hum Reprod. 2012; 41(6): 574–583. Available from: <doi:10.1016/j.jgyn.2012.06.001>

5. Royal College of Obstetricians and Gynaecologists (RCOG), Impey, LWM, Murphy DJ, Griffiths, M, Penna LK. The management of breech presentation Green-top guideline No. 20b. Br J Obstet Gynaecol. 2017;124:e151-e177. [Accessed 10 July 2023]. Available from: https://obgyn.onlinelibrary.wiley.com/doi/epdf/10.1111/1471-0528.14465

6. Obeidat N, Zayed F, Alchalabi H. Umbilical cord prolapse: a 10-year retrospective study in two civil hospitals, North Jordan J Obstet and Gynaecol. 2010; 30 (3): 257–260. Available from: <doi:10.3109/01443610903474330>

7. Royal College of Obstetricians and Gynaecologists (RCOG) Chebsey CS, Bristol BS, Fox R, Draycott TJ, Siassakos D, Winter C. Royal College of Obstetricians and Gynaecologists Umbilical Cord Prolapse Green-top Guideline No. 50.257. 2014 Nov. [Accessed 17 July 2023]. Available from: www.rcog.uk

8. Layden, EA, Thomson, A, Owen, P, Madhra, M, Macgowan, BA. Clinical obstetrics and gynaecology. 5th ed. Amsterdam: Elsevier; 2023.

9. Burns R, Dent K. editors Managing medical obstetric emergencies and trauma. Chichester: John Wiley and Sons; 2022.

10. Pagan, M, Eads, L, Sward, L, Manning, N, Hunzicker, A, Magann, EF. Umbilical cord prolapse: a review of the literature. Obstet Gynecol Surv. 2020; 75(8): 510–518. Available from: <doi:10.1097/OGX.0000000000000818>

11. Chapman V. Cord prolapse and cord presentation. In: Chapman V, Charles C, editors. The midwife's labour and birth handbook. Chichester: John Wiley and Sons; 2017. P. 315–338.

12. Sayed Ahmed, WA, Hamdy, MA. Optimal management of umbilical cord prolapse. Int J Womens Health. 2018; 10: 459–465

13. Bord I, Gemer O, Anteby EY, Shenhav S. The value of bladder filling in addition to manual elevation of presenting fetal part in cases of cord prolapse. Arch Gynecol Obstet. 2011 May; 283(5):989–91. Available from: <doi:10.1007/s00404-010-1509-y>

14. World Health Organisation, United Nations Population Fund, UNICEF, The World Bank Managing complications in pregnancy and childbirth: a guide for midwives and doctors. 2nd ed. 2017. [Accessed 10 July 2023]. Available from: https://apps.who.int/iris/handle/10665/255760

15. Wong, L. Tse, WT, Lai, CY, Hui, ASY, Chaemsaithong, P, Sahota, DS, Poon. LC, Leung, TY. Bradycardia-to delivery interval and fetal outcomes in umbilical cord prolapse. Acta Obstet Gynecol Scand. 2020; 100 (1): 170–177. Available from: <doi:10.1111/agos.13985>

16. Nursing and Midwifery Council. The Code – Professional standards of practice and behaviour for nurses, midwives and nursing associates. (2015 updated 2018) London: NMC; 2015 updated 2018.

17. Calvert KL, McGurgan PM, Debenham EM. Emergency obstetric simulation training: how do we know where we are going, if we don't know where we have been? Aust N Z J Obstet Gynaecol. 2013; 53(6):509–51. Available from: <doi:10.1111/ajo.12120>

18. Black, SE. Obstetric emergencies: enhancing the multidisciplinary team through

simulation. Br J Midwifery. 2018; 25 (2): 96–102 Available from: <doi:10.12968/bjom.2018.26.2.96>

19. Chebsey C, Siassakos D, Draycott T. A review of umbilical cord prolapse and the influence of training on management Fetal Matern Med Rev. 2012; 23 (2): 120–130. Available from: <doi:10.1017/S0965539512000058>

20. Calvert K, Raman P, Nathan E, Epee M. The effect of a multidisciplinary obstetric emergency team training program, the In Time course, on diagnosis to delivery interval following umbilical cord prolapse – a retrospective cohort study. The Royal Australian and New Zealand College of Obstetricians and Gynaecologists. 2016;57(3):327–333. Available from: <doi:10.1111/ajo.12530>

10

Shoulder dystocia

DEBRA SLOAM

Introduction	152	Summary of midwifery responsibilities	160
Pathophysiology	153	Further reading and resources	160
Risk/predisposing factors	153	References	161
Clinical features	154		

BOX 10.1: Shoulder Dystocia

The current definition of shoulder dystocia includes the following: [1,2,3,4,5]

- Shoulder dystocia occurs during a vaginal birth in cephalic presentation.
- After the baby's head is born, the shoulders fail to deliver spontaneously using routine axial traction alone.
- Additional obstetric manoeuvres are required to successfully deliver the baby's shoulders and complete the birth.

Other parameters, such as a documented head-to-body interval of greater than one minute have been suggested to aid diagnosing shoulder dystocia. [5]

INTRODUCTION

Shoulder dystocia is a birth emergency that is difficult to predict and has the potential for serious short- and long-term health consequences for both mother and infant (Figure 10.1). Noted to be increasing in frequency in recent years, inappropriate management can worsen outcomes with significant cost to the woman and her family, the midwifery and maternity team, and the wider NHS.

The Royal College of Obstetricians and Gynaecologists (RCOG) defines shoulder dystocia 'as a vaginal cephalic delivery that requires additional obstetric manoeuvers to deliver the fetus after the head has delivered and gentle traction has failed' (p. 2).[2] Other authorities have slightly different definitions or criteria for diagnosing shoulder dystocia, but they all recognise normal measures undertaken to support the birth of the infant are not sufficient and additional manoeuvres are required.[1,3,4,5]

There can be variation in the reported rate of shoulder dystocia (SD) due to several factors, with the definition and recognition of shoulder dystocia influenced by training, competence, and experience of the healthcare providers involved.[6,7,8,9,10] Therefore, the reported rates of shoulder dystocia vary across studies and countries. Deneux-Thoraux and Delorme conducted a systematic review in France and other resource-rich countries and reported a rate of 0.5–1% of vaginal births being complicated by shoulder dystocia.[4] Other studies from different countries have reported rates such 0.33% of births in Sweden and 0.4% of births in a study by Riggs et al. in the US to just over 3% of births are complicated by shoulder dystocia in the UK.[6,11,12]

DOI: 10.4324/9781003382195-10

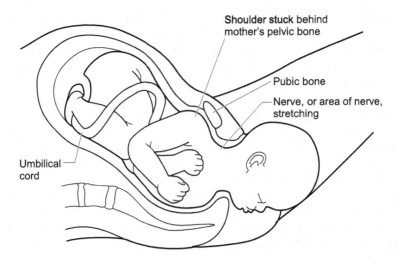

Figure 10.1 Shoulder dystocia (reproduced from the Royal College of Obstetricians and Gynaecologists Patient information leaflet Shoulder Dystocia (2012). London: RCOG, with the kind permission of the Royal College of Obstetricians and Gynaecologists)

Midwives play a pivotal role in childbirth, attending the majority of births and facilitating over 55% of births in the UK.[13] Consequently, midwives are often at the forefront of managing shoulder dystocia when it occurs. It is essential midwives have a thorough understanding of the risk factors and warning signs of shoulder dystocia. Accurate assessment and timely, evidence-informed intervention can make a significant difference when managing this obstetric emergency and minimising potential complications.

The impact of shoulder dystocia extends beyond the physical aspects of the emergency. It can have a lasting psychological effect on the woman, her family, and the healthcare professionals involved.[14,15,16] These often serious and long-lasting psychological and emotional repercussions can influence many facets of both personal and professional lives.[1,14,17,18,19,20] It is important to recognise and address the effects of shoulder dystocia on all individuals involved, to provide appropriate support, care and follow up.

Continuing education, training, and professional development for midwives and the maternity team can help enhance their knowledge and skills in managing shoulder dystocia and provide them with the tools to effectively support women and their families and the wider maternity team during and after this challenging obstetric emergency.

PATHOPHYSIOLOGY

In a typical labour without shoulder dystocia, the fetal shoulders enter the pelvic brim in an oblique or transverse diameter, allowing them to pass relatively easily through the pelvis. However, in cases of shoulder dystocia, the bisacromial diameter is aligned in the direct anterior-posterior (A-P) position. This alignment results in the impaction of the anterior shoulder above the symphysis pubis as the fetus enters the pelvic inlet during labour. In some instances, the posterior shoulder may become impacted on the sacral promontory. Rarely, both shoulders may become trapped above the brim of the pelvis, preventing the fetus from passing through the pelvis.

Subsequent management of shoulder dystocia aims to create more space for the fetus to manoeuvre through the pelvis. This can involve external and/or internal manoeuvres that aim to flatten the sacral promontory to widen the anterior-posterior diameter of the pelvic inlet or dislodge the shoulders under the symphysis pubis.

RISK/PREDISPOSING FACTORS

Findings consistently indicate that although certain risk factors can be identified, they are, at best, weakly or poorly predictive of shoulder dystocia. While some studies, including retrospective studies like Larad et al. and prospective studies like Bouchghoul et al., have attempted to identify specific characteristics or risk factors for shoulder dystocia, the predictive value of these characteristics remains weak even when they cluster together.[21,22,23,24,25,26] Ultrasound measurements of the fetus have been explored as a potential predictor, but studies such as Shinohara et al. have found that these measurements are not able to predict shoulder dystocia accurately.[27,28,29]

However, certain factors have been identified that can increase the risk of a birth being complicated by shoulder dystocia (see Box 10.2).

There has been a growing awareness of the increase in frequency of shoulder dystocia, perhaps attributed to changes within the population of childbearing women.[31,33] These changes include factors such as increased maternal age, higher rates of obesity, and an increase in the incidence of conditions like gestational diabetes, which are known to be associated with larger birth weights and an increased risk of shoulder dystocia. However, the increase in shoulder dystocia frequency may also be due, at least in part, to a well-established awareness of the emergency and systematic training. With improved recognition and awareness of shoulder dystocia, maternity staff may be more vigilant in identifying and documenting

cases, leading to an apparent increase in reported frequency.[6,7,8,9,10,34]

Maternal diabetes, both gestational and chronic, can influence the risk of shoulder dystocia in several ways. While the overall weight of the fetus may not be significantly greater in these cases, the growth pattern can be asymmetric, and the trunk may be more solid with wider shoulders. This can be attributed to the distribution of excess fat on the trunk due to the higher levels of glucose exposure in utero. The rates of macrosomia in large infants also vary in different studies. Reported rates of shoulder dystocia in infants weighing 4kg, 4.5kg, or even 5kg (and some studies using the 90th centile for weight parameters) can be as high as 21–23%.[31] Macrosomia, combined with any risk factor(s) such as maternal diabetes, prolonged pregnancy, obesity, increased age, and previous shoulder dystocia, is associated with higher rates of shoulder dystocia.[4,21-31] Their occurrence together does not reliably predict shoulder dystocia, and even with the presence of these risk factors, the majority of births will not be complicated by shoulder dystocia.

CLINICAL FEATURES

Preconception/antenatal care

For women with a previous history of shoulder dystocia, counselling is essential, as they may have a higher risk of shoulder dystocia in subsequent births.[35,36,37] For women with diabetes, good glycemic control is important, but tighter glycemic control during pregnancy does not appear to significantly impact the fetal size or peripartum outcomes related to shoulder dystocia.[38] However, it is associated with an increased likelihood of hypoglycemic episodes in the antenatal period.[38] In cases of short stature, macrosomia, prolonged second stage, and fetal weight >4kg, or any other factor that may increase the risk of shoulder dystocia, careful consideration should be given to the place of birth.[21,22] The causes and contributing factors to shoulder dystocia are multifactorial and likely to be influenced by a combination of maternal, fetal, and environmental factors. In cases where there are risk factors for shoulder dystocia, in the antenatal period, the midwife can discuss this possibility with the woman and refer her to an obstetrician to plan the birth. Consideration of the birthplace, the appropriateness of induction of labour, and ensuring skilled help is readily available should be part of the planning process. While

---

BOX 10.2: Risk/Predisposing factors for shoulder dystocia[4,21-31]

- Previous shoulder dystocia
- Maternal diabetes
- Maternal obesity (BMI greater than 30)
- Short stature
- Prolonged pregnancy
- Induction of labour
- Augmentation of labour
- Assisted vaginal birth (forceps or suction cup/kiwi)
- Fetal macrosomia**
- Older mothers*
- Multiparous mothers*
- Fertility treatment*
  (*Likely to be associated with older age, maternal obesity and/or fetal macrosomia)
  (**>90th centile customised growth chart or >4.5kg (with maternal diabetes) or 5kg without comorbidities[32])

caesarean sections (CS) may sometimes be necessary to mediate the risk of shoulder dystocia, unnecessary CS can have both short-term and long-term consequences for both the mother and the infant.[39] Informed consent is crucial in discussing and making decisions related to CS or any other interventions, and midwives should ensure open communication with the woman during this process.[2,40]

Labour care

Since shoulder dystocia is difficult to predict, it is essential for all midwives and medical staff supporting women in the intrapartum period to be prepared for its potential occurrence. Recognising the signs of shoulder dystocia enables timely intervention (see Box 10.3).

When any signs of potential shoulder dystocia are present, undertaking diagnostic axial traction will determine if the birth will progress normally or if additional manoeuvres are required. If shoulder dystocia is diagnosed, it is important the woman stops pushing, any oxytocin infusion is halted, and excessive or downward traction and fundal pressure are avoided throughout, as these interventions can exacerbate the entrapment and risk further complications.

Calling for help and activating a structured, systematic approach to managing the emergency is essential. Training programmes play a significant role in preparing the multidisciplinary team to handle shoulder dystocia and other maternity emergencies.

Within the training, aspects of communication, teamwork, management techniques, medication, and assessment tools are covered to ensure the safe care of both the woman and her infant during emergencies. These programmes have been widely adopted in National Health Service (NHS) maternity units in the UK and beyond.[6,7,8,11,34,41] The multidisciplinary team is encouraged to train together, enhancing teamwork and coordination during emergencies that occur rarely. By following a structured algorithm or mnemonic, maternity staff can work cohesively, ensuring each member knows their role and responsibilities. There is a strong emphasis on the importance of evidence-based practice and standardised protocols.

Once shoulder dystocia has been recognised, call for help promptly to ensure the appropriate team members are present to manage the emergency effectively. In the United Kingdom, a universal 'crash call' number 2222 has been in use since 2004 as a strategy to quickly gather the necessary team members during emergencies, including shoulder dystocia (see Box 10.4).[42]

BOX 10.3: Signs of potential shoulder dystocia

- Prolonged first and/or second stage
- Slow descent of the head through the Curve of Carus
- Slow birth of the head and face
- The presence of the turtle sign (head retracting against the perineum)
- Lack of head restitution after birth

BOX 10.4: Multidisciplinary team present at shoulder dystocia

Clearly state the emergency as 'shoulder dystocia' to ensure everyone understands the urgency and nature of the situation.

The following team members would be expected to attend:

- Senior midwife: Their experience and expertise can be valuable in managing the emergency with knowledge of staff skill mix and acuity.
- Senior obstetrician: Provide expertise and support during the emergency, including operative interventions if required.
- Anaesthetist: Provide analgesia and/or anaesthesia. Skilled at managing resuscitation.
- Neonatal team: The infant is likely to need resuscitation and an examination to identify any injury after birth.
- Extra midwifery help: Additional midwives can provide support in various roles, such as scribing important information, preparing third-stage drugs, assisting with the management of postpartum haemorrhage (PPH), and assisting with preparing the neonatal resuscitation area and support.

One member of the team to undertake the 'helicopter' role: The 'helicopter' role involves coordinating the team's actions and ensuring effective communication and organisation during the emergency.

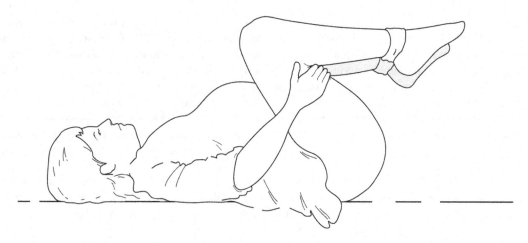

Figure 10.2 McRoberts position

Noting the time when the baby's head is born can provide valuable information to guide the overall management of the emergency. The longer the duration of the shoulder dystocia, the more likely there will be fetal injury, especially fetal hypoxia or hypoxic-ischemic encephalopathy (HIE).[43] A head-to-body birth timing of up to five minutes is considered less likely to result in fetal hypoxia or HIE.[44,45,46] As such, undertaking internal and/or external manoeuvres shown to rectify shoulder impaction as quickly as is safe to do so is recommended. Thus, monitoring the time of head-to-body birth allows the team to assess the duration of the emergency and make decisions accordingly. The caveat to the five-minute guide will always depend on the condition of the fetus prior to the shoulder dystocia. If there are concerns regarding the fetal heart rate pattern, such as signs of fetal distress, there may be less than five minutes to facilitate the birth of the fetus.[47]

In any case of shoulder dystocia, the midwife should be prepared to provide immediate resuscitation and other necessary interventions to support the baby's well-being once the infant is born.

McROBERTS POSITION

The McRoberts manoeuvre is an effective approach to managing shoulder dystocia with a very high success rate of as high as 90%.[2] McRoberts is the least invasive manoeuvre with a low complication rate and therefore employed first. The back of the bed is lowered, pillows are removed, and the mother lies flat. If the woman is in lithotomy, her legs are simultaneously removed, brought together, straightened, and then moved back into McRoberts. It is important to observe this step to reduce the risk of symphyseal diathesis with or without transient femoral neuropathy.[48,49] The woman's thighs are positioned next to the abdomen, bringing her knees up towards her shoulders (see Figure 10.2). This manoeuvre:

- Straightens the maternal lordosis.
- Flattens the sacral promontory.
- Brings the symphysis pubis superiorly and widens the AP diameter of the pelvis.
- Flexes the fetal spine and allows the posterior shoulder to move past the sacrum into the posterior hollow.

SUPRAPUBIC PRESSURE

The addition of suprapubic pressure at this point can nudge the anterior shoulder from above the symphysis pubis into the wider oblique diameter if McRoberts has not corrected the impaction alone. First, palpation for the symphysis pubis and locate the approximate position of the fetal shoulder superiorly to the bone. Place hands together in a 'CPR' position (see Figure 10.3) and apply pressure with the heel of the hand to the posterior aspect of the anterior shoulder. Firm pressure is applied downward and laterally to free the impacted shoulder. When suprapubic pressure is applied, there is no evidence that rocking over continuous pressure is more effective. The key point to remember is that this is a time-limited emergency; therefore,

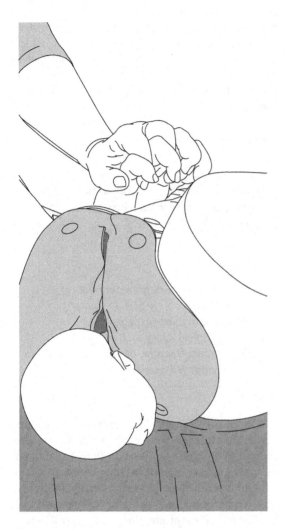

Figure 10.3 Suprapubic pressure

pressure would be applied for no more than 30 seconds.[2] Routine axial traction is applied throughout the external manoeuvres. If there is no movement, then continue with subsequent manoeuvres.

INTERNAL MANOEUVRES

While an episiotomy does not directly address the bony impaction in cases of shoulder dystocia, it might provide better access for internal manoeuvres, making them easier to perform. Episiotomy, when undertaken at times other than to facilitate assisted vaginal birth, appears to increase the risk of OASIS (Obstetric Anal Sphincter Injury).[45,50] Women who experience shoulder dystocia during childbirth appear to be at a higher risk of OASIS, and the use of episiotomy may contribute

to this risk.[51] It has been demonstrated that episiotomy is being performed less frequently in cases of shoulder dystocia than previously.[52] This could indicate a move away from undertaking this procedure due to the significant increase in morbidity for the mother when it is performed and uncertainty regarding episiotomy in resolving shoulder dystocia.[53]

1. *Delivery of the posterior arm*: This is now commonly recommended as the first-line management approach; however, it is suggested that the person undertaking the manoeuvres makes the decision on which manoeuvre to try first, depending on which they feel will be most effective. The manoeuvre involves carefully gaining access to the vagina with a cone-shaped hand (using the hand on the anterior side of the fetus), into the sacral hollow, moving along the fetal humerus, and then gently flexing the posterior fetal arm at the antecubital fossa (A. Figure 10.4). The hand/wrist is then grasped (B. Figure 10.4), and the arm is pulled straight through, thus delivering the posterior arm and shoulder (C. Figure 10.4). This should then allow the anterior shoulder to slip under the maternal symphysis pubis. Applying routine axial traction to the fetal head should then facilitate the birth of the baby. Care should be taken not to pull or hook the upper arm to avoid fracturing the fetal humerus.

2. *Moving the disacromial diameter:* If it is not possible to reach the posterior arm, other internal manoeuvres focus on moving the shoulders into the oblique or transverse diameter. This is achieved by carefully gaining access to the vagina, then with the hand, applying pressure to the anterior aspect of the posterior shoulder, with additional help adding suprapubic pressure in a CPR-like movement (down and across to dislodge the entrapped shoulder). When applying suprapubic pressure, it is crucial to work with the internal rotation rather than against it (pressure to the posterior aspect of the anterior shoulder (externally). If any movement is noted as a result of the manoeuvres, gentle axial traction can be applied to deliver the baby. If there is no movement, the first hand can be removed, and the opposite hand moved into the vagina, again via the

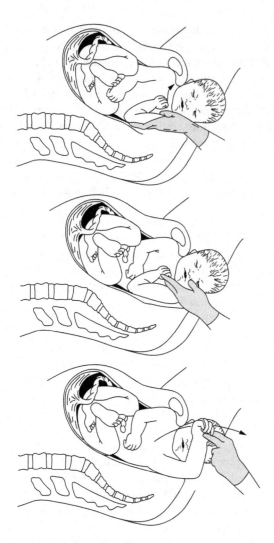

Figure 10.4 Release of the posterior arm

approach.[2,35,54,55] The all-fours position involves the woman being on her hands and knees, which allows for adjustments to the maternal pelvis and sacrum, widening the inlet of the pelvis and potentially facilitating the birth of the posterior shoulder.

Postnatal Care

> ### BOX 10.5: Possible maternal complications following a shoulder dystocia[17,20,45,48,49,53]
>
> - Bruising
> - Bladder injury
> - Third- or fourth-degree perineal laceration
> - Postpartum haemorrhage
> - Psychological injury such as PTSD
> - Dislocation, fracture, or nerve damage (esp. symphysis pubis or hip)

The rate of maternal morbidity is significantly higher among births with shoulder dystocia (14.7%) compared to those without it (8.6%). Shoulder dystocia is associated with an increased risk of adverse outcomes for mothers during childbirth, most commonly third- or fourth-degree perineal laceration.[53] Prompt identification, careful suturing, analgesia, and appropriate follow-up care are important. The increased risk of PPH underpins initial midwifery care, with careful observation of blood loss, uterine tone, and maternal vital signs important (see Chapter 12).

If suprapubic pressure was used, there is a possibility of maternal bladder damage, and observation of fluid balance and renal function should be made. The woman may have an increased need for analgesia after undertaking physical manoeuvres. If the woman presents with continuing pain in the anterior pelvis or across the sacroiliac joints, especially when mobilising, prompt assessment to rule out symphysis pubis diathesis should be undertaken. On-going observation for infection should also be undertaken, especially if internal manoeuvres were used.

For the woman, fear of future childbirth could result from a traumatic birth experience, especially

sacral hollow, to apply pressure to the posterior aspect of the posterior shoulder to attempt to move the disacromial diameter into the wider oblique. If any movement is noted as a result of the manoeuvres, gentle axial traction can be applied to deliver the baby.

It must be noted that Suprapubic pressure should never be applied from the anterior aspect of the infant. This will widen the disacromial diameter, further impacting the posterior shoulder.

In circumstances when a woman is mobile, such as in a home birth setting, and shoulder dystocia occurs, encouraging the woman to adopt an all-fours position can be an effective and safe

BOX 10.6: Possible infant complications following a shoulder dystocia[56,57,58,59,60]

- <7 Apgar score
- Soft tissue damage – bruising, contusion
- Fracture, especially clavicle or humerus
- Brachial Plexus Injury – paraparesis or paralysis of nerves C5-T1 such as Erb's or Klumpke Palsy
- Hypoxic Ischemic Encephalopathy
- Stillbirth or neonatal death

if it involved unexpected outcomes and impacted the mother or the infant. Shoulder dystocia has been found to be three times more likely to result in fear of childbirth compared to other emergencies like emergency caesarean section (CS) or neonatal resuscitation. Therefore, offering psychological support is crucial following shoulder dystocia.[20] A loss of control during childbirth can have a significant impact on a woman's long-term perception of the event.[17,45] Births that involve emergency interventions increase the risk of postnatal post-traumatic stress disorder (PTSD). See Chapter 16 for a discussion concerning mitigating this risk.

Most infants will not suffer any injury during a birth complicated by shoulder dystocia.[6,21,61] However, it is likely, even for the shoulder dystocia that resolves relatively quickly (with external manoeuvres only, for example), the infant may need resuscitation.[57] This could be due to compression of the fetal chest and a subsequent reduction in cardiac output during the emergency. The resulting hypovolemia contributes to a depressed Apgar score and the need for resuscitation following birth.[57,58,59] Infants born following shoulder dystocia may have umbilical cord gases within the normal range pH (set at >7.1) and yet have severely depressed Apgar scores and require resuscitation. Consequently, umbilical arterial pH may not be a reliable guide to the risk of developing Hypoxic Ischemic Encephalopathy (HIE) following shoulder dystocia. Early neonatal gas analysis is indicated to assist in the assessment of the baby's condition, particularly when shoulder dystocia has occurred and the Apgar score is <7 at five minutes.[62] This additional assessment can provide more information to guide appropriate medical management and interventions, even when cord gas results might appear relatively normal.[59]

It is uncommon for there to be soft tissue injury and fracture of the humerus and/or clavicle. However, physical assessment of the neonate should be a priority following all births that require additional manoeuvres to facilitate the birth, regardless of the need for resuscitation.[56] Full assessment of the infant by an experienced clinician such as a Neonatologist should be undertaken to assess for injury, including Brachial Plexus Injury (BPI).

The brachial plexus is a network of nerves that originates from the cervical and upper thoracic spinal nerves and supplies motor and sensory innervation to the upper limb. Its complex course and branching allow it to control movement and sensation in the shoulder, arm, forearm, and hand.

If there is excessive stretching or compression of the brachial plexus, it can lead to various degrees of injury ranging from mild stretching (neuropraxia) to more severe damage, such as rupture or avulsion of the nerve roots.[63] The nerve damage can result in loss or diminished elbow flexion, shoulder external rotation, finger flexion and/or wrist extension.[64] Most BPI involve injury to cervical spine C5-C6 nerve roots (Erb's palsy), and most will resolve within a year following birth.[65,66,67] With injury sustained to the cervical spine-thoracic vertebrae C8-T1 nerve roots (Klumpke palsy) long-term loss of function is more likely to persist.[65,66] There is a correlation between the difficulty in resolving shoulder impaction and the increased likelihood of BPI. Births involving internal manoeuvres and clavicle fractures during shoulder dystocia are associated with a higher risk of brachial plexus injury.[60] The risk of BPI does not solely lie with births complicated by shoulder dystocia and can be present following caesarean section or breech birth or rarely following birth where no difficulty was reported.[68] Accurate documentation (including which shoulder was anterior when the SD was diagnosed) would support identification and early treatment as well as avoid underreporting of BPI and risk of further distress to families.[69]

It is important to provide appropriate care and support to the neonate during their transition to extra-uterine life, with initiation of breastfeeding, skin-to-skin, and relationship building undertaken when safe to do so. Vital signs should be undertaken in the early hours and days following birth, especially for at-risk infants. While most newborns may only require short-term surveillance, certain groups are at higher risk of developing complications during the perinatal period, such as infants following shoulder dystocia. In the general observation of the neonate, the midwife might note unusual crying or movements, which may indicate an undiagnosed injury, prompting referral to a neonatologist. Using a monitoring tool such as 'NEWTT2' to record the well-being of the infant is advised to support early recognition of deterioration and facilitate escalation of concerns as appropriate.[70] This assessment tool incorporates parental concerns, recognising that parents often have valuable insights into their child's well-being and can provide valuable information to the midwife and neonatal staff.[70]

The use of proformas in recording obstetric emergencies like shoulder dystocia allows maternity staff to document the events as they happen, ensuring accurate and contemporaneous documentation throughout the emergency (see Chapter 1 for an example of information that should be included in records made during a shoulder dystocia).

SUMMARY OF MIDWIFERY RESPONSIBILITIES

- Due to the unpredictable nature of shoulder dystocia, midwives and other healthcare staff supporting women during labour and birth must remain aware of the potential for shoulder dystocia to occur at any birth.
- Recognise that risk factors, even combined, are poorly predictive. Referral and escalation of concerns in the antenatal or intrapartum period should be undertaken as appropriate.
- Note the time of the birth of the fetal head.
- Early recognition enables a timely response to the emergency. State 'shoulder dystocia' clearly when gathering assistance.
- Undertake manoeuvres as appropriate according to your local policy or guidance.
- Traction applied should be routine strength only and in line with the fetal spine (axial).
- Throughout the birth, ensure fundal pressure and excessive or lateral traction are avoided.
- Delegation of tasks should be undertaken at the earliest opportunity. Include a scribe to ensure accurate records can be taken and maintained. Using a 'proforma' for the emergency can aid accurate documentation.

- Communicate with and advocate for the woman and her birth partner throughout.
- Recognise the effects of a traumatic experience and mitigate this during the emergency if possible. An opportunity should be offered for reflection after the birth (see Chapter 16).
- Attend training and practice manoeuvres via 'skills drills' whenever possible. Simulation-based training can improve individual and team performance and reduce the incidence of permanent BPI[71] (see Chapter 1 for more details).
- Undertake a personal reflection and consider Restorative Clinical Supervision to manage your own well-being.
- Carry out risk assessments and reporting requirements in line with local maternity unit guidance.

FURTHER READING AND RESOURCES

Prompt manual – Module 10. Available from: https://assets.cambridge.org/97811084/30296/frontmatter/9781108430296_frontmatter.pdf

Prompt Shoulder Dystocia video. Available from: www.youtube.com/watch?v=UTz2eliZOL8

Prompt Shoulder Dystocia Powerpoint. Available from: www.youtube.com/watch?v=9jlhg-zl3po

BAPM Deterioration of the newborn –A framework for practice. Available from: www.bapm.org/resources/deterioration-of-the-newborn-newtt-2-a-framework-for-practice

RCOG green top guidance. Available from: www.rcog.org.uk/guidance/browse-all-guidance/green-top-guidelines/shoulder-dystocia-green-top-guideline-no-42/

   The purpose of this guideline is to review the evidence related to shoulder dystocia and focus on prediction, prevention, and management of shoulder dystocia. There is a strong emphasis on skills training to manage shoulder dystocia. Although published in 2012, much remains unchanged with regard to women most at risk, that shoulder dystocia remains unpredictable, and an evidence-based approach involving the well-trained MDT is advised should this emergency occur.

RCOG patient information leaflet. Available from: www.rcog.org.uk/for-the-public/

browse-all-patient-information-leaflets/
shoulder-dystocia-patient-information-leaflet/

This leaflet can be given to women following an explanation and discussion regarding their individual risk of shoulder dystocia. It will provide a recap of the pertinent points and something for the woman to refer back to when making choices about place or mode of birth.

REFERENCES

1. Politi S, D'emidio L, Cignini P, Giorlandino M, Giorlandino C. Shoulder dystocia: an Evidence-Based approach. J Prenat Med 2010;4(3):35–42.

2. Royal College of Obstetricians and Gynaecologists. Shoulder dystocia: green-top guideline 42. Clinical Guideline. 2012 Mar. Available from: <doi:10.1111/1471-0528.12002>; https://www.rcog.org.uk/guidance/browse-all-guidance/green-top-guidelines/shoulder-dystocia-green-top-guideline-no-42/

3. Hansen A, Chauhan SP. Shoulder dystocia: definitions and incidence. Semin Perinatol 2014;38(4):184–188.

4. Deneux-Tharaux C, Delorme P. [Epidemiology of shoulder dystocia]. J Gynecol Obstet Biol Reprod (Paris) 2015;44(10):1234–1247.

5. Davis DD, Roshan A, Canela CD, Varacallo M. Shoulder dystocia. In: StatPearls. Treasure Island, FL: StatPearls Publishing LLC; 2023.

6. Crofts JF, Lenguerrand E, Bentham GL, Tawfik S, Claireaux HA, Odd D, et al. Prevention of brachial plexus injury-12 years of shoulder dystocia training: an interrupted time-series study. BJOG: An International Journal of Obstetrics & Gynaecology 2016;123(1):111–118.

7. Dahlberg J, Nelson M, Dahlgren MA, Blomberg M. Ten years of simulation-based shoulder dystocia training- impact on obstetric outcome, clinical management, staff confidence, and the pedagogical practice – a time series study. BMC Pregnancy Childbirth 2018;18(1):N.PAG.

8. Olson DN, Logan L, Gibson KS. Evaluation of multidisciplinary shoulder dystocia simulation training on knowledge, performance, and documentation. Am J Obstet Gynecol MFM 2021;3(5):100401.

9. Chou WK, Ullah N, Arjomandi Rad A, Vardanyan R, Shah V, Zubarevich A, et al. Simulation training for obstetric emergencies in low- and lower-middle income countries: a systematic review. Eur J Obstet Gynecol Reprod Biol 2022 September 01;276:74–81.

10. Heinonen K, Saisto T, Gissler M, Kaijomaa M, Sarvilinna N. Rising trends in the incidence of shoulder dystocia and development of a novel shoulder dystocia risk score tool: a nationwide population-based study of 800 484 Finnish deliveries. Acta Obstet Gynecol Scand 2021;100(3):538–547.

11. Mollberg M, Ladfors LV, Strombeck C, Elden H, Ladfors L. Increased incidence of shoulder dystocia but a declining incidence of obstetric brachial plexus palsy in vaginally delivered infants. Acta Obstet Gynecol Scand 2023 January 01;102(1):76–81.

12. Riggs K, Roberts A, Ibarra C, Stafford IA. Has the incidence of hemorrhage after shoulder dystocia changed in the last three decades? AM J OBSTET GYNECOL 2022;226(1):S209.

13. NHS Digital. Compendium of maternity statistics, England, April 2015. 2018. [Accessed 14 January 2023]. Available from: https://digital.nhs.uk/data-and-information/publications/statistical/compendium-of-maternity-statistics/compendium-of-maternity-statistics-england-april-2015

14. Handelzalts JE, Hairston IS, Muzik M, Matatyahu Tahar A, Levy S. A paradoxical role of childbirth-related posttraumatic stress disorder (PTSD) symptoms in the association between personality factors and mother-infant bonding: a cross-sectional study. Psychol Trauma Theory Res Pract Policy 2022;14(6):1066–1072.

15. Chen J, Lai X, Zhou L, Retnakaran R, Wen SW, Krewski D, et al. Association between exclusive breastfeeding and postpartum post-traumatic stress disorder. Int Breastfeed J 2022;17(1):78.

16. Buttigieg GG, Micallef-Stafrace K. Shoulder dystocia: updating some medico-legal issues. Medico Legal Journal. 2022;90(1):13–16.

17. Slade P, Balling K, Sheen K, Houghton G. Establishing a valid construct of fear of childbirth: findings from in-depth interviews with women and midwives. BMC Pregnancy Childbirth 2019;19(1):96.

18. Minooee S, Cummins A, Foureur M, Travaglia J. Catastrophic thinking: is it the legacy of traumatic births? Midwives' experiences of shoulder dystocia complicated births. WOMEN BIRTH 2021;34(1): e38-e46.

19. Raoust GM, Bergström J, Bolin M, Hansson SR. Decision-making during obstetric emergencies: a narrative approach. PLoS One 2022;17(1).

20. Vaajala M, Liukkonen R, Kuitunen I, Ponkilainen V, Mattila VM, Kekki M. Factors associated with fear of childbirth in a subsequent pregnancy: a nationwide case-control analysis in Finland. BMC Womens Health 2023 January 24,;23(1):34-7.

21. Larad R, Ishaque U, Korb D, Drame S, Coutureau C, Graesslin O, et al. Evaluation of obstetric management of women with macrosomic foetuses in two Level 3 maternity hospitals in France and identification of predictive factors for obstetric and neonatal complications. Eur J Obstet Gynecol Reprod Biol 2022;274:34-39.

22. Bouchghoul H, Hamel J, Mattuizzi A, Ducarme G, Froeliger A, Madar H, et al. Predictors of shoulder dystocia at the time of operative vaginal delivery: a prospective cohort study. Sci Rep 2023;13(1):2658.

23. Athukorala C, Crowther CA, Willson K. Women with gestational diabetes mellitus in the ACHOIS trial: risk factors for shoulder dystocia. AUST NZ J OBSTET GYNAECOL 2007;47(1):37-41.

24. Øverland EA, Vatten LJ, Eskild A. Pregnancy week at delivery and the risk of shoulder dystocia: a population study of 2 014 956 deliveries. BJOG: An International Journal of Obstetrics & Gynaecology 2014;121(1):34-42.

25. Moraitis AA, Shreeve N, Sovio U, Brocklehurst P, Heazell AEP, Thornton JG, et al. Universal third-trimester ultrasonic screening using fetal macrosomia in the prediction of adverse perinatal outcome: a systematic review and meta-analysis of diagnostic test accuracy. PLoS Medicine 2020;17(10):1-15.

26. MacDonald TM, Robinson AJ, Hiscock RJ, Hui L, Dane KM, Middleton AL, et al. Accelerated fetal growth velocity across the third trimester is associated with increased shoulder dystocia risk among fetuses who are not large-for-gestational-age: a prospective observational cohort study. PLoS ONE 2021;16(10):1-12.

27. Shinohara S, Okuda Y, Hirata S. Risk assessment of shoulder dystocia via the difference between transverse abdominal and biparietal diameters: a retrospective observational cohort study. PLoS ONE 2021;16(2):1-9.

28. Duewel AM, Doehmen J, Dittkrist L, Henrich W, Ramsauer B, Schlembach D, et al. Antenatal risk score for prediction of shoulder dystocia with focus on fetal ultrasound data. Obstet Gynecol 2022;227(5):753.

29. La Verde M, De Franciscis P, Torre C, Celardo A, Grassini G, Papa R, et al. Accuracy of fetal biacromial diameter and derived ultrasonographic parameters to predict shoulder dystocia: a prospective observational study. Int J Environ Res Public Health 2022;19(9).

30. Ouzounian JG, Gherman RB. Shoulder dystocia: are historic risk factors reliable predictors? . . . includes discussion. AM J OBSTET GYNECOL 2005;192(6):1933-1938.

31. Youssefzadeh AC, Tavakoli A, Panchal VR, Mandelbaum RS, Ouzounian JG, Matsuo K. Incidence trends of shoulder dystocia and associated risk factors: a nationwide analysis in the United States. Int J Gynaecol Obstet. 2023 Jan 27;162(2):578-589.

32. Gardosi J, Francis A, Turner S, Williams M. Customized growth charts: rationale, validation and clinical benefits. Am J Obstet Gynecol 2018;218(2):S609-S618.

33. Grossman L, Pariente G, Baumfeld Y, Yohay D, Rotem R, Weintraub AY. Trends of changes in the specific contribution of selected risk factors for shoulder dystocia over a period of more than two decades. J Perinat Med 2020;48(6):567-573.

34. Wagner SM, Mendez-Figueroa H, Chauhan SP. Interventions to decrease complications

after shoulder dystocia: a systematic review and Bayesian meta-analysis: a response. Am J Obstet Gynecol 2022;226(6):875–876.

35. Jevitt CM. Shoulder dystocia: etiology, common risk factors, and management. J Midwifery Womens Health 2005;50(6):485–549.

36. Usta IM, Hayek S, Yahya F, Abu-Musa A, Nassar AH. Shoulder dystocia: what is the risk of recurrence? Acta Obstet Gynecol Scand 2008;87(10):992–997.

37. Overland EA, Spydslaug A, Nielsen CS, Eskild A. Risk of shoulder dystocia in second delivery: does a history of shoulder dystocia matter? AM J OBSTET GYNECOL 2009;200(5):506.e1–6.

38. Crowther CA, Samuel D, Hughes R, Tran T, Brown J, Alsweiler JM. Tighter or less tight glycaemic targets for women with gestational diabetes mellitus for reducing maternal and perinatal morbidity: a stepped-wedge, cluster-randomised trial. PLoS Medicine 2022;19(9):1–17

39. Costa-Ramón A, Kortelainen M, Rodríguez-González A, Sääksvuori L. The Long-Run Effects of Cesarean Sections. J Hum Resour 2022;57(6):1–39.

40. Heinonen K, Saisto T, Gissler M, Kaijomaa M, Sarvilinna N. Pitfalls in the diagnostics of shoulder dystocia: an analysis based on the scrutiny of 2274 deliveries. Arch Gynecol Obstet. 2023 April 3;309(4):1401–1409.

41. John W. Beasley MD, James R. Damos MD, Richard G. Roberts M, JD, Thomas S. Nesbitt MD. The Advanced Life Support in Obstetrics Course. A National Program to Enhance Obstetric Emergency Skills and to Support Maternity Care Practice. Arch Fam Med 1994 December;3:1037–1041.

42. Ranger C. National Patient Safety Agency. Safety in numbers: moving to a standard crash-call number. CLIN GOVERNANCE INT J 2004;9(4):267–269.

43. Spain JE, Frey HA, Tuuli MG, Colvin R, Macones GA, Cahill AG. Neonatal morbidity associated with shoulder dystocia maneuvers. AM J OBSTET GYNECOL 2015;212(3):353.e1–5.

44. Leung TY, Stuart O, Sahota DS, Suen SSH, Lau TK, Lao TT. Head-to-body delivery interval and risk of fetal acidosis and hypoxic ischaemic encephalopathy in shoulder dystocia: a retrospective review. BJOG: An International Journal of Obstetrics & Gynaecology 2011;118(4):474–479.

45. Dajani NK, Magann EF. Complications of shoulder dystocia. Semin Perinatol 2014;38(4):201–204.

46. Antelo LF, Williams S, Krishnamoorthy K, Powell KA, Apuzzio J, Gittens-Williams L. Head-to-body interval and neonatal outcomes after shoulder dystocia [A225]. Obstetrics & Gynecology. 2022;139:65S.

47. Habek D, Prka M, Luetic AT, Marton I, Medic F, Miletic AI. Obstetrics injuries during shoulder dystocia in a tertiary perinatal center. Eur J Obstet Gynecol Reprod Biol 2022 November 01;278:33–37.

48. Gherman RB, Ouzounian JG, Incerpi MH, Goodwin TM, Gherman RB, Ouzounian JG, et al. Symphyseal separation and transient femoral neuropathy associated with the McRoberts' maneuver. AM J OBSTET GYNECOL 1998;178(3):609–610.

49. Seidman AJ, Siccardi MA. Postpartum Pubic Symphysis Diastasis. StatPearls 2022.

50. Royal College of Obstetricians and Gynaecologists. Third- and fourth- degree perineal tears, management: green top guideline 29. Clinical Guideline. 2015 June. Available from: <doi:10.1111/1471-0528.17003>; https://www.rcog.org.uk/guidance/browse-all-guidance/green-top-guidelines/third-and-fourth-degree-perineal-tears-management-green-top-guideline-no-29/

51. Levaillant M, Loury C, Venara A, Hamel-Broza J, Legendre G. Is there still an indication for episiotomy? Results from a French national database analysis. Int J Gynaecol Obstet 2023 March 01;160(3):880–885.

52. Stitely ML, Gherman RB. Shoulder dystocia: management and documentation. Semin Perinatol 2014;38(4):194–200.

53. Mendez-Figueroa H, Hoffman MK, Grantz KL, Blackwell SC, Reddy UM, Chauhan SP. Shoulder dystocia and composite adverse outcomes for the maternal-neonatal dyad. American Journal of Obstetrics & Gynecology MFM 2021;3(4).

54. Bruner JP, Drummond SB, Meenan AL, Gaskin IM. All-fours maneuver for reducing

shoulder dystocia during labor. J Reprod Med 1998;43(5):439–443.

55. Bothou A, Apostolidi D, Tsikouras P, Iatrakis G, Sarella A, Iatrakis D, et al. Overview of techniques to manage shoulder dystocia during vaginal birth. Eur J Midwifery. 2021;5:48.

56. Rogers EK, Bolger S, Paul SP. Managing neonates with clavicle fractures. Midwives 2015;18(3):50–52.

57. Menticoglou S, Schneider C. Resuscitating the Baby after Shoulder Dystocia. Case Reports in Obstetrics & Gynecology 2016:1–3.

58. Cesari E, Ghirardello S, Brembilla G, Svelato A, Ragusa A. Clinical features of a fatal shoulder dystocia: the hypovolemic shock hypothesis. Med Hypotheses 2018;118:139–141.

59. Battin MR, van den Boom J, Oben G, McDonald G. Shoulder dystocia, umbilical cord blood gases and neonatal encephalopathy. Aust N Z J Obstet Gynaecol 2021;61(4):604–606.

60. Elmas B, Ercan N, Ersak DT, Ozdemir EU, Celik IH, Tapisiz OL, et al. Risk factors for brachial plexus injury and permanent sequelae due to shoulder dystocia. Niger J Clin Pract 2022 December 01;25(12):2016–2023.

61. Ouzounian JG. Risk factors for neonatal brachial plexus palsy. Semin Perinatol 2014;38(4):219–221.

62. Stoke R, Schreiber V, Hocking K, Jardine L, Kumar S. Perinatal antecedents of moderate and severe neonatal hypoxic ischaemic encephalopathy: an Australian birth cohort study. Aust N Z J Obstet Gynaecol 2023 March 27.

63. Evans-Jones G, Kay SPJ, Weindling AM, Cranny G, Ward A, Bradshaw A, et al. Congenital brachial palsy: incidence, causes, and outcome in the United Kingdom and Republic of Ireland. ARCH DIS CHILD FETAL NEONAT ED 2003;88(3):185.

64. El-Gammal T, El-Sayed A, Kotb MM, Saleh WR, Ragheb YF, Refai OA, et al. Long-Term Results of Microsurgical Brachial Plexus Reconstruction in Late-Presenting Cases of Brachial Plexus Birth Injury. J Hand Surg Am 2023;48(2):126–133.

65. Alfonso I, Alfonso DT, Papazian O. Focal upper extremity neuropathy in neonates. Semin Pediatr Neurol 2000;7(1):4–14.

66. Ojumah N, Ramdhan RC, Wilson C, Loukas M, Oskouian RJ, Tubbs RS. Neurological neonatal birth injuries: a literature review. Cureus 2017;9(12):e1938.

67. Gherman R. Are there specific interventions that may reduce the incidence of neonatal brachial plexus palsy? Dev Med Child Neurol 2020;62(6):662.

68. Van der Looven R, Le Roy L, Tanghe E, Samijn B, Roets E, Pauwels N, et al. Risk factors for neonatal brachial plexus palsy: a systematic review and meta-analysis. Dev Med Child Neurol 2020;62(6):673–683.

69. Hersey AE, Wagner SM, Gupta M, Chang K, Yang L, Chauhan SP. Utilizing International Classification of Diseases Codes to Identify Shoulder Dystocia and Neonatal Brachial Plexus Injury. Pediatr Neurol 2023;144:115–118.

70. British Association of Perinatal Medicine. Deterioration of the newborn (NEWTT 2): a framework for practice. Practice framework. 2023 Jan. Available from: <doi:10.1136/archdischild-2022-320331>; https://www.bapm.org/resources/deterioration-of-the-newborn-newtt-2-a-framework-for-practice

71. Kaijomaa M, Gissler M, Ayras O, Sten A, Grahn P. Impact of simulation training on the management of shoulder dystocia and incidence of permanent brachial plexus birth injury: an observational study. BJOG. 2023 Jan 1;130(1):70–77.

11

Uterine complications

MARIE HALL

UTERINE RUPTURE	165	Introduction	171
Introduction	165	Pathophysiology	172
Pathophysiology	166	Risk/pre-disposing factors	172
Risk/pre-disposing factors	166	Clinical features	173
Clinical features	169	Care	174
Care	170	Follow-up/long-term issues	175
Follow-up/long-term issues	170	Summary of midwifery responsibilities	176
Summary of midwifery responsibilities	171	References	176
UTERINE INVERSION	171		

Uterine rupture is a serious complication of pregnancy and labour in which the wall of the uterus tears. It is classified as either being complete (full), which represents a potential catastrophic event that can result in severe maternal morbidity and mortality as well as possible fetal death, or incomplete (partial), which occurs when the tear does not extend through the full thickness of the uterine wall. A complete rupture is most likely to occur after 32 weeks gestation and predominantly where there is a uterine scar. An incomplete rupture is more common, also occurring when there is an existing scar (scar dehiscence), but rarely resulting in extensive maternal or fetal complications. Although common in resource-poor countries, in the UK, rupture of the unscarred pregnant uterus is a rare event.

BOX 11.1: Uterine rupture

Uterine rupture is a serious complication of pregnancy and labour in which the wall of the uterus tears. It is classified as either being complete (full) or incomplete (partial).

INTRODUCTION

A *complete rupture* of the uterus represents a potentially catastrophic event that can result in severe maternal morbidity and mortality, as well as possible fetal death. When occurring in pregnancy, it is more likely to be after 32 weeks gestation and predominantly where there is an existing classical (longitudinal) uterine scar.[1]

An *incomplete rupture* or *partial rupture* occurs when the tear does not extend through the full thickness of the uterine wall. In those with a scarred uterus, it may result in scar dehiscence. This is a more common event and rarely results in extensive maternal or fetal complications.

The incidence of uterine rupture varies extensively throughout the literature. In the UK, a national case-control study over a one-year period estimated the incidence of uterine rupture was 0.2 per 1,000 maternities overall.[2] Consistent with previous studies, it was found to be higher in those women with a previous caesarean birth who were planning a vaginal birth or repeat elective caesarean section quoting the estimated incidence as 2.1 and

DOI: 10.4324/9781003382195-11

0.3 per 1,000 maternities, respectively.[2] This risk was increased when associated with labour induction, the use of oxytocin and an increased number of previous caesarean sections. A perinatal mortality rate of 124 per 1,000 births was identified.[2]

The RCOG[3] suggests that women should be informed that planned VBAC (vaginal birth after caesarean) is associated with an approximately 1 in 200 (0.5%) risk of uterine rupture.

It has been reported that the number of women attempting vaginal birth after CS birth (VBAC) is decreasing in many countries with an associated increase in the caesarean section rates.[4] The World Health Organisation has reported that caesarean sections account for more than 1:5 (21%) of births and is continuing to increase.[5] This has fundamentally been driven by reports implying the compounded risk of maternal and fetal complications related to VBAC, including uterine rupture. A study by Knight[6] ascertained that, from 143,970 women who had their first baby by caesarean section between 2004 and 2011, just over half (52%) attempted a vaginal birth after caesarean section (VBAC) for their second baby, with approximately two-thirds (63%) having a successful vaginal birth. A population-based survey in Norway conducted by Al-Zirqi[7] concluded that the incidence of rupture of both scarred and unscarred uteri over four decades appeared to be on the increase, with obstetric interventions contributing to this increase.

In resource-poor countries, uterine rupture is a more serious problem with an overall rate of 0.1–1%, with reports indicating that 75% of uterine ruptures occurred on an unscarred uterus[4] possibly associated with higher parity, longer labours, operational practices and a higher frequency of contracted pelves in these areas, together with poor access to emergency obstetrical facilities.[8]

In resource-rich countries, rupture of the unscarred pregnant uterus is a rare event, estimated to occur in 0.3–2.0/10,000 maternities.[3,9,7]

PATHOPHYSIOLOGY

A *complete* uterine rupture is a full-thickness tear of all three layers of the uterus (endometrium, myometrium and perimetrium). This can extend to the broad ligament and/or bladder, and the uterine contents can escape into the peritoneal cavity.

An *incomplete* or *partial* uterine rupture occurs when the tear does not extend through the full thickness of the uterine wall and the peritoneum remains intact. This is most commonly seen in

> ### BOX 11.2: Risk/pre-disposing factors for uterine rupture
>
> - Previous uterine surgery (CS as well as minimally invasive procedures)
> - Pharmacological induction of labour/ augmentation of labour
> - Grand multiparity
> - Multi-fetal pregnancy
> - Macrosomic fetus
> - Previous uterine rupture
> - Abnormal placentation (in particular PAS)
> - Certain medical conditions
> - Congenital uterine anomalies
> - Trauma to the abdomen
> - Intrauterine manipulation or interventional procedures
> - External cephalic version
> - Prolonged labour
> - Obstructed labour

those with a scarred uterus involving scar dehiscence. It generally presents with less acute symptoms and less significant bleeding from the edges of the pre-existing uterine scar[1] and may well be found inadvertently. The fetus, placenta and umbilical cord remain inside the uterine cavity.

It is vital that these two events are distinctly differentiated as the clinical management and outcomes are considerably different.

RISK/PRE-DISPOSING FACTORS

Spontaneous uterine rupture happens most often during labour in the context of a scarred uterus. Nonetheless, it can occur in an unscarred uterus and even with no discernible associated risk factors, although this is rare. Uterine rupture before or during labour in women with no preceding uterine surgery is an event which can lead to potentially life-threatening complications.[10] There are several risk factors that pre-dispose to a uterine rupture. Familiarity and understanding of these features may assist midwives in not only being aware of them but also anticipating through correct interpretation of the signs and symptoms, ensuring appropriate and timely escalation.

The vast majority of documented evidence in the literature identifies previous caesarean section as the predominant risk factor for uterine rupture. Other factors have been attributed to its occurrence (see Box 11.2).

Previous caesarean section

It is widely accepted in the literature that a woman has an increased possibility of sustaining a uterine rupture if she has a scarred uterus.[1,11] Predominately, this will arise from a previous caesarean section. However, other forms of uterine surgery, such as myomectomy, must also be taken into account.

The consequence of previous caesarean birth on the risk of uterine rupture has been studied extensively, yet it is difficult to precisely measure the risk it has as evidence within the literature varies considerably. In the UK, around 10–15% of the obstetric population has experienced previous caesarean delivery. The risk of perinatal death or severe morbidity should uterine rupture happen is higher with a trial of vaginal birth than with elective repeat caesarean section (ERCS).[12] There is virtually no risk of uterine rupture in women undergoing ERCS; however, additional complications that are associated with a CS birth exist.[13] These findings complicate the decision-making process as clinicians and women try to weigh up the risks involved. It is fundamental that antenatal counselling should comprise of an individualised assessment of the risks and benefits of ERCS and planned VBAC so that women are fully informed with the most up-to-date evidence.[3]

PREVIOUS CLASSICAL (LONGITUDINAL) INCISION

The incidence of a uterine rupture occurring when the scar from a previous caesarean section is in the lower segment is relatively low as this is the segment of the uterus that does not contract.[12] However, although caesarean section birth with a classical (longitudinal) incision is relatively uncommon in the modern era (representing 0.3%-0.4% of deliveries), it does pose a significant risk of rupture with subsequent pregnancies.[14] Available data recommend that a planned caesarean section at 36–37 weeks optimises both maternal and fetal outcomes in these cases.[15] Among women with previous longitudinal scars, it is suggested that uterine rupture or uterine scar dehiscence is neither predictable nor preventable; one-third of these occurred before the onset of labour.[14]

Pregnancy interval

Short interpregnancy interval increases the risk for uterine rupture and other major morbidities twofold to threefold in those women having a VBAC.[16] The timing between pregnancies appears to be an important predictor.[17] An interpregnancy interval of less than 12 months seems to be independently associated with uterine rupture in women with prior CS, but does not appear to influence risk in women with an unscarred uterus.[18] An earlier study by Bujold[19] found that the risk of uterine rupture was significantly higher in women with an inter-birth interval of less than 18 months (4.8%) than in women with an interval of 24 months or longer. The rates of uterine rupture for an interval of 24 months or more were 1.3%, and between 18 and 24 months, 1.9%.

Previous labour or vaginal birth

Those women who have had a prior vaginal birth appear to have a considerably lower risk of uterine rupture than women without a previous vaginal birth.[3,20]

The number of previous caesarean sections

The more caesarean births a woman has seems to increase the risk of uterine rupture,[6] but there remains uncertainty within the literature as to the number. A study by Fitzpatrick et al.[2] found that women with two or more previous caesarean sections had an increased risk of uterine rupture compared to those with only one previous caesarean. Ruptures were also found to occur more frequently during the time before active labour in those who had multiple or unusual uterine scars.[7] If the woman has previously had a successful vaginal birth, this will reduce her risk.[3]

Previous wound closure

There are many studies suggesting that the types of uterine closure methods, either single or double layer, have an impact on the rates of uterine rupture,[21,22,23] but although closure of the CS uterine incision in two layers seems to be practiced more widely, there is no clear guidance.

Previous wound healing

Delayed wound healing with or without associated sepsis at the time of caesarean birth may increase the risk of uterine rupture in subsequent pregnancies as there may be a weakness in the scar due to poor wound healing secondary to the infection.[17]

Previous surgical procedures

It is possible that any previous surgical intervention on the uterus, such as myomectomy, dilatation and curettage (D&C) or hysteroscopy, may cause weakness of the uterus and pre-dispose to uterine rupture. However, studies have suggested that uterine rupture following laparoscopic myomectomy is rare as long as women meet certain criteria.[3]

Parity

It has been suggested that multiparity is considered a contributing factor to uterine rupture. However, studies on the incidence of this vary widely. It was a customary belief within obstetrics that a "primigravida did not rupture". Nonetheless, it is important to be aware that uterine rupture in primiparous women can occur even when no contributing risk factors have been identified.[24,25,26] There is a higher rate of mortality for the primiparous women who sustain a uterine rupture compared to the multiparous. The rupture of an unscarred uterus is a more dangerous event than rupture through a previous scar, as the area of rupture is more vascular. This has been identified as a mortality rate of 26% compared to 11.7%, respectively, with a higher rate of hysterectomy also noted in primiparous women.[27] It has also been suggested that since suspicion is greater, perhaps diagnosis and, therefore, treatment is instigated far more quickly for the multiparous woman, so delays may occur for those who are primigravid. It is, therefore, paramount that clinicians are aware that uterine rupture can occur in primiparous women, and the outcome can be catastrophic.[28]

Abnormal placentation

The incidence of abnormal placenta implantation, as in placenta accreta syndrome (PAS) (see Chapter 4, Box 4.2), is rising due to the increase in caesarean sections within modern-day obstetric practice. One of the most severe complications of placenta percreta is uterine rupture with a haemoperitoneum. It has been documented that uterine rupture from percreta can occur in the early trimester periods. The contributing factor is thought to be an absence in the decidua basalis, which allows chorionic villus invasion of the myometrium. Once the woman has been diagnosed with abnormal placentation, careful and frequent monitoring must be undertaken throughout pregnancy, with a concise plan of management in her notes.

Medical conditions

There are no direct links associated with medical conditions and uterine rupture; however, they can be a contributing risk factor. Hypertensive disorders have been previously linked to uterine rupture, but there is no contemporaneous evidence to support this.[29] There has been a suggested association with women who have a connective tissue disorder such as Ehlers-Danlos syndrome as well as those with on-going steroid use.[9,24]

Pharmacological induction/ augmentation: oxytocin and/or prostaglandin

The use of prostaglandin E2 gel and intravenous Syntocinon® for women with a previous caesarean section is listed as a contraindication in use by the manufacturers' guidelines of both agents. Despite this, both are used for either the induction or augmentation of labour for women with a previous caesarean scar. It is well documented in the literature that induction of labour for women with a previous caesarean section carries an increased risk of uterine rupture.[30,31,32] It is also worth remembering that induction of labour following a vaginal birth with an unscarred uterus can double the risk of uterine rupture.[33] In today's practice, the use of prostaglandin and oxytocin is routine; however, caution should always be displayed when using these drugs for all women.

Trauma to abdomen

Uterine rupture is reported to occur in up to 0.6% of blunt abdominal trauma cases in pregnancy.[34] Motor vehicle crashes, domestic violence and falls are the most common causes of blunt trauma in pregnancy. Trauma can also occur through obstetric interventions,[11] such as external cephalic version, internal podalic version, mid to high instrumental vaginal delivery, manual removal of the placenta, manoeuvres performed in shoulder dystocia, as well as unstable lies and fetal malpresentation. Penetrating trauma to the abdomen is usually sustained through either gunshot wounds or stabbing with a sharp instrument such as a knife. However, these types of injuries are uncommon.

CLINICAL FEATURES

Signs and symptoms

The initial signs and symptoms of uterine rupture largely depend on the timing, site and degree of the uterine defect but can be nonspecific and vary vastly, which makes the diagnosis difficult and sometimes delays fundamental treatment. Uterine rupture at the site of a previous uterine scar is typically less harrowing than a spontaneous or traumatic rupture because of the decreased vascularity of scar tissue.[1] The warning signs and symptoms of uterine rupture can be inconsistent and may have similarities with those of a concealed abruption. It is also worth bearing in mind that some signs and symptoms may be concealed due to medical conditions (such as pre-eclampsia) or certain prescribed drugs masking tachycardia, as well as the use of epidural infusions potentially masking pain.

FETAL HEART RATE ABNORMALITIES

The most consistent early indicator of uterine rupture is an abnormal fetal heart rate pattern, with bradycardia being the most common fetal heart rate abnormality, especially if it is profound, persistent and prolonged.[35,36] It is, therefore, understandable why the majority of hospitals, in conjunction with national guidelines[37] recommend that women labouring with a previous caesarean section scar have continuous fetal heart monitoring in labour. Studies have noted that abnormal fetal heart rates were present in 66–76% of uterine rupture cases.[3]

BOX 11.3: Potential signs and symptoms of uterine rupture

- Fetal heart rate abnormalities
- Diminished or slowing of uterine contractility
- Pain
- Bleeding
- Bandl's ring (pathological constriction ring in labour)
- Change in maternal vital signs

DIMINISHED OR SLOWING OF UTERINE CONTRACTILITY

The slowing down or sudden cessation of previously effective uterine contractions is often an indication that there is a problem. No particular pattern of uterine activity is diagnostic of uterine rupture.[11,38] The uterine contractility pattern may vary depending on the presence or absence of a pre-existing scar or the location and direction of rupture.[35] However, there has been one case report describing the 'staircase sign' as characteristic of uterine rupture. This sign classically illustrates on the CTG monitor a stepwise gradual decrease in amplitude of the contraction succeeded by the sudden onset of profound and prolonged fetal bradycardia.[35] The RCOG and the ACOG do not recommend the use of intrauterine pressure catheters as a tool for early detection of uterine rupture,[3,36] as they appear to have no added significance over clinical or CTG observation.

PAIN

Sudden or atypical maternal abdominal pain occurs less frequently than abnormal fetal heart abnormalities; however, the onset of severe continuous abdominal pain should never be ignored and gives rise to suspicion of uterine rupture.[37] The pain is usually of sudden onset and above and beyond that of normal labour pain, and the abdomen will be rigid and tender to touch. In the scarred uterus, tenderness in the abdomen may be apparent before the rupture takes place. Chest pain or shoulder tip pain (Kehr's sign) has also been observed in some cases. These are valuable signs of intraperitoneal blood in the sub-diaphragmatic region, although it is important to appreciate that it may take up to 24 hours or longer after the bleeding has occurred for the blood to track up under the diaphragm – however, referred pain can be of great diagnostic significance.[37] Any woman post birth (either vaginal or by caesarean section) who has severe pain not relieved by opiate analgesia should be investigated for possible uterine rupture if all other sources have been ruled out.

BLEEDING

Vaginal bleeding during uterine rupture is a rare occurrence; a case-controlled study of 159 cases of uterine rupture reported only 29% presented with vaginal bleeding.[2]

As bleeding is usually behind the presenting part, it may not be visualised until after the birth as a postpartum haemorrhage.[11] Bleeding into the abdomen can be profuse, especially if the tear is longitudinal rather than transverse, with the woman displaying signs of shock or even sudden collapse. Haematuria is often seen, especially if a urinary catheter is present, as the bladder may be adherent to a previous uterine scar and be the first indication of a rupture.

ABDOMINAL PALPATION

A Bandl's ring is a pathological constriction ring and may be palpable – it is described as a late warning sign of impending rupture.[38] Following a uterine rupture, on examination, a loss of uterine contour may be identified and two swellings may be prominent; one is the fetus lying in the abdominal cavity, and the other is the contracted and retracted uterus. The fetal parts may then be easily palpable with a change in the fetal presenting part.[39] Examination will also be very painful for the woman.

MATERNAL VITAL SIGNS

Changes in vital signs from tachycardia to hypovolaemic shock may be the first indication of uterine rupture.[37,40] The changes that may be observed are dependent on the extent of rupture. The woman may initially be restless before any visual signs of shock are evident. The necessity of midwives using all of their senses to create a general assessment of the woman is vital. A previously fit and healthy woman who states she feels unwell must never be ignored, and tachypnoea and breathlessness are frequently the first signs of acute illness.[41] In most cases of maternal collapse, the cause is usually apparent, but concealed haemorrhage from a ruptured uterus should not be ruled out.[3] The majority of cases will usually see a progressive deterioration in basic vital signs.

Incomplete Rupture

Incomplete rupture is also referred to as uterine dehiscence, whereby the uterine muscular layer is lost, but the uterine serosa is preserved. This can occur in the unscarred primigravid uterus even without etiological or risk factors.[42] An incomplete rupture can be asymptomatic and signs may initially be quite subtle. Diagnosis is usually made during the process of caesarean section or other surgical intervention for bleeding.[43,44]

CARE

Prediction

It has been proposed that thinning of the lower uterine segment (LUS) measured by ultrasonography could be a potential predictor of uterine rupture.[45] Assessment of the LUS thickness may become routine antenatal practice in the future.[46,47]

Actions if uterine rupture is suspected

- Summon urgent help immediately. Like all obstetric emergencies, this should comprise an MDT approach, with a senior obstetrician, anaesthetist and midwife in attendance. If at home, the emergency response team should be called (dial 999 in the UK) for immediate transfer to hospital.
- Commence resuscitation (see Chapter 3), administer facial oxygen and treat shock as necessary: cannulation, a blood specimen sent for x-match, intravenous fluids as necessary and monitoring of vital signs (including FH).
- If an oxytocin infusion is in use, this must be stopped and disconnected.
- Preparation for surgical delivery or laparotomy – gaining consent in whatever is an appropriate method at the time of the emergency.

FOLLOW-UP/LONG-TERM ISSUES

It is important that the woman and her family not only have on-going explanations throughout the event but also have access to professionals after its conclusion so they can feel they have a full understanding of what happened and why actions were taken. This may take several discussions, and the woman should also be able to have questions answered after she leaves hospital. Many maternity units have a "Birth Reflections" service that a woman can access when she feels it necessary to discuss her experiences.

It is essential that careful consideration and planning are undertaken with regards to subsequent pregnancies and, indeed, a planned caesarean section may be recommended. Repair of the uterus is by and large possible for the majority of women; however, it does carry an increased risk of recurrence.[47] In others, haemorrhage from the extension of the rupture into the broad ligament or extensive damage to the uterus requires a hysterectomy, and it may be that a hysterectomy is required to save the woman's life.[37] A study in Scandinavia[48] reported that the rate of peripartum hysterectomy following uterine rupture was 3.5:10,000 births, although higher numbers have been suggested.[11]

SUMMARY OF MIDWIFERY RESPONSIBILITIES

- Uterine rupture can occur in an unscarred uterus as well as in a primiparous woman. Midwives, therefore, need to be vigilant when caring for all women while also being aware of the potential risk factors, longer labours and the prolonged use of oxytocin infusions.
- Midwives need to maintain an up-to-date knowledge of risk factors and management of uterine rupture and also ensure that knowledge and skills of IOL and augmentation are maintained. This should include an understanding of drug doses and potential side effects. Maintaining proficiency in basic life support by attending mandatory skills and drills updates is vital.
- It is essential that hospitals have evidence-based guidelines and policies that staff are familiar with and that are adhered to. This will ensure the safety of women who choose to have a vaginal birth after a previous caesarean section by increased vigilant observation, careful monitoring in labour and the implementation of strict interventional criteria standards.
- Women at risk of uterine rupture should be identified as soon as possible and appropriate referrals made.
- Women choosing to have a VBAC need to have a discussion concerning their individual characteristics. Many maternity units have a 'VBAC clinic' or similar, and midwives are usually part of the team supporting these women. Women who have been advised against VBAC but still wish to proceed with a vaginal birth continue to require support and careful management from senior obstetricians and midwives. At no time should their choice be met

with disapproval, as this may only drive them away from care and a setting that can provide safe treatment in the event of an emergency.

- Midwives should ensure that women are educated on the signs and symptoms of scar tenderness.
- Women choosing a VBAC should have an agreed plan of care documented in their notes relating to the management of labour, plus whether the use of prostaglandins and/or oxytocin is to be considered.
- Caution should be applied during oxytocin augmentation, especially in slow-progressing multiparous women and those with a history of previous caesarean section.
- When caring for a woman undertaking a VBAC, the midwife should pay particular attention to prolonged labour, scar tenderness, fetal distress or any sign that may indicate imminent scar dehiscence or uterine rupture.
- If a uterine rupture occurs, the midwife must work effectively within the multidisciplinary team, ensure excellent record keeping and communicate with the woman and her family during and after the event, arranging long-term access to relevant agencies if necessary.

UTERINE INVERSION

BOX 11.4: Uterine inversion

Uterine inversion is described as the passage of the uterine fundus through the endometrial cavity and cervix, turning the uterus inside out. It can occur either spontaneously, through mismanagement of the third stage or in the postpartum period. It requires rapid diagnosis with immediate clinical intervention to prevent maternal morbidity and mortality.[49]

INTRODUCTION

Uterine inversion is a rare but extremely serious obstetric emergency, and without swift management, the woman can become profoundly shocked. The incidence of uterine inversion occurring varies within the literature. It has been cited as between

1:1,000 to 1:50,000,[40,50,51] and it has been suggested most are seen in 'low risk' births.[50] This variation is likely due to geographic location, reporting of incidence and how the third stage of labour is managed.

The high incidence of uterine inversion in resource-poor areas is believed to be associated with the absence of active management of the third stage of labour and the lack of skilled or trained birth attendants. Suitable education and training regarding the third stage of labour, specifically focussing on safe physiological management of the third stage, as well as diagnosis and management of uterine inversion, should be made available to traditional birth attendants and family physicians so that this potentially life-threatening emergency can be avoided.[52]

In a recent MBRRACE-UK report,[53] two women died from haemorrhage associated with uterine inversion. It would appear that the incorrect practice of third-stage management was directly responsible. However, this was compounded by the fact that prompt replacement of the uterus did not appear to be undertaken.

PATHOPHYSIOLOGY

The pathophysiology of uterine inversion involves a part of the uterine wall prolapsing through the dilated cervix, relaxation of the uterine wall and downward traction of the fundus – caused by inappropriate third-stage management or spontaneously from the weight of the placenta – which leads to the inversion. The resulting stretching of the pelvic parasympathetic nerves can contribute to the shock symptoms in the woman, which are also caused by haemorrhage.

Uterine inversion can be classified according to either *timing* of the inversion or *degree* (anatomical severity).

Timing

- *Acute uterine inversion*: occurs either at the third stage of labour or within 24 hours of birth.
- *Subacute inversion*: occurs after 24 hours and within four weeks after birth.
- *Chronic inversion*: occurs after 30 days postpartum and is rare.

Severity

The severity of uterine inversion is classified either in stages or degrees.

- *First degree* (also referred to as incomplete): the inverted fundus extends to, but not through, the cervix.
- *Second degree*: the inverted uterus extends through the cervix but remains within the vagina.
- *Third degree* (complete): the inverted uterus extends down outside the vagina to the introitus.
- *Fourth degree* (total): the vagina and uterus are inverted.

RISK/PRE-DISPOSING FACTORS

Several risk factors/causes have been linked to uterine inversion[40,49] (see Box 11.5), but often, there is no suggestion of mismanagement of the third stage of labour. In about 50% of cases, no risk factors were identified, and it is, therefore, in essence, regarded as unpredictable.[9]

The most commonly reported iatrogenic factor associated with uterine inversion is mismanagement of the third stage of labour that involves:

BOX 11.5: Risk/pre-disposing factors for uterine inversion

- Mismanagement of third stage of labour
- Fundal implantation of the placenta
- Connective tissue disorders (for example, Marfan's syndrome)
- Congenital abnormalities of the uterus (for example, bicornuate/unicornuate uterus)
- Retained placenta and abnormal adherence of the placenta (PAS)
- Short umbilical cord
- Excessive fundal pressure
- Primigravida
- Decompression of an overstretched uterus as in the case of polyhydramnios, macrosomia or multiparity
- Certain drugs, such as those promoting tocolysis

- Excessive and/or premature controlled cord traction (CCT) before signs of placental separation.
- Carrying out controlled cord traction on a relaxed uterus.
- The use of fundal pressure with or without cord traction.

Controlled cord traction (CCT) must never be carried out on a relaxed uterus. At the time of uterine contraction, CCT with counter traction must be applied to support and stabilise the uterus. It is worth noting that CCT is not intended to separate the placenta from the uterine wall but to facilitate its removal only. In both of the women who died from uterine inversion, MBRRACE-UK[53] commented that "it was clear that the placenta had not separated but clinicians persisted with controlled cord traction" (p. 62). Midwives need to be mindful of this when managing the third stage of labour as well as the dangers of combining active and physiological third-stage management.[53,54] Active management of the third stage of labour done correctly is currently deemed best practice and is now potentially perceived as the worldwide standard of care.

CLINICAL FEATURES

Many signs and symptoms associated with uterine inversion (see Box 11.6) are the same as those which have a more common explanation. Nevertheless, uterine inversion should always be considered as a potential cause, until a definite diagnosis is made.

Pain: is usually in the pelvic region and can be described as severe cramping or lower back pain accompanied by a bearing down sensation. This is due to the traction on the infundibulopelvic ligaments, round ligaments and the ovaries.[51]

Shock: occurs in approximately 40% of cases, with the signs usually sudden and acute and may be inconsistent with the amount of blood loss visualised. This is generally thought to be due in part to the parasympathetic response to traction of the uterine suspensory ligaments and is often accompanied by profound bradycardia.[51] Ultimately, shock will be a result of haemorrhage, and, therefore, inversion should always be eliminated in cases of acute postpartum collapse with or without visualised haemorrhage.

BOX 11.6: Signs and symptoms

The main fundamental signs of uterine rupture are shock, severe pain and bleeding, along with clinical findings.[51,53,55] Pain is not only apparent when other symptoms appear but is also present when attempting to deliver the placenta.[53] Other clinical indications include:

Signs	Symptoms
Lump in the vagina	Severe abdominal pain
Abdominal tenderness	Sudden cardiovascular collapse: shock
Absence of uterine fundus on palpation (or 'dimpling')	Postpartum haemorrhage
Polypoidal red mass in the vagina with placenta attached	

Diagnosis

Uterine inversion is rare and, therefore, may not be immediately considered; as a result, healthcare professionals must be vigilant as it can be a life-threatening obstetric emergency. The clinical presentation and diagnosis depend on the classification and severity, of obesity, making the diagnosis slightly more difficult. A first-degree inversion is also more difficult to diagnose and can be missed as the fundus of the uterus is not visible or palpable at the cervix. Abdominal examination, however, may demonstrate dimpling of the uterine fundus, and a bi-manual examination will aid in confirming the diagnosis.[56] Further diagnostic tools, such as imaging studies, may be considered.

The diagnosis in both second and third-degree inversion is clinical in nature, with clear signs of the uterine fundus in the vagina or beyond.[49] In a third-degree uterine inversion, the uterine endometrium with or without the attached placenta may be visible.[56] On abdominal palpation, there is an absence of the uterine fundus or the existence of a noticeable defect. These findings require immediate intervention.

As shock is a prime indication of an acute event, it is necessary to eliminate any other clinical conditions. Differential diagnosis includes pulmonary embolism, uterine rupture, amniotic fluid embolism and acute myocardial infarction, concealed bleed or marked uterine atony.[57]

CARE

Uterine inversion is a rare but extremely serious obstetric emergency, with the most commonly reported cause being fundal placentation with excessive cord traction in the third stage of labour.[41,53] All types of uterine inversion denote a need for rapid diagnosis and correction.

A prompt vaginal and abdominal examination will confirm the presence of uterine inversion, and, once confirmed, it is crucial to take action immediately to minimise maternal morbidity and mortality. Delayed treatment will cause the uterus to become swollen and congested and may also lead to the formation of a contraction ring, all of which will impede the replacement of the uterus and compromise the overall clinical status of the woman.[49] In both women who died following uterine inversion, reported in a recent MBRRACE-UK report,[53] there appeared to be no attempt to replace the uterus, and this delay led to significant deterioration in the women's conditions.

Immediate actions

As with all obstetric emergencies, assistance is required, and this is activated with the emergency call system specific to each maternity unit. This ensures all relevant MDT members, including a consultant obstetrician and anaesthetist, are present.

The management consists of two vital components:[9,57,49]

- The immediate treatment of shock.
- The replacement of the uterus.

Any oxytocin infusion must be stopped immediately once inversion has been confirmed and withheld until correction has taken place. Replacement of the uterus is the quickest way to treat neurogenic shock.

REPLACEMENT OF THE UTERUS

This should be attempted whether the placenta has separated or not. Gentle manipulation is instigated to try and return the uterus to the vagina if it has prolapsed outside the introitus – **no attempt should be made to remove the placenta manually if it has not separated.** This would only exacerbate clinical shock and contribute to further massive haemorrhage.[9,57] It is thought that the attached placenta prevents bleeding because the uterine sinuses are not exposed.

Manual repositioning of the uterus

If the uterine fundus can be felt or indeed is visible, then the uterus should be replaced manually. If possible, this should be done under a general anaesthetic.[9]

This procedure is commonly referred to as the *Johnson's manoeuvre*. The midwife or obstetrician inserts their hand into the vagina and cups the fundus of the uterus in the palm of their hand. Pressure is then applied back up and along the long axis of the vagina towards the posterior fornix of the vagina.[9,40,58] When feeding the uterus back through the cervix, it is fundamental to reposition the last section of the uterus that inverted first to avoid overlapping tissue at the cervix which would further compound the oedema and congestion. Counter support must also be applied as the uterus is put back by placing the other hand over the abdomen. Once the uterus is reverted, it is essential that the clinician's hand remains inside the uterine cavity for several minutes until contraction takes place to ensure the uterus remains in the pelvis.

Following repositioning, uterotonic drugs such as intravenous oxytocin should be administered to promote uterine tone and prevent the recurrence of the inversion. If this procedure is performed before oedema and the development of a contraction ring, then it should be successful, allowing the cervix to reform.[58]

In some circumstances, the clinician will use myometrial relaxant medication to assist with the replacement of the uterus. Magnesium sulphate, terbutaline and salbutamol are the most commonly prescribed drugs due to their availability and frequent administration. There have been reports of good results with the use of nitroglycerin, with benefits cited as the quicker onset of uterine relaxation and quick dissipation of the effect, obviating the need for reversal, as well as less effect on haemodynamics than with magnesium sulphate. These medications will not only relax the uterus but will also relax a cervical contraction ring.[9,58,59]

Once the uterus has been successfully replaced, manual removal of the placenta is necessary – this will generally take place in theatre under a general anaesthetic due to the risk of postpartum haemorrhage.

Hydrostatic methods

If manual replacement fails, the hydrostatic method should be used as recommended by the World Health Organisation.[60] Before this method is attempted, uterine rupture must be excluded. The procedure is performed in the operating theatre with the woman in the lithotomy position. The hydrostatic pressure involves warm sterile water or isotonic sodium chloride solution being rapidly instilled into the vagina via a rubber tube or intravenous giving set while the clinician's hand blocks the introitus. The fluid flows into the posterior aspect of the vagina and pushes the fundus upwards into its natural position by hydrostatic pressure. The bag of fluid should be elevated approximately 100–150 cm above the level of the vagina to ensure sufficient pressure. A problem associated with this method is the intricacy of maintaining a tight seal at the introitus. However, there are reports that this can be overcome by the use of a silastic ventouse cup positioned just inside the vagina, with tubing connected to the fluid, although a hand may still be necessary to ensure a tight seal. Despite large volumes of fluid being used, there has been no reported incidence of embolus or pulmonary oedema.[52,60]

There is some evidence in the literature that the use of an intrauterine balloon tamponade device can be successful in preventing recurrence once the uterus has been manually repositioned. This will enable the maintenance of the structural integrity of the uterine body following repositioning. The balloon insertion ensures that the balloon conforms to the contours of the uterine cavity to prevent reinversion of the uterus as a spherical body exerting pressure on the cavity. When inserting the balloon, it should be lifted up as much as possible into the cavity using placental forceps, ensuring that the uterine supporting ligaments are then extended, thus creating a combination of both Johnson's method and hydrostatic pressure. In addition, this method also has a haemostatic effect against haemorrhage, which is its primary role.[61,62]

If immediate replacement is not possible, the woman's condition should be stabilized, and she must be taken to theatre urgently for a general anaesthetic. Manual replacement may then be possible, and if not, then surgical intervention in the form of a laparotomy will be required.

CARE WHEN MEDICAL ASSISTANCE IS NOT IMMEDIATELY AVAILABLE

No attempt should be made to remove the placenta for the reasons stated previously.

- *Assistance*: call the emergency services (in the UK, dial 999) and arrange for an immediate transfer to hospital by ambulance. The nearest consultant-led obstetric unit should be contacted and made aware of the transfer and acuteness of the situation. While awaiting emergency services, the following procedures should be carried out.
- *Resuscitation and treatment of shock*: even though a woman may not display signs of shock initially, IV cannulation and fluid replacement must be commenced as the condition of these women can deteriorate suddenly.
- *Replacement of the uterus*: an attempt to replace the uterus using the Johnson's manoeuvre described previously should be undertaken as soon as possible. If this is unsuccessful and the uterus is inverted outside the vulva, efforts should be made to return it into the vagina gently to prevent further shock. If this is not deemed possible, then the uterus should be covered in sterile gauze that is soaked with either warm saline or water. It is useful to place a plastic bag over the gauze to retain the heat and moisture. This can then be further wrapped in a towel to preserve warmth and potentially delay the onset of shock. Reassurance and support must be given to the woman at all times.

FOLLOW-UP/LONG-TERM ISSUES

Care following uterine inversion needs to take place in either an intensive care environment or an obstetric high-dependency unit, depending on the amount of intervention that occurred. It is vital there is an adequate antibiotic cover, and close observation of haemoglobin and clotting levels should be carried out in the immediate hours post-partum. An oxytocin infusion may continue, and regular checking of the uterine fundus and blood loss is crucial. A senior obstetrician must have regular input into care and a referral to physiotherapy is also required. Time must be made to enable adequate discussion of the events with the woman and her family at times suitable for them. It might be appropriate to ensure the midwife involved in the case is included in this meeting.

The woman will also require some counselling regarding the possibility of recurrence of uterine inversion in a subsequent labour, and a discussion of this and recommendations concerning place and mode of birth must be undertaken.

SUMMARY OF MIDWIFERY RESPONSIBILITIES

- Ensure management of the third stage is always exemplary.
- Maintain up-to-date knowledge of signs, symptoms and actions necessary for uterine inversion.
- Be aware of local policies and guidelines related to the management of uterine inversion.
- If uterine inversion is suspected, call for help immediately if in hospital, or arrange emergency transfer if at home.
- Maintain knowledge of Johnson's manoeuvre for replacing the uterus, as the speed of replacement is vital.
- Be aware of hydrostatic methods of replacement of the uterus, to enable efficient assistance to be given to the obstetrician.
- Ensure clear and contemporaneous documentation is maintained.
- Communicate with the woman and her family throughout and after the emergency.

FURTHER READING AND RESOURCES

Royal College of Obstetricians and Gynaecologists (RCOG). Birth after previous caesarean birth. Green-top guideline no. 45. London: RCOG; 2015.

Burns R, Dent K, editors. Managing medical and obstetric emergencies and trauma. 4th ed. Oxford: Wiley Blackwell; 2022.

- Chapter 31 Uterine Inversion
- Chapter 32 Ruptured Uterus

REFERENCES

1. Nahum GG. Uterine rupture in pregnancy. Medscape. 2015. Available from: http://reference.medscape.com/article/275854-overview
2. Fitzpatrick KE, Kurinczuk JJ, Alfirevic Z, Spark P, Brocklehurst P, Knight M. Uterine rupture by intended mode of delivery in the UK: a national case-control study. 2012. Available from: http://journal.plo.org/plosmedicine/aricale?id+10.371/journal.pmed100118
3. Royal College of Obstetricians and Gynaecologists (RCOG). Birth after previous caesarean birth: green-top guideline no. 45. London RCOG; 2015.
4. Homer CSE, Johnson R, Foureur M. Next birth after caesarean section: changes over a nine-year period in one Australian state. Midwifery. 2011;27(2):165–169.
5. World Health Organisation. Caesarean section rates continue to rise, amid growing inequalities in access. Departmental News, 2021 June 16.
6. Knight HE, Gurol-Urganci, van der Meulen JH, Mahmood TA, Richmond D H, Dougall A, Cromwell D A. Vaginal birth after caesarean section: a cohort study investigating factors associated with its uptake and success. BJOG An International Journal of Obstetrics & Gynaecology. 2013;121(2):183–192.
7. Al-Zirqi I, Stray-Perdersen B Forsén L, Daltveit LK, Vangen S. Uterine rupture: trends over 40 years. BJOG. [Epub ahead of print]. 2015 Apr 2. Available from: <doi:10.1111/1471-0528.13394>
8. Hofmeyer GJ, Say L, Gülmezoglu A. WHO systematic review of maternal mortality and morbidity: the prevalence of uterine rupture. BJOG. 2005;112(9):1221–1228.
9. Burns R, Dent K, editors. Chapter 31 uterine inversion and Chapter 32 ruptured uterus in managing medical and obstetric emergencies and trauma. 4th ed. Oxford: Wiley Blackwell; 2022. p. 267–274.
10. Zhao P, Su C, Wang C, Xu J, Bai X. Clinical characteristics of uterine rupture without

previous Cesarean section: a 25-year retrospective study. J Obstet Gynaecol Res. 2021;47:2093–2098. Available from: <doi:10.1111/jog.14761>

11. Togioka BM, Tonismae T. Uterine rupture. In: StatPearls [Internet]. Treasure Island (FL): StatPearls Publishing. [Updated 2023 Jul 29]; Available from: www.ncbi.nlm.nih.gov/books/NBK559209/

12. Talaulikar V, Arulkumaram S. Vaginal birth after caesarean section. Obstetrics, Gynaecology and Reproductive Medicine. 2015;25(7):195–202. Available from: <doi:10.1016/j.ogrm.2015.04.005>

13. Sandall J, Tribe R, Avery L, Mola G et al. Short-term and long-term effects of caesarean section on the health of women and children. Lancet. 2018;392(10155): 1349–1357. Available from: <doi:10.1016/S0140-6736(18)31930-5>. PMID: 30322585.

14. Kan A. Classical Cesarean Section. Surg J (NY). 2020 Feb6;6(Suppl 2):S98-S103. Available from: <doi:10.1055/s-0039-3402072.

15. Landon MB, Lynch CD. Optimal timing and mode of delivery after cesarean with previous classical incision or myomectomy: a review of the data. Seminars in Perinatology 2011;35(5):257–261.

16. Stamilio DM, DeFranco E, Emmanuelle P, Odibo AO, Peipert JF et al. Short interpregancy interval: risk of uterine rupture and complications of vaginal birth after cesarean section Obstetrics & Gynecology. 2007;110(5):1075–1082.

17. Caughey AB. Vaginal birth after cesarean section. Medscape. 2013. Available from: https://emedicine.medscape.com/article/272187-overview

18. Cunningham S, Algeo C, DeFranco E. Influence of interpregnancy interval on uterine rupture. J Matern Fetal Neonatal Med. 2021;34(17):2848–2853. Available from: <doi:10.1080/14767058.2019.1671343>. Epub 2019 Oct 1. PMID: 31570033.

19. Bujold E, Gauthier RJ. Risk of uterine rupture associated with an inter-delivery between 18 and 24 months Obstetrics & Gynecology. 2010;115:1003–1006. Available from: <doi:10.1097/AOG.0b013e3181d992fb>

20. Mantal A, Aine G, Wolimann C & Stephansson O. Previous preterm cesarean delivery and risk of uterine rupture in subsequent trial of labor – a national cohort study. American Journal of Obstetrics & Gynecology 2020;224(4). Available from: <doi:10.1016/j.ajog.2020.09.040>

21. Vachon-Marceau C, Demers S, Bujold E, Roberge S, Gauthier RJ, Pasquier JC, Girard M, Chaillet N, Boulvain M, Jastrow N. Single versus double-layer uterine closure at cesarean: impact on lower uterine segment thickness at next pregnancy. Am J Obstet Gynecol. 2017 Jul;217(1):65.e1–65.e5. Available from: <doi:10.1016/j.ajog.2017.02.042>. Epub 2017 Mar 3.

22. Humphries G. The suture debate ICAN (international caesarean awareness network). 2014. Available from: www.ican-online.org/wp-content/uploads/2014/06/The-Suture-Debate.pdf

23. Roberge S, Demers S, Berghella V, Chaillet N, Moore L, Bujold E. Impact of single-vs double layer closure on adverse outcomes and uterine scar defect: a systematic review and meta-analysis. AJOG. 2014;211(5):453–460.

24. Mourad WS, Bersano DJ, Greenspan PB, Harper DM. Spontaneous rupture of unscarred uterus in a primigravida with preterm prelabour rupture of membranes. BMJ Case Rep. 2015 Jun 8;2015:bcr2014207321. Available from: <doi:10.1136/bcr-2014-207321>. PMID: 26055584; PMCID: PMC4460412.

25. Trivedi, Kiran; Anand, Shikha; Monalisa. Case series of unscarred uterine rupture in primigravida. Journal of Family Medicine and Primary Care 11(7):p 4079–4082, July 2022. | Available from: <doi:10.4103/jfmpc.jfmpc_2325_21>

26. Mizutamari E, Honda T, Ohba T, Katabuchi H. Case report: spontaneous rupture of an unscarred uterus in a primigravid woman at 32 weeks of gestation case reports. Case Rep Obstet Gynecol. 2014. Available from: <doi:10.1155/2014/209585>

27. Walsh CA, O'Sullivan RJ, Foley ME. Unexplained prelabor uterine rupture in a term primigravida. Obstetrics & Gynecology. 2006;108(3):725–727.

28. Halassy S, Eastwood J & Prezzato J. Uterine rupture in a gravid, unscarred uterus: a case report. Case Reports in Women's Health. 2019;24:e00154 Available from: <doi:10.1016/j.crwh.2019.e00154>

29. Ronel D, Wiznitzer A, Sergienko R, Zlotnik A, Sheiner E. Trends, risk factors and pregnancy outcome in women with uterine rupture. Archives Gynecology & Obstetrics. 2012;285(2):317–321. Available from: <doi:10.1007/s00404-011-1977-8>

30. Wallstrom T, Bjorklund J, Frykman J, Jarnbert-Pettersson H, Akerud H, Darj E, Gemzell-Danielsson K, Wiberg-Itzel E. Induction of labor after one previous Cesarean section in women with an unfavorable cervix: a retrospective cohort study. PLoS One. 2018 Jul 2;13(7):e0200024. Available from: <doi:10.1371/journal.pone.0200024>. PMID: 29965989; PMCID: PMC6028115.

31. West HM, Jozwiak M, Dodd JM. Methods of term labour induction for women with a previous caesarean section. Cochrane Database of Systematic Reviews 2017, Issue 6. Art. No.: CD009792. Available from: <doi:10.1002/14651858.CD009792.pub31>

32. Dy J, DeMeester S, Lipworth H & Barrett J. SOGC Clinical Practice No.382-Trial of Labour After Caesarean. Journal of Obstetrics and Gynaecology Canada. 2018;41:7. Available from: <doi:10.1016/j.jogc.2018.11.008>

33. Harper LM, Cahill AG, Boslaugh S, Odibo AO, Stamilio DM, Roehl KA, Macones GA. Association of induction of labor and uterine rupture in women attempting vaginal birth after cesarean: a survival analysis. Am J Obstet Gynecol. 2012 Jan;206(1):51.e1–5. Available from: <doi:10.1016/j.ajog.2011.09.022>. Epub 2011 Sep 24. PMID: 22000899; PMCID: PMC3246100.

34. Tang A, Bellal J, Coc C, Rhee P. Trauma. In: van de Velde M, Schofield H, Plante LA, editors. Maternal critical care: a multidisciplinary approach. Cambridge: Cambridge University Press; 2013.

35. Matsuo K, Scanlon JT, Atlas RO, Kopelman JN. Staircase sign: a newly described uterine contraction pattern seen in rupture of unscarred gravid uterus Journal of Obstetric Gynaecology Research. 2008;34:100–104.

36. Vlemminx MW, de Lau H, Oei SG. Tocogram characteristics of uterine rupture: a systematic review. Arch Gynecol Obstet. 2017 Jan;295(1):17–26. Available from: <doi:10.1007/s00404-016-4214-7>. Epub 2016 Oct 8. PMID: 27722806; PMCID: PMC5225169.

37. Harris CM. Trauma and pregnancy. In: Foley MR, Storng TH, Gartie TJ, editors. Obstetric intensive care manual. 3rd ed. New York: McGraw-Hill Medical; 2011.

38. Gupta R, Nageeb EM, Minhas I, Dang N, Mock SA, Rivera J, Ballas DA. Emergent cesarean section in a Bandl's ring patient: an obstetrics and gynecology simulation scenario. Cureus. 2018 Dec 31;10(12):e3800. Available from: <doi:10.7759/cureus.3800>. PMID: 30868014; PMCID: PMC6402741.

39. Manoharan M, Wuntakal R, Erskine K. Review uterine rupture: a revisit. The Obstetrician & Gynaecologist. 2011;12:223–230. Available from: <doi:10.1576/toag.12.4.223.27613>

40. Francois K, Foley M. Antepartum and postpartum hemorrhage. Chapter 18 in: Gabbe SG, Niebyl JR, Simpson JL, Landon MB, Galan HL, Jauniaux ERM, Driscoll DA, Berghella V, Grobman WA, editors. Obstetrics: normal and problem pregnancies. 7th ed. London: Elsevier; 2017. p. 395–424.e3, ISBN 9780323321082, Available from: <doi:10.1016/B978-0-323-32108-2.00018-4>; www.sciencedirect.com/science/article/pii/B978032332108 2000184

41. Francois K. Postpartum haemorrhage. In: Foley MR, Storng TH, Gartie TJ, editors Obstetric intensive care manual. 3rd ed. New York: McGraw-Hill Medical; 2011.

42. Matsubara S, Shimada K, Kuwata T, Usui R, Suzuk M. Thin anterior wall with incomplete uterine rupture in a primigravida detected by palpation and ultrasound: a case report. Journal of Medical Case Reports. 2011;5(14):1752–1947 Available from: <doi:10.1186/1752-1947-5-14>

43. Zhu Z, Li H, Zhang J. Uterine dehiscence in pregnant with previous caesarean delivery. Ann Med. 2021 Dec;53(1):1265–1269.

Available from: <doi:10.1080/07853890.2
021.1959049>. PMID: 34309465; PMCID:
PMC8317916.

44. Ahmadi F, Siahbazi S, Akhbari F. Incomplete
Cesarean Scar Rupture. Journal of
Reproductive Infertility 2013;14(1):43–45.
PMID: 23926561; PMCID: PMC3719360.

45. Kok N, Wiersma IC, Opmeer IC, De Graaf
IM, Mol BW, Paikrit E. Sonographic measurement of lower uterine segment thickness to
predict uterine rupture during a trial of labor
in women with previous Cesarean section:
a meta-analysis Ultrasound Obstetrics &
Gynecology. 2013;42(2):132–139. Available
from: <doi:10.1002/uog.12479>

46. Hatstat LM. Sonographic assessment of
uterine dehiscence during pregnancy in
women with a history of cesarean section: a
case series. Journal of Diagnostic Medical
Sonography. 2016;32(5):283–286. Available
from: <doi:10.1177/8756479316661246>

47. Siraj SHM, Lional KM, Tan KH, et al. Repair
of the myometrial scar defect at
repeat caesarean section: a modified
surgical technique. BMC Pregnancy
Childbirth. 2021;21:559. Available from:
<doi:10.1186/s12884-021-04040-9>

48. Colmorn LB, Petersen KB, Jakobsson
M, Lindqvist PG, Klungsoyr K, Källen K,
Bjarnadottir RI, et al. The Nodic Obstetric
Surveillance Study: a study of complete
uterine rupture, abdominal invasive placenta, peripartum hysterectomy and severe
blood loss at delivery. Acta Obstetricia et
Gynecologica Scandinavia. 2015;94(7):734–
744. Available from: <doi:10.1111/
aogs.12639>

49. Leal RFM, Luz RM, Branco RCC. Total and
acute uterine inversion after delivery: a case
report Journal of Medical Case Reports.
2014;8:347.

50. Thakur M, Thakur A. Uterine inversion. In:
StatPearls [Internet]. Treasure Island, FL:
StatPearls Publishing; [Updated 2022 Nov
28]. 2023 Jan. Available from: www.ncbi.
nlm.nih.gov/books/NBK525971/

51. Kumari S, Singh V, Ray A, Swain A. Postpartum complete acute uterine inversion:
a coordinated multi-disciplinary approach
ameliorates an obstetric nightmare, a
case report. J Family Med Prim Care.

2022 Feb;11(2):793–795. Available from:
<doi:10.4103/jfmpc.jfmpc_1164_21>. Epub
2022 Feb 16. PMID: 35360782; PMCID:
PMC8963637.

52. Ojabo OA, Adesiyun AG, Ifenne DI,
Hember-Hilekan S, Umar H. Acute uterine inversion: a case report and literature
review. Archives of International Surgery.
2015;5:52–55.

53. Tuffnell D, Knight M, On Behalf of the
MBRRACE-UK Haemorrhage and AFE
Chapter-Writing Group. Chapter 7: les-
sons for care of women with haemorrhage
or amniotic fluid embolism. In: Knight M,
Bunch K, Tuffnell D, Shakespeare J, Kotnis
R, Kenyon S, Kurinczuk JJ, On Behalf
of MBRRACE-UK, editors. Saving lives,
improving mothers' care – lessons learned
to inform maternity care from the UK and
Ireland confidential enquiries into maternal
deaths and morbidity 2016–18. Oxford:
National Perinatal Epidemiology Unit,
University of Oxford; 2020. p. 58–63.

54. Ganges F, Beck D, Engelbecht. Prevention
of postpartum haemorrhage: implement-
ing active management of the third stage
of labour. A reference manual for health
care providers. Seattle path. 2007. Available
from: https://media.path.org/documents/
MCHN_popphi_amtsl_ref_man.pdf

55. Zaki-Metias K, Hosseiny M, Behzadi
F & Balthazar P. Uterine Inversion.
Radiographics 2023;43(6). PMID: 37200219.
Available from: <doi:10.1148/rg.230004>

56. Saxena R. Postpartum haemorrhage. In:
Saxena R, editor. Bedside obstetrics &
gynecology. 2nd ed. New Delhi: Jaypee
Medical; 2014.

57. Davis G. Collapse in the puerperium. In:
Hollingworth T, editor. Differential diag-
nosis in obstetrics & gynaecology. 2nd ed.
London: CRC Press; 2015.

58. Kaur A, Singh B. Acute uterine inversion – a complication revisited; a case
series and review of literature. Case
Reports in Perinatal Medicine.
2022;11(1):20200081. Available from:
<doi:10.1515/crpm-2020-0081>

59. Sunjaya AP, Dewi AK. Total uterine inversion post partum: case report and management strategies. J Family Reprod Health.

2018 Dec;12(4):223–225. PMID: 31239851; PMCID: PMC6581659.

60. Bonner S. Uterine inversion. In: MacLennan K, Robinson C, editors. Obstetric decision-making and simulation. Cambridge: Cambridge University Press; 2019. p. 57–65. Available from: <doi:10.1017/9781108296793.011>

61. Haeri, S., Rais, S. and Monks, B. Intrauterine tamponade balloon use in the treatment of uterine inversion. BMJ Case Reports. 2015;pii:brc2014206705. Available from: <doi:1136/bcr-2014-206705>. PubMed PMID:25564634;PubMed Central PMCID: PMC4289782.CrossRefGoogle ScholarPubMed

62. Ida A, Ito K, Kubota Y, Nosaka M, Kato H, Tsuji Y. Successful reduction of acute puerperal uterine inversion with the use of a Bakri postpartum balloon case reports. Obstetrics and Gynecology. 2015;Article ID 424891. Available from: <doi:10.1155/2015/424891>

12

Primary postpartum haemorrhage

JESSICA SCOBLE

Introduction	181	Care	183
Pathophysiology	182	Summary of midwifery responsibilities	191
Risk/predisposing factors for PPH	182	Further reading and resources	192
Clinical features	183	References	192

BOX 12.1: Definition

Primary postpartum haemorrhage (PPH) is defined as the loss of 500ml or more of blood from the genital tract within 24 hours of the birth of the baby[1] or any blood loss that results in signs and symptoms of hypovolaemia.[2]

PPH in caesarean section is usually defined as a blood loss in excess of 1000ml.[3]

PPH can be classified as 'minor' (500–1000ml) or 'major' (more than 1000ml and/or maternal compromise). Major PPH can be further divided into moderate (1001–2000ml) and severe (more than 2000ml).

Note that women who weigh less than 60kg can become clinically compromised with a relatively small blood loss.

INTRODUCTION

Postpartum haemorrhage is one of the most common emergencies a midwife may encounter during their career and can be frightening when it occurs. Bleeding can be sudden and obvious; however, it can also be a slow trickle that, over time, results in maternal deterioration. It is essential that the midwife can recognise a PPH and understand the actions that need to be taken to stop the hemorrhage and save the woman's life.

Whilst PPH is the leading cause of maternal mortality in low-income countries and globally causes 70,000 maternal deaths,[4] in the UK, maternal death from haemorrhage is rare – between 2018 and 2020, there were 16 direct deaths from haemorrhage accounting for just below 0.8 per 100,000 maternities.[5] However, whilst mortality is low, there can be short and long-term physical and psychological consequences for the woman and her family, therefore, knowledge of the risk factors and the actions to be taken when bleeding occurs is necessary.

In order to reduce morbidity and mortality, not only is prompt recognition of the severity of any bleeding needed, but excellent communication and teamwork skills in the subsequent management of the situation are required. This is aided by regular, multidisciplinary simulation training, which has been shown to improve knowledge, practical skills, communication and team performance.[6] Every maternity unit should have a multidisciplinary protocol for managing PPH[7] with which all staff should be familiar.

During any PPH, it is important that a helicopter view is taken, where one senior clinician has an overview of the situation enabling them to identify ongoing deterioration and direct the necessary actions.

PATHOPHYSIOLOGY

Once the baby has been born, the uterine muscles continue to contract and retract to expel the placenta and membranes and control the bleeding. Any factor that interferes with this physiological process can result in excessive blood loss. During pregnancy, blood volume increases by 45–50%, and at term, the placental circulation is 450 to 700 ml/min,[8] therefore, when bleeding occurs, it can be sudden and potentially catastrophic.

BOX 12.2: Causes of PPH

- Placental abruption.
- Placenta praevia.
- Ruptured uterus.
- Cervical or vaginal lacerations.
- Atonic uterus, with or without retained products (placenta, membrane and/or blood clot).
- Haematoma in the vagina or broad ligament.

Any combination of the causes (see Box 12.2) or predisposing factors (see Box 12.4) will increase the risk of PPH, although it must be remembered that PPH can occur in women with no identifiable risk factors, therefore, vigilance is needed.

Postpartum haemorrhage can be classified in terms of 'the four Ts' (See Box 12.3), and some women will develop more than one of these.

BOX 12.3: The 4 T's

Tone – Uterine atony (poor uterine contraction) is the most common cause at 70–90% of PPHs.[9] Caused when the uterus fails to contract and retract correctly.

Trauma – To the uterus (rupture), cervix (tear), or vagina/perineum (haematoma, tear or episiotomy).

Tissue – Any tissue that prevents uterine contraction, e.g., retained placental tissue, membrane or blood clots.

Thrombin – Blood coagulation failure caused by coagulation abnormalities, either due to conditions that deplete clotting factors such as antepartum hemorrhage or conditions such as pre-eclampsia, HELLP syndrome or retained dead fetus.

RISK/PREDISPOSING FACTORS FOR PPH

BOX 12.4: Risk factors for PPH

Pre-pregnancy or antenatal factors:

- Maternal age >35.
- Grand multiparity.
- BMI > 35kg/m2.
- Previous PPH.
- Previous caesarean: scarring of the uterus is a risk factor for placenta praevia and accreta.
- Anaemia: Haemoglobin (Hb) less than 90g/l is associated with greater blood loss at delivery and postpartum[10] due to weakened uterine muscular strength.
- Multi-fetal pregnancy, polyhydramnios, fetal macrosomia: due to uterine over-distension leading to poor retraction. Multi-fetal pregnancies and fetal macrosomia can also have a larger placental site, which increases the risk of haemorrhage.
- Retained placenta and fibroids: prevents the uterus from contracting effectively.
- Pre-eclampsia/hypertensive disease: pre-eclampsia and hypertensive disease can increase the risk of induction and operative delivery. There can also be a complication of coagulopathy.
- Chorioamnionitis: due to inefficient contraction and retraction.

- Placenta praevia.
- Placenta accreta.

Factors associated with labour:

- Prolonged first/second/third stage, induced or augmented labour: due to inefficient contraction and retraction.
- Episiotomy-perineal laceration.
- General anaesthesia.
- Caesarean section: a risk factor due to the amount of tissue incised to reach the baby, and if an elective caesarean, there will not be circulating Oxytocin immediately available.
- Mismanagement of the third stage of labour: can cause PPH as it interferes with the normal rhythmic contractions of the myometrium and can cause only partial separation of the placenta. Mismanagement includes inappropriate massaging of the uterus or over strong cord traction on an unseparated placenta.

CLINICAL FEATURES

Postpartum haemorrhage can be diagnosed following delivery by estimating the volume of blood that has come out of the vagina, although this can be challenging, especially in cases of concealed haemorrhage. Visual estimation of blood loss is known to be inaccurate, with estimation becoming increasingly inaccurate with the larger the blood loss.[11] There is no evidence to support one method of estimating blood loss over another, for example, visual estimation, weighing the blood loss or using calibrated drapes to assess the loss.[12]

Pictorial guidelines may help midwives estimate blood loss;[1] however, clinical signs and symptoms of hypovolaemia should be included when assessing blood volume lost (see Table 12.1).

Midwives must remember that due to the physiological increase in circulating blood volume in pregnancy, the signs of hypovolemic shock become less sensitive. Young, fit pregnant women compensate when bleeding occurs, and therefore, normal clinical observations can provide false reassurance. Pulse and blood pressure do not change until blood loss exceeds 1000ml, whilst a systolic blood pressure below 80mmHg, worsening tachycardia, tachypnoea and altered mental state indicate blood loss in excess of 1500ml.[1] Other symptoms of maternal shock include poor peripheral perfusion, low urine output and unexplained metabolic acidosis.[13] It is also worth remembering that women of small stature may show signs of hypovolaemic shock with a relatively small blood loss due to their lower circulating blood volume.[14]

Women who present with abdominal pain or high levels of perineal discomfort could also have PPH considered as a cause, as this could be due to retained placental tissue or a haematoma. This is a pool of blood which can collect in the tissue of the perineum or broad ligament caused by a ruptured or bleeding vein.

The slow, steady trickle of blood after delivery of the placenta can be the most dangerous of all if it is not closely monitored. Changes of shift, failure to add up the total blood loss and frequent changes of inco pads may lead midwives to underestimate the situation, and the woman may slowly deteriorate into hypovolemic shock.

If the midwife is unsure of the severity of the blood loss, it is wise to call for help sooner rather than later.

CARE

Antenatal and labour

There are several steps that can be taken to prevent or reduce the chance or severity of PPH.

Any woman who is identified as high risk for PPH should have early multidisciplinary involvement from the senior obstetrician, anaesthetist and haematologist to discuss plans of care in conjunction with the woman. She should also be advised to have a hospital birth where immediate and effective treatment can be provided, such as the provision of a range of drugs, blood products and cell salvage.

Anaemia is a risk factor for PPH and should be treated in the antenatal period as anaemia (Hb less

Table 12.1 Maternal symptoms of primary PPH by amount of blood loss[15,10]

Average proportion lost of total blood volume (=6litres) of a pregnant woman	Amount of blood lost	Degree of shock in a woman with BMI 20–25	Physiological effects	Signs and symptoms a health professional will notice
20%	1200ml	Mild	Decreased perfusion of non-vital organs and tissues, e.g., bone, fat and skeletal muscle	Pale and cool skin Woman starts to complain of thirst Clamminess Possible mild tachycardia and a small drop in blood pressure
20–40%	1200–2400ml	Moderate	Decreased perfusion to vital organs and tissues, e.g., gut, liver and kidneys	Skin on legs starts to mottle Tachycardia more noticeable and further drop in blood pressure Oliguria and/or anuria
40% and more	2400ml+	Severe	Reduced perfusion to heart and brain	Agitation, restlessness, coma Echocardiogram and electrocardiogram abnormalities Metabolic acidosis and, finally, cardiac arrest

than 90g/l) is associated with greater blood loss during birth and postpartum.[9] The woman's blood group and antibody status, as well as haemoglobin levels, should also be checked on admission in labour.

Early intravenous access should be offered to women at risk of PPH as the rapid administration of fluids, drugs and blood products may be required in the management of PPH.[1]

The midwife should ensure that the woman's bladder is regularly emptied, as a full bladder can prevent efficient uterine contractions. The midwife should also monitor the progress of labour and refer to an obstetrician if there are signs of prolonged labour.

Management of the third stage should be discussed to enable the woman to make an informed choice. Active management of the third stage, including the administration of a uterotonic, has been shown to reduce the risk of PPH,[16] although routine early clamping of the umbilical cord is no longer recommended.[1] The midwife should wait for signs of placental separation before starting

controlled cord traction,[14] and once the placenta is delivered, assess the uterus to check it is well contracted. Nipple stimulation or breastfeeding can be commenced as it releases oxytocin; however, there is no clear evidence that it reduces the rate of PPH,[17] and fundal massage should not be used to prevent bleeding.

Regarding which uterotonic drug should be used, it has been shown that the prophylactic use of Oxytocin may reduce blood loss; however, it may also increase the risk of a third stage longer than 30 minutes. Ergot alkaloids can have possible side effects of diastolic hypertension, vomiting and headache.[18] There is evidence that shows the use of Oxytocin and ergometrine together (Syntometrine) may reduce blood loss compared to ergot alkaloids,[18] although this must be balanced against the side effects of ergometrine. There is no evidence to support the use of prostaglandins (Carboprost) or Ergometrine or Tranexamic Acid in the routine prophylaxis of preventing PPH.[1] NICE recommends the administration of 10IU Oxytocin intramuscularly with the birth of the anterior shoulder or after birth and before the cord is clamped.[7] They also recommend waiting at least one minute from the birth of the baby before the cord is clamped. It is worth noting that hospitals may vary in their pharmacological approach to third-stage management and managing PPH, so midwives should always follow their local Trust guidelines.

Management of PPH

A PPH is a stressful and traumatic incident, and whilst there are many actions that should be carried out simultaneously, it is imperative to maintain communication with the woman and her birthing partner, where feasible, informing them of the clinical development and proposed management. Excellent communication is also required within the multidisciplinary team, ensuring the use of a standard form of words and closed-loop communication to reduce misunderstandings. Senior staff should listen to the concerns of more junior staff, and all should be aware of the role of Human Factors in managing an emergency such as a PPH.

One person on the team should take responsibility for recording all actions taken, including personnel present, all events, fluids, drugs, blood components given and vital signs. Most Trusts use a PPH proforma to aid in recording the actions taken.

The discussion of the management of a PPH will be broken down into three sections – bleeding before the delivery of the placenta, minor PPH and major PPH.

BLEEDING BEFORE THE DELIVERY OF THE PLACENTA

If the placenta is not delivered and the woman starts bleeding, an attempt to deliver the placenta with the administration of a third-stage oxytocic drug (if not already given) and controlled cord contraction should be made (although an ergometrine component should not be given as this can close the cervix). If the placenta does not deliver, a retained placenta is diagnosed and urgent help must be sought.

If there is excessive bleeding before the placenta is delivered, then the placenta is partially or completely detached but may be trapped by the cervix or lower uterine segment. It can also be caused by an atonic uterus, which has prevented normal separation, or because of a partially or completely adherent placenta.

Intravenous access should be obtained with consent and the woman's bladder emptied. Blood must be taken for cross-matching and checking the haemaglobin levels. Whilst the routine use of intravenous oxytocic agents should not be used in cases of a retained placenta, if the bleeding is excessive and the placenta is retained, they can be considered.[7]

The need for manual removal of the placenta (see Box 12.5 and Figure 12.1), preceded by a vaginal examination, should be discussed; however, the

---

BOX 12.5: Manual removal of placenta[19]

ENSURE ASEPTIC TECHNIQUE IS USED:

Insert a urinary catheter if not already done.

Hold the cord with the non-dominant hand whilst inserting the dominant hand (using cone-shaped fingers) through the cervix into the uterine cavity, following the cord to the placenta.

Identify the edge of the placenta.

Move the non-dominant hand up to support the fundus externally.

The fingers of the inserted hand remain closed when finding the edge of the placenta.

Move fingers behind the placenta to start gently shearing it off the uterine wall in a side-to-side motion.

As the placenta separates, cup it in the hand.

Once completely separated, rub up a contraction, which should expel the hand containing the whole placenta.

Rub up a contraction.

Commence an oxytocic infusion.

Inspect the placenta and membranes to ensure they are complete.

(a)

(b)

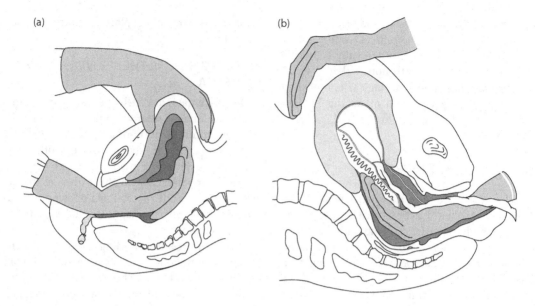

Figure 12.1 Manual removal of placenta (a) stage 1: separation, (b) stage 2: removal

woman should be informed this can be painful and analgesia may be required. If the woman reports inadequate analgesia during a manual removal procedure, it must be stopped and adequate pain relief administered. It is usually the obstetrician who carries out this procedure, although a midwife can do this in an emergency or a community setting (NMC, 2019).

Placenta accreta is a spectrum disorder (PAS) which ranges from an adherent placenta to deeply invasive placenta tissue and can cause catastrophic bleeding once any part of the placenta separates from the uterine wall (see Chapter 4, Box 4.2 for further information). However, a retained placenta, which is merely entrapped in the uterus after childbirth owing to constriction of the cervix, should not be included in the category of PAS disorders, nor should cases where a retained placenta is easily removed within 30 minutes after birth.[20]

MINOR PPH

The following actions should be taken when a minor PPH is diagnosed (see Box 12.1 for a definition). If taken in a timely manner, in most cases, these actions are effective, and the bleeding can be controlled. Depending on the help available, these actions should be taken simultaneously.

Call for help: if in a hospital, the emergency call bell should be used, or if at home, call an emergency ambulance (dial 999 in the UK) for assistance and transfer.

Identify the cause: if the uterus feels soft and 'boggy' it is not contracted, therefore, a contraction should be immediately 'rubbed up' by cupping a hand over the fundus and massaging the uterus with a rotational movement to stimulate a contraction (see Figure 12.2). This should also expel any blood clots or retained products that may be restricting the contraction of the uterus.

The perineum and genital tract should be examined for any lacerations. If a bleeding point is seen, pressure should be applied and suturing should take place as soon as possible.

Observation of the blood loss should be carried out to ensure blood is clotting normally.

First line drugs should be administered: the choice of drug will depend on local Trust policy and the availability of the drugs. See Box 12.6 for examples.

Intravenous access should be obtained: at least one large gauge cannula is necessary in order to obtain blood samples, administer drugs and give replacement fluids. One litre of warmed crystalloid solution should be commenced. An overview of fluid therapy can be found in Box 12.8.

Blood specimens should be taken for urgent group and screen, full blood count, coagulation screen including fibrinogen and any other tests according to local guidelines.

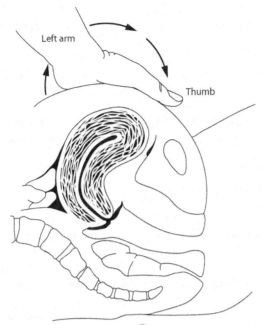

The left hand is cupped over the uterus ( ) and massages it with a firm circular motion in a clockwise direction.

Figure 12.2 Rubbing up a contraction

BOX 12.6: First line drugs[1,10]

One of the following can be considered:

- Oxytocin 5IU by slow intravenous injection.
- Oxytocin 10IU by intramuscular injection.
- Ergometrine 0.5mg by intramuscular injection or slow intravenous injection (contraindicated in women with hypertension and heart/renal disease).
- Intramuscular Syntometrine (Oxytocin 5IU and ergometrine 0.5mg).

In addition to the previous, an intravenous infusion of 40IU Oxytocin in 500ml Sodium Chloride over 4 hours running at 125ml/minute can be commenced, or an Oxytocin infusion according to local Trust Guidelines.

Tranexamic Acid – 1g given by slow intravenous injection over ten minutes. This may be repeated after 30 minutes and works by inhibiting the breakdown of clots.

Close monitoring of the blood loss and maternal condition should be maintained for as long as necessary to identify any further deterioration in the clinical situation.

Documentation should be completed: ensure a Modified Early Warning Obstetric Score (MEOWS) and fluid balance chart is ongoing to compare with future findings. Any other documentation according to the local Trust's guidelines should also be filled out.

Communication with the woman, her partner and the multidisciplinary team should be maintained throughout the emergency.

Regular vital signs should be carried out – pulse, respiratory rate and blood pressure should be checked at least every 15 minutes and temperature hourly. Continuous pulse oximetry (saturations) readings may be a valuable assessment tool.

An indwelling urinary catheter should be inserted to empty the bladder as a full bladder can inhibit uterine contractions.

MAJOR PPH

As soon as a major PPH is recognised, in addition to the previous measures, the following should be carried out, again simultaneously where possible, taking an ABC approach (see Box 12.1 for a definition of PPH).

Call for further help: if in a hospital, the emergency call bell should be used, or call an emergency ambulance (dial 999 in the UK) if at home for urgent assistance and transfer. In most UK hospitals, a MOH (Major Obstetric Haemorrhage) call will notify the consultant obstetrician, senior anaesthetist, haematologist and porters and ensure that theatre staff are on standby.

A helicopter view of the situation should be maintained by one senior clinician, who should coordinate all aspects of care, ensuring all tasks are being done at the same time where possible and a scribe has been allocated. The anaesthetist plays a crucial role in the multidisciplinary team in maintaining haemodynamic stability and, if necessary, administering the most appropriate form of anaesthesia.

Airway, breathing and circulation should be assessed, and if there is any sign of compromise, the woman should be laid flat with attention paid to ensuring the airway is maintained. High-flow oxygen at 10–15lt/min can be administered via a facemask. If the airway is compromised due to impaired consciousness level, this should improve once the circulating volume is restored.

Vital signs (pulse, blood pressure, respirations, oxygen saturations and temperature) should be assessed frequently to monitor the maternal condition. The woman must be kept warm as she can easily become hypothermic, which will exacerbate acidosis.

Continuous assessment of the bleeding, keeping a running total of the amount (weighing blood loss if possible), and maintaining uterine massage if necessary.

Second line drugs should be administered. Again, the choice of drug will depend on local Trust policy and the availability of the drugs. See Box 12.7 for an overview.

Intravenous access and blood tests: if not already done, a second large gauge cannula should be inserted. Any additional or repeat blood tests should be taken according to Trust guidelines, and blood should be cross-matched and dispatched from the blood bank according to need.

Fluid replacement is continued, using rapid fluid warming equipment and pressure bags where possible. It is important that fluids are warm as the infusion of cold fluids can impair clotting and

---

BOX 12.7: Second line drugs[1]

- Carboprost 0.25mg by intramuscular injection repeated at 15-minute intervals to a maximum of 8 doses.
- Misoprostol 800 to 1000 ug given rectally.
- Tranexamic Acid – 1g in 10mls given by slow intravenous injection over ten minutes – can be repeated 30 minutes after the first dose.

---

cause potentially lethal cardiac arrhythmias.[21] The woman should be kept warm at all times.

The cornerstone of resuscitation is to restore blood volume and oxygen-carrying capacity. The anaesthetist will take the lead in managing the fluid therapies to be used, but accurate and contemporaneous fluid balance records and monitoring of the woman's condition are needed as large volumes of clear fluids may dilute clotting factors and therefore interfere with the effectiveness of coagulation.[22] See Box 12.8 for an overview of the fluids that may be administered.

Fluid assessment: if not already done, an indwelling urinary catheter with a urometer should be inserted, as urine output needs to be monitored at least hourly to check renal function and ensure an accurate fluid balance.

Bimanual compression should be carried out in a timely manner if the bleeding continues or if help is not available and the midwife is on their own. Whilst being effective, it is also invasive and painful; therefore, it should be discussed with the woman and her birthing partner so consent can be given. See Box 12.9 and Figure 12.3

Another option is Abdominal Aortic Compression, which can be used in an emergency as a short-term measure. This involves the midwife pacing a fist above the umbilicus and fundus and pushing down to compress the aorta against the spine to reduce blood flow to the uterus.[10]

If bleeding continues, the woman may need to be transferred to theatre for more invasive procedures. An overview of the potential interventions follows:

- *Cell salvage* should be considered for emergency use in both vaginal births and caesarean delivery. It is a process in which the blood that

BOX 12.8: Fluid overview[1]

- A maximum of 2L or crystalloid can be given, followed by up to 1.5L of colloid whilst waiting for packed red cells.
- Whilst there are no firm criteria for administering blood transfusion, the decision to do so should be based on both haematological and clinical assessment, as women with an acute PPH can have normal haemoglobin levels.
- Whilst waiting for cross-matched blood, most maternity units will have Group O rhesus-negative blood available for emergencies, and this can be warmed and administered.
- The administration of other blood products will be decided in conjunction with the haematologist and may include fresh frozen plasma, platelets, fibrinogen, cryoprecipitate and recombinant factor VIIa. Note – four units of fresh frozen plasma should be given if bleeding continues after four units of red blood cells have been administered.
- Dilutional coagulopathy and fluid overload may occur if large volumes of clear fluids and blood are given without consideration of these blood products.

BOX 12.9: Bimanual compression

- Using cone-shaped fingers, gently insert the hand into the anterior fornix of the vagina.
- Form a fist and apply pressure to the anterior wall of the uterus.
- The external hand dips down behind the uterus and pulls it forwards towards the symphysis. The hands are pushed together, compressing the uterus and placental site.
- Continue the pressure until the bleeding is under control.
- External bimanual compression can also be done by squeezing the uterus between the hands without entering the vagina.

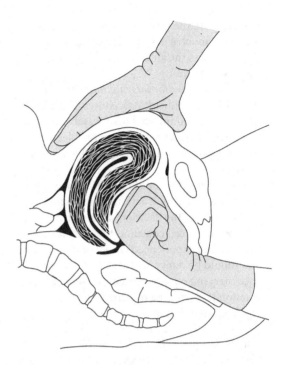

Figure 12.3 Internal bimanual compression

is being lost is collected, filtered and washed to produce red blood cells to be transfused back into the woman. It has been shown to be safe and effective in women at high risk of PPH during both elective and emergency caesarean sections where haemaglobin levels are less than 80g/L during the operation.[23]

- *Interventional radiology*: whilst difficult to perform in an emergency situation due to the specialised equipment and personnel needed, it can be useful in cases of continuing bleeding.
- *Intrauterine tamponade*: the insertion of a hydrostatic balloon catheter (e.g., Bakri [Cook Medical] or Rusch [Teleflex Medical] balloon) is seen as the first-line surgical intervention. If the bleeding is controlled following insertion, then laparotomy is not generally required;[1] however, if bleeding continues, then laparotomy is required so that surgical methods can be used to stop the bleeding.
- *Haemostatic suturing*: various techniques of haemostatic suturing are available, such as B-lynch suture and modified B-lynch suture; however, there is no evidence that any one method is better than another.[24] They work by compressing the uterus to stop the bleeding;

some require the uterine cavity to be opened, and some involve parallel or vertical sutures that compress the anterior uterine wall against the posterior wall.

- *Uterine vessel and/or internal iliac artery ligation*: although difficult procedures, the uterine, ovarian and internal iliac vessels can all be ligated in an attempt to stop the bleeding. A senior vascular surgeon should be informed and involved.
- *Hysterectomy*: this should be performed sooner rather than later in situations of uncontrollable bleeding. The decision should be made by an experienced consultant, ideally involving a second experienced clinician if possible and should be done by a surgeon with experience carrying out the procedure. Whilst the decision to perform a hysterectomy can be challenging, it is important not to delay the decision until the woman is in an advanced state of compromise.[1]

Invasive monitoring may be considered during and after a MOH. A central venous pressure (CVP) line can be used to monitor fluid replacement and to avoid fluid overload, and an arterial line may be used to monitor the condition of the woman and to take arterial blood to assess blood gases. These lines would be inserted by an anaesthetist.

Good documentation is vital to ensure an accurate record of all actions taken, drugs and fluids given, personnel involved and the ongoing condition of the woman is recorded. This is important for further clinical management, continuity of care and teamwork, and most Trusts use a proforma to record this information. The midwife should complete their documentation in line with their Trust's policies, ensuring a Modified Early Warning Obstetric Score (MEOWS) and fluid balance records are clear.

An incident report should also be completed as all cases of PPH greater than 1500ml should be subject to a formal incident review to ensure learning is taken from the incident.[7]

Communication should be maintained with the multidisciplinary team, and the woman and her family should be kept informed of events in an appropriate and sensitive manner. Consideration should be given to the traumatic nature of a PPH and the psychological impact this can have on the family and everyone involved (see Chapter 16). A debrief should be considered for the team when appropriate.

Postnatal care

Women should be closely monitored following a PPH for signs of further blood loss and ongoing clinical deterioration. See Box 12.10 for potential complications following a Major Obstetric Haemorrhage. Transfer to an intensive care unit or high-dependency unit is possible, especially if central venous pressure lines or arterial lines are still required to monitor fluid balance and the woman's condition.

Blood pressure, pulse, respirations, oxygen saturations and temperature should be regularly monitored and recorded on a MEOWS chart. Fluid balance should be accurately recorded and the woman should be kept warm and pain-free.

BOX 12.10: Risks for women who have had a massive obstetric haemorrhage

Women who have had a massive obstetric haemorrhage are at risk of:

- Renal impairment due to poor perfusion of the kidneys.
- Respiratory compromise – secondary to fluid overload or transfusion reactions.
- Venous thromboembolism due to infused clotting agents and rebound hypercoagulable state.
- Iron deficiency if not adequately treated.
- Infection due to invasive procedures carried out and likely anaemia.
- Further bleeding due to deranged coagulation.
- Sheehans' syndrome – a rare but serious complication in which infarctions of the pituitary gland occur as a result of hypovolaemia. The damage can lead to poor lactation, amenorrhoea, infertility, hypothyroidism and adrenal cortex failure. The breasts and genital organs can also atrophy.

BOX 12.11: Disseminated Intravascular Coagulation (DIC)

DIAGNOSIS

An acute history of a predisposing condition (e.g., placental abruption).

Bleeding from orifices, e.g., nose, mouth, venepuncture site, haematuria.

Blood loss does not immediately clot.

Torrential haemorrhage.

Signs of circulatory obstruction, e.g., cyanosis in fingers, cerebrovascular accident (stroke) or renal failure.

Blood test results: low haemoglobin, abnormal clotting study results (prothrombin time, abnormal levels of platelets, fibrinogen and FDPs).

MANAGEMENT[25]

Request urgent medical attendance when DIC is suspected.

Give ongoing explanations and emotional support to the woman and her partner as necessary.

Refer to the local protocol, which should include how DIC should be managed.

Look for the underlying cause if it is not known (DIC is never a primary disease), although the woman's condition will need to be stabilised before the condition is treated (or the baby delivered when the condition occurs in pregnancy).

Urgent blood test results will dictate the course of management, including full blood count, clotting studies and time taken to group and cross-match blood. Replacement of blood cells and clotting factors will be required with fresh frozen plasma, platelet concentrates and, ultimately, red blood cells.

Maintain frequent and accurate observations of the woman's vital signs. Invasive monitoring with a central venous pressure and/or arterial line may be necessary; however, the woman's coagulation status must be considered. The bladder should be catheterised, and fluid balance vigilantly monitored.

Transfer to ICU is likely.

Disseminated Intravascular Coagulation (DIC) can occur after severe blood loss due to coagulation factors being rapidly used up and the fibrinolytic system is activated. This causes disruption to the control of the balance between coagulation and fibrinolysis and can cause bleeding from wounds and venous puncture sites. If this continues, physiological haemostasis may no longer be possible.[10] Prompt diagnosis and management are vital for maternal survival. See Box 12.11 for details.

Women who have experienced a major PPH should be offered a debrief and an opportunity to discuss the events at a time appropriate to them. Major PPH can be traumatic to women and their families and has been linked to the subsequent development of post-traumatic stress disorder.[26] See Chapter 16 for a more in-depth discussion of this subject.

SUMMARY OF MIDWIFERY RESPONSIBILITIES

- Be aware of the maternity unit's PPH protocol.
- Ensure an ongoing knowledge of drugs and techniques used to treat PPH/MOH, as these are subject to change.
- Participate in regular multidisciplinary training.
- Be aware of the causes and risk factors of PPH.
- Recognise a PPH when it is happening, call for appropriate help and initiate initial measures to stop the bleeding.
- Act as the woman's advocate.
- Be mindful of the traumatic nature of a major PPH on both the woman and her family, as well as a potential effect on all participating staff.

FURTHER READING AND RESOURCES

Royal College of Obstetricians and Gynaecologists (RCOG). Prevention and management of postpartum haemorrhage. Green top guideline no. 52. London. RCOG; 2016. Available from: <doi:10.1111/1471-0528.14178>

Manual removal of the placenta video. Available from: www.youtube.com/watch?v=4iHSXADzc98

Sheehan syndrome video. Available from: https://youtu.be/1exN1kFX2wl

Placenta accreta video. Available from: https://youtu.be/x3EMTQQjoA0

REFERENCES

1. Royal College of Obstetricians and Gynaecologists (RCOG). Prevention and management of postpartum haemorrhage. Green top guideline no. 52. London. RCOG; 2016. Available from: <doi:10.1111/1471-0528.14178>
2. Evensen A, Anderson J, Fontaine P. Postpartum haemorrhage: prevention and treatment. American Family Physician. 2017;95(7):442–449. PMID: 28409600.
3. Fawcus S, Moodley J. Postpartum haemorhage associated with caesarean section and caesarean hysterectomy. Best Practice and Research Clinical Obstetrics and Gynaecology. 2013;27(2):233–224. Available from: <doi:10.1016/j.bpobgyn.2012.08.018>
4. World Health Organisation (WHO). WHO postpartum haemorrhage (PPH) summit. Current Project Brief. WHO; 2022.
5. Knight M, Bunch K, Patel R, Shakespeare J, Kotnis R, Kenyon S, Kurinczuk J., On Behalf of MBRRACE-UK Saving Lives, editors. Saving lives, improving mothers' care: core report: lessons learned to inform maternity care from the UK and Ireland confidential enquiries into maternal deaths and morbidity 2018–20. Oxford: National Perinatal Epidemiology Unit, University of Oxford; 2022.
6. Daniels K, Auguste T. 2013. Moving forward in patient safety: multidisciplinary team training. Semin Perinatol, 37(3):146–150. Available from: <doi:10.1053/j.semperi.2013.02.004>
7. National Institute for Health and Care Excellence. CG 190 intrapartum care for health women and babies. 2014, updated 2022. [Accessed 16 July 2023]. Available from: www.nice.org.uk/guidance/cg190
8. Stables D, Rankin J. Physiology in childbearing: with anatomy and related biosciences. 4th ed. London: Elsevier; 2017.
9. Winter C, Crofts J, Draycott T. Major obstetric haemorrhage, module 8, practical obstetric multiple professional training course manual. 3rd ed. Cambridge: Cambridge University Press; 2017.
10. Kavle J.A, Stoltzfus RJ, Witter F, Tielsch JM, Khalfan SS, Caulfield LE. Association between anaemia during pregnancy and blood loss at and after delivery among women with vaginal births in Pemba Island, Zanzibar, Tanzania. Journal of Health and Population and Nutrition. 2008;26:232–240. PMC2740668.
11. Hancock A, Weeks AD, Lavender DT. Is accurate and reliable blood loss estimation the 'crucial step' in early detection of postpartum haemorrhage: an intergrative review of the literature. BMC Pregnancy Childbirth. 2015;15:230. Available from: <doi:10.1186/s12884-015-0653-6>
12. Diaz V, Abalos E, Carroli G. Methods for blood loss estimation after vaginal birth (Review). Cochrane Database of Systematic Reviews. 2018;9. Available from: <doi:10.1002/14651858.CD010980.pub2>
13. Paterson-Brown S, Howell C. Managing obstetric emergencies and trauma. 3rd ed. Cambridge: Cambridge University Press; 2014.
14. Tuffnell D, Knight M, On Behalf of the MBRRACE-UK Haemorrhage Working Group. Lessons for care of women with haemorrhage or amniotic fluid embolism. In: Knight M, Bunch K, Tuffnell D, et al., editors. Saving lives, improving mothers' care – lessons learned to inform maternity care from the UK and Ireland confidential enquiries into maternal deaths and morbidity 2016–2018. Oxford: National Perinatal Epidemiology Unit, University of Oxford; 2020.

15. Mukherjee S, Arulkumaran S. Postpartum haemorrhage. Obstetrics, Gynaecology and Reproductive Medicine. 2009;19(5):121–126 .

16. Begley CM, Gyte, GML, Devane D, McGuire W, Weeks A, Biesty LM. Active versus expectant: management for women in the third stage of labour. Cochrane Database of Systematic Reviews. 2019;2. Available from: <doi:10.1002/14651858.CD007412.Pub5>

17. Abedi P, Jahanfar S, Namvar F, Lee J. Breastfeeding or nipple stimulation for reducing postpartum haemorrhage in the third stage of labour. Cochrane Database of Systematic Reviews. 2016;1. Available from: <doi:10.1002/14651858.CD010845.Pub2>

18. Salati JA, Leathersich SJ, Williams MJ, Cuthbert A, Tolosa JE. Prophylactic oxytocin for the third stage of labour to prevent postpartum haemorrhage (Review). Cochrane Database of Systematic Reviews. 2019;4. Available from: <doi:10.1002/14651858.CD001808.pub3>

19. Gunawardane K, Ratnayake C. Retained placenta. In: Chandraharan E, Arulkumaran S, editors. Obstetric and intrapartum emergencies: a practical guide to management, 2nd ed. Cambridge: Cambridge University Press; 2021.

20. Jauniaux E, Chantraine F, Silver RM, Langhoff-Roos J. FIGO consensus guidelines on placenta accreta spectrum disorders: epidemiology, Int J Gynecol Obstet. 2018;140(3):265–273. Available from: <doi:10.1002/ijgo.12407>

21. Freedman RL, Lucas DN. MBRACE-UK: saving lives, improving mothers' care – implications for anaesthatists. International Journal of Obstetric Anesthia. 2015;24(2):161–173. Available from: <doi:10.1016/j.ijoa.2015.03.004>

22. Gillessen A, van den Akker T, Caram-Deelder C. Association between fluid management and dilutional coagulopathy in severe postpartum haemorrhage: a nationwide retrospective cohort study. BMC Pregnancy Childbirth. 2018;19:1–9. Available from: <doi:10.1186/s12884-018-2021-9>

23. Lei B, Guo M, Deng X, He S, Lu X, Wang Y, Wang L. Intraoperative cell salvage as an effective intervention for postpartum hemorrhage – evidence from a prospective randomised controlled trial. Frontiers in Immunology. 2022;13:1–10. Available from: <doi:10.3389/fimmu.2022.953334>

24. Kellie FJ, Wandabwa JN, Mousa HA, Weeks AD. Mechanical and surgical interventions for treating primary postpartum haemorrhage. Cochrane Database of Systematic Reviews. 2020;7. Available from: <doi:10.1002/14651858.CD013663>

25. Erez O. Disseminated intravascular coagulation in pregnancy: new insights. Thrombosis Update. 2022;6:100083.

26. de Graaff LF, Honig A, van Pampus MG, Stramrood CAI. Preventing post-traumatic stress disorder following childbirth and traumatic birth experiences: a systematic review. Acta Obstet Gynecol Scand. 2018;97:648e656. Available from: <doi:10.1111/aogs.13291>

13

Amniotic fluid embolism: (Anaphylactoid syndrome of pregnancy)

MAUREEN BOYLE

Introduction	194	Follow-up/long-term issues	200
Pathophysiology	195	Summary of midwifery responsibilities	200
Risk/pre-disposing factors	196	Further reading and resources	200
Clinical features	196	References	201
Care	198		

BOX 13.1: Amniotic Fluid Embolism (AFE)

AFE usually includes a sudden cardiovascular collapse, DIC (disseminated intravascular coagulation) and hypoxia, often manifesting as an altered mental state.

Although many definitions involve the timing of AFE restricted to occurrence in labour and immediately postnatal, there are cases that have been reported in the second trimester,[1] after trauma[2] and postnatally.[3] Also, rarely, cases have been reported antenatally after first-trimester termination and following amniocentesis.[4]

INTRODUCTION

Amniotic fluid embolism is a rare obstetric emergency that is impossible to predict. It offers few, if any, warning signs and frequently has a tragic outcome.

AFE was first mentioned in 1926; however, the description in 1941 by Steiner and Lushbaugh of maternal pulmonary embolism by amniotic fluid, after finding amniotic fluid in the pulmonary vessels at autopsy following a collapse during delivery with symptoms mimicking pulmonary embolism, is seen as the first publication in English acknowledging its importance.[5] Knowledge of the condition has only developed slowly since then due to its rarity. However, in 1988, a central registry recording women suffering from amniotic fluid embolism in the USA was set up, and reports from this group have contributed to awareness.[6] In the UK, a similar registry was set up in 2000.[7] The collection of data is now undertaken by UKOSS (UK Obstetric Surveillance System), their latest report on AFE being in 2012,[8] although UKOSS data was used in a study by Fitzpatrick et al.[9] more recently in 2015.

Currently, all cases of suspected AFE are submitted to UKOSS,[8] and deaths from AFE continue to be reported on with the analysis contributing to clinical recommendations by the Confidential Enquiries into Maternal Deaths, now under the umbrella of MBRRACE-UK (Mothers and Babies: Reducing Risk through Audits and Confidential Enquiries across the UK).[10]

When assessing the rates of maternal deaths, it is difficult to make comparisons between countries

DOI: 10.4324/9781003382195-13

as there are variations in the methodology of data collection as well as in definitions. However, in all countries that keep comprehensive records, AFE is identified as one of the most significant contributors to maternal mortality. Much knowledge of AFE worldwide continues to be gained from the review of case reports or case studies and, due to the differences in reporting these events, analysis may be challenging. Agustin Conde-Agudelo and Roberto Romero[11] have identified the need for a worldwide registry based on uniform diagnostic criteria and reports.

In the UK, recent research[9] covering 2005–2014 demonstrated AFE being diagnosed in 1.7:100,000 births. In the UK, in the years 2016–2018, eight women died from AFE, a mortality rate of 0.33, which was not statistically significantly different from the previous triennium. Six of the women died shortly after their initial collapse and resuscitation efforts. Two women were admitted to ITU after resuscitation but subsequently died.[10]

Other studies have also identified women dying early despite resuscitation. Rath[12] suggested that 56% of women don't survive more than two hours. The highest mortality in women appears to be very soon following the initial collapse in the acute stage, and chances of survival may be good with appropriate on-going supportive care.[13]

Alongside the mortality rate, it has also been noted that long-term morbidity is frequently associated with AFE survivors.[3,14] Extensive recent research[9] has suggested significant long-term morbidity, including permanent neurological injury. Recent analysis of the American International Registry[15] suggested a maternal death rate of 10% and a neurologically intact survival rate of 46%.

If the fetus is still alive when the AFE occurs, it is estimated that there may be a 70% survival rate for the infants,[3] but this will, of course, be related directly to the gestation and the time from maternal collapse to the birth of the baby. Although it has been suggested in the past that surviving infants commonly have neurological damage, it is likely that better care is decreasing this number.[9]

PATHOPHYSIOLOGY

The pathophysiology of AFE is unclear. It seems that amniotic fluid may enter the maternal circulation without causing problems,[13] but once this occurs, there are thought to be a number of haemodynamic, humoral and coagulopathic changes that may occur in some women and lead to the signs and symptoms of AFE. In these women, it seems an inflammatory response can develop, causing a rapid collapse similar to anaphylaxis or septic shock. There remains uncertainty about why this response occurs, but it is clear that the effect on the woman can be devastating and usually includes a sudden cardiovascular collapse, DIC (disseminated intravascular coagulation) and hypoxia, often manifesting as an altered mental state or respiratory arrest.

Obvious times of risk for entry of amniotic fluid and its constituents are during caesarean section or uterine rupture, but since amniotic fluid embolism can occur without these scenarios, it is also suggested that there may be small injuries during labour that allow the fluid access to maternal circulation through cervical veins, placental attachment or uterine surgical incisions/injury. Amniotomy is an intervention that may cause injury, and many studies report the majority of women had ruptured membranes at or before AFE presentation. The suggestion that placenta praevia and abruption[16] may be pre-disposing factors for AFE, together with more recent research implicating PAS (placenta accreta spectrum),[17] a further indication that the breakdown of the maternal/fetal barrier may be significant. However, it is clear that in some cases, the damage may occur spontaneously.

It is suggested that fetal antigens in the amniotic fluid could stimulate a cascade of endogenous immune mediators, producing a reaction similar to anaphylaxis.[18] It has been proposed that the immune reaction, when triggered, could result in the activation of the complement system generated by fetal antigens.[19,20] Others have suggested that bioactive chemicals present in the amniotic fluid cause these reactions directly.[21,22] It is possible that it is the amount of amniotic fluid, the chemical composition or the individual woman's susceptibility that causes the AFE, or perhaps a combination of these or other unknown factors.

The initial haemodynamic result is acute pulmonary vessel vaso-restriction, resulting in acute right heart failure, dilation of the right ventricle and significant tricuspid insufficiency.[12] This will lead to respiratory failure, cardiac arrest and other acute signs and symptoms.

As AFE is now seen as a maternal response to the amniotic fluid and/or fetal debris in the circulation, rather than the fluid itself causing a blockage, this is represented in the suggested new name: **Anaphylactoid Syndrome of Pregnancy**. Various other names have also been suggested in the literature, such as 'anaphylactoid lung of pregnancy' and 'sudden obstetric collapse syndrome'; however, the term Amniotic Fluid Embolism continues to be widely used.

RISK/PRE-DISPOSING FACTORS

> ### BOX 13.2: Possible risk/pre-disposing factors for AFE[3,15,23,24]
>
> - 'Tumultuous' contractions
> - Age (primigravida > 35 years old)
> - Multiple pregnancy/Large fetus (uterine overdistension)
> - Meconium
> - Long labour
> - Abruption/placenta praevia/PAS
> - Multiparity
> - Induction/augmentation
> - Caesarean section
> - Invasive interventions in labour
> - Abdominal trauma
> - Medical history of allergy or atopy
> - Fetal distress
> - Fetal death

Amniotic fluid embolism appears to be more common with increasing age, specifically over 35 years old.[9,20] Interestingly, in a large study (where almost three million hospital records over five years were reviewed), age and, in particular, older primigravid women were significantly more likely to experience an AFE.[16] However, there were no deaths in this category. This is particularly relevant as it is assumed this group would be more likely to have an induction of labour, caesarean section and other interventions. It could be hypothesised that perhaps increased surveillance led to quicker recognition and treatment and, therefore, a better outcome.

Induction of labour with prostaglandins or oxytocin or augmentation with oxytocin or artificial rupture of membranes (ARM) are often considered to be associated with amniotic fluid embolism,[20] and UKOSS[8] identified induction as a significant risk factor. In the most recent Confidential Enquiries, all of the eight women who died had induction of labour, and it was identified that for some of the women, the reason for induction was unclear.[10]

'Tumultuous' labour was described in 28% of women in one American report,[16] and abnormally strong contractions have also been noted by previous Confidential Enquiries in the UK.[25] Multiparity has been identified as a common factor in many studies.[3,17,23] If the strength of contractions is considered to have an influence over the occurrence of AFE, multiparous women could be assumed to frequently have very strong contractions and, therefore, be at increased risk.

However, it is also possible that the reported intense/tumultuous contractions are not the cause of the AFE but a reaction to it. It is a common characteristic of mammals when a sudden threatening pathophysiological event occurs for the body to make a desperate attempt to rid itself of the pregnancy in order to survive. This could be a normal reaction of the woman's body to try and survive the acute insult of the AFE.

When interpreting risk factors from reports, caesarean section/instrumental delivery are usually high on the list,[9,11] but analysis of the studies should be made as frequently the intervention was a result of the signs and symptoms of AFE, rather than the signs and symptoms occurring for the first time following the delivery.

Identification of risk factors is common throughout the literature; however, these are not yet specific enough to allow AFE to be predicted or even anticipated. Although the roles of different risk factors are uncertain, they do serve to highlight the range of women who may suffer AFE and the necessity for the midwife to keep the possibility of an occurrence in mind.

CLINICAL FEATURES

Signs and symptoms

The first symptoms seen may be shortness of breath, with or without altered mental status, followed by cardiovascular collapse and DIC. However, haemorrhage may be the first symptom, or in some cases, fetal bradycardia. Seizures are a less common presenting symptom. AFE should always be suspected if a previously asymptomatic healthy woman develops cardiac or respiratory failure during labour, caesarean section or immediately after.

Analysis of the American Registry showed that the symptoms of women diagnosed with amniotic fluid embolism were as follows, given in the order in which they most commonly occurred:[6]

- Hypotension
- Fetal distress

BOX 13.3: UKOSS[8] case definition for AFE

Either: *clinical diagnosis*, such as maternal collapse with one or more of the following features:

Cardiac arrest, acute hypotension, acute hypoxia, cardiac arrhythmias, seizures, haemorrhage/coagulopathy, premonitory symptoms, sudden fetal compromise

OR: *pathological diagnosis*:

The presence of fetal squames or hair in the lungs.

In the absence of any other potential explanation for the signs and symptoms.

- Pulmonary oedema
- Cardiopulmonary arrest
- Cyanosis
- Coagulopathy
- Respiratory distress
- Seizures
- Uterine atony
- Bronchospasm

However, in individual women, these symptoms can appear alone, in combination and, of course, in any order. Diagnosis is made on clinical symptoms after the exclusion of other possible causes. UKOSS[8] who have been monitoring AFE occurrences since 2005, define AFE clinically, using set criteria for diagnosis (see Box 13.3).

Coagulation problems affect about 80% of those developing AFE.[3] It has been noted by a UK Confidential Enquiries report[26] that the small number of women who did not demonstrate DIC all died quickly, suggesting that the coagulopathy effect perhaps had not yet commenced. In a French study, it was reported that ten of the 11 women diagnosed with AFE had DIC, necessitating massive blood and blood products transfusion.[27] The cause of this coagulopathy is not well understood. It is known that amniotic fluid is a procoagulant,[28,29] but this may not be enough to cause the often catastrophic haemorrhage. The coagulopathy may also be a result of complement system activation.[19] It has been noted that there may be increased coagulation pathology when meconium is present.[3] The DIC is likely to be consumptive rather than fibrinolytic as amniotic fluid contains active coagulation factors II, VII and X.[13]

Fetal distress may occur as maternal catecholamine release can involve shunting of uterine blood from the uterus and placenta to the maternal circulation to maintain blood pressure, and this would adversely affect the oxygenation of the fetal heart. This may precede cardiopulmonary symptoms in the woman.[30]

There is a suggestion that women may present with vague 'premonitory' signs and symptoms such as breathlessness, chest pain, light-headedness, nausea/vomiting, distress or panic immediately or up to four hours prior to AFE.[31] Many women, especially in advanced labour, become agitated and commonly display non-specific symptoms, especially related to hyperventilation which often occurs at this time. It is difficult to see how these suggested 'premonitory' signs can translate to normal midwifery care in labour; however, it could be that early recourse to oxygen saturation monitoring would be minimally disruptive to the labour, reassuring to the midwife and serve to identify a woman with hypoxia in the very rare circumstances that this occurs.

Traditionally, diagnosis of amniotic fluid embolism was only made on post-mortem examination when fetal cells or debris were found during histological analysis of the maternal lungs. Diagnosis has also been made in women who have survived, for example, following special staining of blood from the mothers' pulmonary vessels or after finding fetal squames in sputum. However, these cells may be due to contamination and adult and fetal squames often cannot be distinguished histologically[11] and have, in fact, been found in even non-pregnant women.[29] Of course, these tests are usually carried out only when the woman's physical condition is compromised. It should also be noted that evidence of fetal debris in maternal lungs may not be present at autopsy if she survived for several days.[31]

The finding of squamous cells is considered more significant if they are present in large numbers, are coated with neutrophils and/or are accompanied by other fetal debris.[11,18] It is a difficult diagnosis as fetal squames may be found in maternal circulation in those who don't die or, in fact, are not unwell.[26]

Most authorities agree that an unexplained sudden onset of a triad of severe symptoms, namely **hypotension**, **hypoxia** and **coagulopathy**, are highly suspicious of AFE. These can involve:[6,29]

- Acute hypotension or cardiac arrest
- Acute hypoxia (cyanosis, dyspnoea or respiration arrest)
- Coagulopathy
- Acute fetal compromise
- Onset during labour or within 30 minutes of delivery
- No other clinical conditions or possible diagnoses for signs and symptoms

CARE

Since it is not yet possible to clearly identify those women who are at risk of AFE or to prevent it, the focus must be on providing those women who collapse with prompt and competent basic care prior to a speedy transfer to where they can receive expert support and treatment, usually in an intensive care unit. This can improve their chances not only of survival, but also of a complete recovery.

Treatment aims

- Respiratory support
- Circulatory support
- Correct coagulopathy

Immediate care following collapse

This will be the same whether at home or in hospital and includes the following:

- Call for emergency help (in hospital: emergency call bell, at home: emergency paramedics – phone 999 in the UK)
- Ventilation: oxygen administration, manual ventilation with an ambubag or intubation, depending on the site and availability of equipment or personnel
- Cardiac compressions as necessary
- Intravenous access X 2 and consideration of fluids

(See Chapter 3 for further details of basic CPR.)

On-going care

Following the arrival of help in hospital or the woman's arrival at hospital, the priorities of care in response to treatment aims continue, many occurring simultaneously:

Respiratory support

- Early endotrachael intubation is recommended[30]
- Maintain oxygenation via intermittent positive pressure ventilation (IPPV) as required
- Oxygen saturation should be commenced to monitor respiratory function
- If still pregnant, peripartum caesarean section may be necessary for successful resuscitation, and the midwife needs to anticipate this
- Trigger MOH protocol at the same time as the decision to proceed to perimortem caesarean section is made, or earlier if any indication[10]

Maintain circulation

- Administer fluids to support circulation (may be blood, fresh frozen plasma, cryoprecipitates, crystalloids or platelets, depending on availability and the woman's need)
- Fluids are given to maintain BP and respond to haemorrhage – note that there is a danger of overload leading to pulmonary oedema, so careful fluid balance and renal assessment (including inserting an indwelling urinary catheter at the earliest opportunity) must be maintained

Treat coagulopathy

- Coagulation abnormalities and major maternal haemorrhage should be anticipated – blood and blood product transfusion with fresh frozen plasma, cryoprecipitate and platelets are often required as indicated by laboratory results and advised by the haematologist. Early involvement of the haematologist is advised[10]
- Control any uterine haemorrhage: initially, routine assessment of the uterus/uterine massage as necessary, and the usual drugs (oxytocics, ergometrine, prostaglandins, tranexamic acid) and/or surgically (tamponade by intrauterine balloon, brace suture), including

bimanual compression (see Chapter 12 for more detail)

- Hysterectomy may be necessary, and it has been reported that about one-quarter of women may need a hysterectomy to stop the bleeding[13]
- Monitor clotting and correct coagulopathy
- Uterine artery embolisation to inhibit coagulopathy may be used if available

Assessment

- Initial blood tests should include a full blood count, group and cross-match, electrolytes, coagulation studies including prothrombin time, partial thromboplastin time, fibrin degradation products, D-Dimer and anti-thrombin III levels, plus venous/arterial blood gases (see Box 13.4 for a full list of potential investigations)
- Monitor maternal condition, initially with continuous pulse oximetry to assess the respiratory system, continuous cardiac telemetry to detect arrhythmias and frequent blood pressure monitoring
- Central venous pressure, arterial lines or pulmonary artery catheters, as appropriate, may be used to guide therapy, but coagulopathy may restrict the ability to use invasive monitoring
- The effect of blood/fluid replacement and supportive treatment should be continuously monitored by signs and symptoms of adequate oxygen delivery and tissue perfusion

Drugs

- In addition to drugs to treat haemorrhage (as listed previously under coagulopathy), medication such as epinephrine, dopamine, milrinone or noradrenaline may be used to support the cardiovascular system[3,18]
- Treatment of anaphylaxis with salbutamol, aminophylline and hydrocortisone may be appropriate

Additional treatments

Several treatments have been suggested but are not currently in widespread use.

BOX 13.4: Potential investigations

Blood tests:

- Clotting factors are assessed frequently, as well as FBC for levels of Hb and platelets
- Urea & Electrolytes and VBG/ABG assessments are carried out to evaluate the renal and respiratory systems
- Sialyl (fetal glycoprotein) may be elevated, and complement levels may be decreased

INVESTIGATIONS WHICH MAY EXCLUDE/CONFIRM DIAGNOSES INCLUDE:

- *Chest x-rays* (usually non-specific in AFE but may show diffuse lung opacity)
- *Twelve-lead ECG* (which may show changes from the right ventricular strain)
- *Echocardiograms* (may confirm right or left ventricular failure or severe pulmonary hypertension)
- *Lung V/Q scan* (may show non-specific perfusion defects)

However, no tests should delay basic, comprehensive and on-going resuscitation: a previous Confidential Enquiries[31] noted sub-standard care in two cases where resuscitation was delayed as the women were sent for unnecessary diagnostic scans.

- Heparin, either unfractionated or low molecular weight, has been reported to be used but is not yet established as recommended care[32]
- Pulmonary vasodilators, for example, inhaled nitric oxide, intralipids and cardio-pulmonary bypass, have all been suggested as potential treatments in some circumstances[26,29]
- Plasma exchange transfusion may be used, in theory, to remove cellular debris, coagulation by-products and cytokines, and may also help correct acidosis[13]
- Extracorporeal membrane oxygenation (ECMO) use has been reported to be of use[29,33]
- Therapeutic hypothermia has been suggested, with the aim of maintaining a normal neurological outcome[34]

FOLLOW-UP/LONG-TERM ISSUES

Support and care for partners and others must not be neglected, and consideration of psychological support for women who survive this life-threatening situation is necessary. See Chapter 16 for further discussion on this important matter.

Most commonly, after an AFE the woman will be initially stabilised and then transferred to an Intensive Care facility for supportive care. Midwives will usually only care for this woman again when she has been moved back to the maternity critical care unit, and it is likely her needs will mainly involve the same elements as women recovering from a massive haemorrhage (see Chapter 12).

Although there are very limited numbers to base this on, there are indications that recurrence of AFE is unlikely in subsequent pregnancies.[29,35]

SUMMARY OF MIDWIFERY RESPONSIBILITIES

- If a woman collapses at home or in hospital, prompt, effective emergency support can improve her chance of complete recovery.
- The resuscitation trolley needs to contain equipment (pre-mounted scalpel blade, gloves and cord clamps at a minimum) to undertake perimortem caesarean section wherever necessary.
- All maternity units should have regular resuscitation 'skills drills', and it should be mandatory for all those working within midwifery and obstetrics to update regularly – emergencies happen too infrequently for any midwife or doctor to be complacent about their abilities. It is also particularly useful (although admittedly challenging to arrange) if at least some of these 'skills drills' take place on the labour ward itself. This can help to ensure all personnel know how to access relevant drugs and equipment.
- Labour, and especially transition, is often a time of mood change and uncharacteristic maternal behavior, and midwives are very familiar with this scenario. However, given that confusion and/or behavior/mood change can be the first sign of hypoxia, it would be useful if the midwife could assess

this quickly with an oxygen saturation reading, so she can be reassured or, in the unlikely event hypoxia is present, summon help immediately ensuring as early action as possible is obtained. Until there is further knowledge of the meaning and reliability of these noted 'premonitory' signs, there seems little else the midwife can do other than ensure she remains alert.

- The strong association between induction and AFE is clear, and, therefore, particular care needs to be taken in the use of prostaglandins and oxytocins, particularly in those women with other possible risk factors, for example, age, multiparity and obstetric complications, and that other obstetric interventions, such as amniotomy, should be used only when necessary. Despite their common use, prostaglandin and oxytocin should always be treated with respect, and all women receiving these drugs should be monitored carefully.
- The use of midwifery skills to augment slow labour (including support, mobilisation, water and comfort strategies) may help to avoid amniotomy and oxytocin use.
- Effective resuscitation may depend on the birth of the baby (see Chapter 3), and during the resuscitation, the midwife may be the member of the team who is delegated to assess times and remind those undertaking resuscitation of the time scales. It is noted in a recent MBRRACE-UK report[26] that no woman received perimortem CS within five minutes. The midwife may also need to call the neonatal team.
- If the baby was born before the collapse, appropriate care for the infant must be undertaken.
- Ensure the partner and other family/friends present are informed and given support as appropriate (see Chapter 3).

FURTHER READING AND RESOURCES

Amniotic Fluid Embolism Foundation is a collaboration between private and academic institutions established to assist patients and families, provide education and promote research. www.afesupport.org

REFERENCES

1. Crissman HP, Loder C, Pancaro C, et al. Case report of amniotic fluid embolism coagulopathy following abortion; use of viscoelastic point-of-care analysis. BMC Pregnancy Childbirth. 2020;20:9. Available from: <doi:10.1186/s12884-019-2680-11>

2. Ellingsen C et al. Amniotic fluid embolism after blunt abdominal trauma. Resuscitation 2007;75(1):180–183.

3. Kaur K, Bhardwaj M, Kumar P, Singhal S et al. Amniotic fluid embolism. J Anaesthesiol Clin Pharmacol 2016;32(2):153–159. Available from: <doi:10.4103/0970-9185.173356>

4. Panda S, Das A, Sharma N, et al. (April 26, 2022) Amniotic Fluid Embolism After First-Trimester Abortion. Cureus 14(4): e24490. Available from: <doi:10.7759/cureus.2449>

5. Benson M. Amniotic fluid embolism: the known and not known. Obstetric Medicine 2014;7(1):17.21 Available from: <doi:10.1177/1753495X13513578>

6. Clark S, Hankins G, Dudley D et al. Amniotic fluid embolism: analysis of the national registry. Am J Obstet Gynecol. 1995;172(4:1):1158–1169. Available from: <doi:10.1016/0002-9378(95)91474-9>

7. Tuffnell D and Johnson H. Amniotic fluid embolism: the UK register. Hosp Med. 2000;61(8):532–534. Available from: <doi:10.12968/hosp.2000.61.8.1394>

8. Knight M, McClymont C, Fitzpatrick K, et al. United Kingdom obstetric surveillance system (UKOSS) annual report 2012. Oxford: National Perinatal Epidemiology Unit; 2012.

9. Fitzpatrick KE, Tuffnell D, Kurinczuk JJ, Knight M. Incidence, risk factors, management and outcomes of amniotic-fluid embolism: a population-based cohort and nested case – control study. BJOG 2015; Available from: <doi:10.1111/1471-0528.13300>

10. Tuffnell D, Knight M, On Behalf of the MBRRACE-UK Haemorrhage and AFE chapter-writing group. Chapter 7: Lessons for care of women with haemorrhage or amniotic fluid embolism. In: Knight M, Bunch K, Tuffnell D, Shakespeare J, Kotnis R, Kenyon S, Kurinczuk JJ, On Behalf of MBRRACE-UK, editors. Saving lives, improving mothers' care – lessons learned to inform maternity care from the UK and Ireland confidential enquiries into maternal deaths and morbidity 2016–18. Oxford: National Perinatal Epidemiology Unit, University of Oxford; 2020. p. 58–63.

11. Conde-Agudelo A and Romero R. Amniotic fluid embolism: an evidenced- based review. Am J Obstet Gynecol. 2009;201(5):445, e1–13 Available from: <doi:10.1016/j.ajog.2009.04.052>

12. Rath WH, Hoferr S, Sinicina I. Amniotic fluid embolism: an interdisciplinary challenge: epidemiology, diagnosis and treatment. Dtsch Arztebl Int. 2014 Feb 21;111(8): 126–32. Available from: <doi:10.3238/arztebl.2014.0126>. PMID: 24622759; PMCID: PMC3959223.

13. Tuffnell D and Slemeck E. Amniotic Fluid Embolism. Obstetrics, Gynaecology and Reproductive Medicine. 2014;24(5): 148–152. Available from: <doi:10.1016/j.ogrm.2014.04.004>

14. McDonnell N, Percival V and Paech M. Amniotic fluid embolism: a leading cause of maternal death yet still a medical conundrum. International Journal of Obstetric Anesthesia. 2013;22:329–336. Available from: <doi:10.1016/j.ijoa.2013.08.004>

15. Stafford I, Moaddab A, Dildy G, Klassen M, Berra A et al. Amniotic fluid embolism syndrome: analysis of the United States International Registry. Amer J Obsteric Gene. 2020;MFM PMID:33345954 doi:10.1016/j.ajogmf.2019.100083

16. Abenhaim H, Azoulay L, Kramer M & Leduc L. Incidence and risk factors of amniotic fluid embolisms: a population-based study on 3 million births in the United States. Am J Obstet Gynecol 2008;199:49, e1–e8. Available from: <doi:10.1016/j.ajog.2007.11.061>

17. Mazza G, Youssefzadeh A & Klar M et al. Association of pregnancy characteristics and maternal mortality with amniotic fluid embolism. JAMA Netw Open. 2022;5(11):e2242842 doi:10.1001/jamanet-workopen.2022.42842

18. Rudra A, Chatterjee S, Sengupta S et al. Amniotic fluid embolism. Indian Journal of Critical Care Medicine. 2009;13(3):129–135. Available from: <doi:10.4103/0972-5229.58537>

19. Benson M. A hypothesis regarding complement activation and amniotic fluid embolism. Medical Hypotheses 2007;68(5):1019–1025. Available from: <doi:10.1016/j.mehy.2006.09.052>

20. Metodiev Y, Ramasamy P & Tuffnell D. Amniotic fluid embolism. BJA. 2018;18(8):234–238. Available from: <doi:10.1016/j.bjae.2018.05.002>

21. Dedhia J & Mushambi M. Amniotic fluid embolism. Continuing Education in Anaesthesia Critical Care and Pain. 2007;7(5):152–156. Available from: <doi:10.1093/bjaceaccp/mkm031>

22. Abeysundara A, Abayadeera A, Wasala S & Ratnayake C. Early coagulopathy in amniotic fluid embolism. IAIM. 2021;8(2):92–96. ISSN:2394-0026(P) ISSN: 2394-0034 (O) Available online at http://iaimjournal.com

23. Fitzpatrick K, van den Akker T, Bloemenkamp K, Deneuz-Tharauz C, et al. Risk factors, management and outcomes of amniotic fluid embolism: a multicountry, population-based cohort and nested case-control study. PLoS Med. 2019;16(11):e1002962. Available from: <doi:10.1371/journal.pmed.1002962>

24. Hikiji W, Tamura N, Shigeta A et al. Fatal amniotic fluid embolism with typical pathohistological, histochemical and clinical features. Forensic Science International. 2012;226:e16–e19. Available from: <doi:10.1016/j.forsciint.2012.12.008>

25. Department of Health. Why mothers die: report on confidential enquiries into maternal deaths in the United Kingdom 1994–1996. London: The Stationery Office; 1998.

26. Harper A, Wilson R, On Behalf of the MBRRACE-UK Amniotic Fluid Embolism chapter writing group. Caring for women with amniotic fluid embolism. In: Knight M, Kenyon S, Brocklehurst P, Neilson J, Shakespeare J, Kurinczuk JJ, On Behalf of MBRRACE- UK, editors. Saving lives, improving mothers' care – lessons learned to inform future maternity care from the UK and Ireland confidential enquiries into maternal deaths and morbidity 2009–12. Oxford: National Perinatal Epidemiology Unit, University of Oxford; 2014.

27. Guillaume A, Sananes N, Akladios C et al. Amniotic fluid embolism: 10-year retrospective study in a level III maternity hospital. European Journal of Obstetrics & Gynecology and Reproductive Biology. 2013;169:189–192. Available from: <doi:10.1016/j.ejogrb.2013.02.017>

28. Hell L, Wisgrill L, Ay C, spittle et al. Procoagulant extracellular vesicles in amniotic fluid. Translational Research: the Journal of Laboratory and Clinical Medicine 2017;184:1220.e1 Available from: <doi:10.1016/j.trsl.2017.01.003>

29. Burns R, Dent K, editors. Chapter 12, amniotic fluid embolism in managing medical and obstetric emergencies and trauma. 4th ed. Oxford: Wiley Blackwell; 2022. p. 113–118.

30. Clark S. Managing obstetric emergencies: anaphylactoid syndrome of pregnancy (aka AFE). Contemporary OB/GYN. 2018;64(7):14–21.

31. Lewis G, editor. The confidential enquiry into maternal and child health (CEMACH). Saving mothers' lives: reviewing maternal deaths to make motherhood safer 2003–2005. The Seventh Report on Confidential Enquiries into Maternal Deaths in the UK. London: CEMACH; 2007.

32. Uszyński M & Uszyński W. Heparin and other anticoagulants in amniotic fluid embolism (AFE): literature review and concept of the therapy. Open Journal of Obstetrics and Gynecology – Electronic document. 2013 Sep;3(7):573–598. Available from: <doi:10.4236/ojog.2013.37106>

33. Durgam S, Sharma M, Dadhwal R, Vakil A, Surani S. The role of extra corporeal membrane oxygenation in amniotic fluid embolism: a case report and literature review. Cureus 2021;13(2): e13566. Available from: <doi:10.7759/cureus.13566>

34. Barriuso V, Pombar X, Bankowski H. The use of therapeutic hypothermia in the

management of amniotic fluid embolism. Obstetric Medicine. 2013;6(2): 92–93. Available from: <doi:10.1258/OM.2011.110069>

35. Stafford I, Parkes P, Moaddab A, Clark S et al. 177: the risk of amniotic fluid embolism reoccurrence in subsequent pregnancy. Am J Obstet Gynecol. 2018;218(Suppl 1). Available from: <doi:10.1016/j.ajog.2017.10.054>

14

Serious infection

JUDY BOTHAMLEY

SEPSIS	204	Care following admission to hospital	211
Introduction	204	INFLUENZA (flu)	213
Pathophysiology	205	Introduction	213
Risk/predisposing factors	206	Pathophysiology	214
Clinical features	206	Clinical features	214
Care	208	Care	215
COVID-19	209	Follow-up/long-term issues	216
Introduction	209	Summary of midwifery responsibilities	216
Pathophysiology	210	Further reading and resources	217
Clinical features	210	References	218

SEPSIS

BOX 14.1: Definitions

Infection is an invasion by pathogenic organisms that reproduce and multiply, which then generate an immune response. Prevention of infection and early identification and treatment of infection are key in preventing the development of sepsis.

Sepsis is defined as life-threatening organ dysfunction caused by a dysregulated host response to infection.[1] Things to note in this definition are that sepsis is life-threatening and, if not recognised early and managed promptly, can lead to septic shock, multiple organ failure and death.

Septic shock indicates profound deterioration. It is characterised by persistent hypotension requiring vasopressors (drugs to restrict blood vessels) to maintain mean arterial pressure ≥65 mmHg; and serum lactate >2 mmol/L (>18 mg/dL). It is associated with a greater risk of mortality than with sepsis alone.[1]

INTRODUCTION

Sepsis and septic shock are considered medical emergencies and need to be treated promptly.[2] The physiology of pregnancy and the interventions of childbirth make women more susceptible to serious complications of infection. Reports arising from the 'Confidential Enquiry into Maternal Deaths'[3,4] have noted a sustained increase in maternal mortality and morbidity due to sepsis. They have emphasised the need for awareness of the symptoms of sepsis, early recognition and prompt

DOI: 10.4324/9781003382195-14

referral of women with a 'back to basics' approach advocated that includes acknowledgement of risk factors, careful clinical assessment and recording of vital signs. Effective referral by the midwife to enable prompt interventions, including IV antibiotics, will be life-saving.

Sepsis can arise as a complication of infection from various sites in the body, commonly the genital tract and the lungs. Around 4% of live births are complicated by puerperal sepsis, which is an infection in the postnatal period and arising from the genital tract, urinary system, surgical sites or mastitis.[5] In addition, sepsis can arise antenatally, resulting in both maternal and fetal complications. Infection is a cause of miscarriage and preterm delivery and is thought to be associated in up to 25% of cases of stillbirth.[5] However, causes of maternal sepsis are not limited to infections relating directly to childbirth. In recent years, there have been a significant number of deaths from respiratory infections[5,6] (see sections on Covid-19 and Influenza).

PATHOPHYSIOLOGY

Pregnant and postpartum women are vulnerable to developing infections that may lead to sepsis.

In genital tract sepsis, *Escherichia coli* and group B streptococcus are the most common bacteria to cause infection, with the most severe outcomes associated with group A streptococcus (GAS).[7] GAS is a particularly serious, life-threatening organism that women may acquire from family members, particularly children. A concerning feature of GAS infections is that initially, the infection has few symptoms but can progress rapidly to fulminant infection and multi-organ involvement. The Confidential Enquiries report gives examples of the rapid progression of the infection. Even where health professionals recognised the illness and acted promptly, sadly, some women still died, despite excellent care.[8] GAS is normally found in the nasopharynx, and it is a cause of pharyngitis ('strep throat') and scarlet fever as well as genital tract sepsis. Approximately 5–30% of the population are asymptomatic carriers of the organism. Transmission is via aerosolised droplets and occurs more frequently in the winter months. Colonisation of the genital tract may occur via incomplete handwashing with subsequent contamination of the perineum.[9] Midwives should enquire about possible infection amongst family members

and advise women to wash their hands prior to and after using the toilet and/or changing their sanitary pads. For each maternal sepsis death, 50 women had life-threatening morbidity from sepsis.[9]

In sepsis, the normal immune response to infection is exaggerated and 'out of control'.[1] Cells of the immune system, such as macrophages and neutrophils, are activated in response to the presence of an invading pathogenic bacteria and are normally effective at controlling the spread of infection. Noncellular aspects of the immune system, including cytokines, tumour necrosis factor and interleukins, create a hostile environment for the bacteria causing inflammation, vasodilation and a rise in temperature. These responses are effective at controlling infection and/or the features of infection are identified, and antibiotic treatment commenced. However, in situations where there are lots of bacteria, treatment is not started, or the immune regulatory response is out of control and the response to the infection becomes generalised, resulting in sepsis. The inflammatory mediators act on the endothelial lining of blood vessels, causing increased capillary permeability and an increased production of the powerful vasodilator, nitric acid.[2] The blood vessels dilate, and fluid moves into the interstitial space, causing a significant drop in blood pressure and poor tissue perfusion.[5] Anaerobic metabolism due to oxygen deficiency in the cells starts to produce lactic acid. Compensatory mechanisms such as an increased heart rate and an increased respiratory rate aim to increase cardiac output and correct acidosis, but as these compensatory mechanisms fail to work, under-perfusion to the organs occurs and organs such as the kidneys and heart start to fail. The fluid shifts caused by sepsis put the woman at risk of pulmonary oedema. In sepsis, there will be reduced blood flow to the uterus, with consequent reduced oxygenation to the fetus and signs of fetal distress or demise may be evident. The midwife, through regular assessment of vital signs, should recognise and respond to the identification of these compensatory mechanisms.

A second wave of cytokine responses in sepsis involves the release of platelets and stimulation of the coagulation, complement and kinin systems. Platelet aggregation is triggered by endothelial damage. This activation of the coagulation system can result in disseminated intravascular coagulation (DIC).[2] See Chapter 12, Box 12.11 for further information about DIC. The tendency to clot formation on top of already-existing pro-coagulation of pregnancy predisposes pregnant and postpartum women with sepsis to microvascular clot formation. The combination of ischaemia from low blood pressure and clot formation will result in further organ dysfunction.

RISK/PREDISPOSING FACTORS

Interventions in labour, relative immune suppression of pregnancy, enhanced blood supply to the uterus, surgery, wounds and urinary catheterisation are a few reasons why childbirth increases the risk of sepsis. Pre-existing medical conditions such as diabetes, sickle cell disease, HIV and obesity increase vulnerability to infection. See Box 14.2 for a list of risk factors for the development of infection and sepsis. Although risk factors have been identified, it must be remembered that sepsis can occur in previously healthy women following uncomplicated pregnancy.

CLINICAL FEATURES

Sepsis is a complex syndrome, and some of the symptoms can be vague and overlap with other clinical conditions such as ectopic pregnancy, placental abruption and gastroenteritis. Midwives need to be alert to signs of sepsis by performing a regular set of observations, particularly on women who appear unwell and/or have risk factors such as women who have had prolonged rupture of membranes, possible incomplete delivery of the placenta, uterine tenderness or sub-involution (see Box 14.2 for risk factors). The midwife or a family member may note that the woman is 'not quite right', and the response to this intuitive concern should be an objective assessment of the woman. A general examination to identify features of infection, as well as indications that the woman's condition may be deteriorating, and assessment of any progression to sepsis and organ dysfunction must be undertaken. See Box 14.3 for signs and symptoms of sepsis and Box 14.5 for features of sepsis that the midwife may identify during assessment.

An ABCDE (plus BUMP[16])approach is advocated to ensure a systematic and thorough assessment.[17] The midwife will start her examination by asking the woman how she feels. The evaluation of the woman's response to this question covers a number of aspects of an Airway, Breathing and Circulation (ABC) assessment, both in the content

> ## BOX 14.2: Risk factors for development of infection and sepsis[10,11,12]
>
> *Features of the women:*
>
> Medical conditions: Diabetes, HIV, Sickle cell disease, obesity
> Women from minority and poor socio-economic groups
> Women for whom language was a barrier to receiving care
>
> *Pregnancy:*
>
> Septic miscarriage or termination of pregnancy
> Cervical suture
> Prolonged spontaneous rupture of membranes (especially if preterm)
> Amniocentesis or other invasive procedures
>
> *Labour and puerperium:*
>
> Induction of labour
> Preterm birth
> Caesarean section or instrumental vaginal delivery
> Prolonged rupture of membranes or chorioamnionitis
> Retained products of conception
> Urinary tract infection and/or catheterisation
> Mastitis
> Close contact with someone with Group A Streptococcus (GAS) – for example, a child with a throat infection

of her response and the physical aspects of the way she communicates. She may seem unwell, have some difficulty breathing (increased respiratory rate), be in pain, or have characteristics of an infection with or without a temperature.

The midwife will perform and record a basic set of vital signs, including temperature, pulse, respiratory rate, oxygen saturations and blood pressure. Where the midwife is concerned about the woman, it is helpful that the midwife does these observations face-to-face. Subtle changes such as a bounding pulse (subsequent to vasodilation, an inflammatory response) or a thready pulse (a later sign of septic shock as peripheral shutdown occurs to conserve blood pressure) will be felt. When

BOX 14.3: Signs and symptoms of sepsis[12,13,14,15]

Signs

- Temperature <35^0 C or >38^0 C
- Heart rate > 120 beats/min
- Respiratory rate >25 breaths/min
- Oxygen saturations <95% in air
- Systolic BP < 90 mmHG
- Reduced urine output
- Impaired neurological state

Symptoms

- Feeling unwell, anxious, distressed
- Feverish or shivery
- Pain that is out of the ordinary and not responding to analgesia
- Abdominal or pelvic pain
- Diarrhoea
- Vomiting
- Generalised rash

Symptoms related to focus on infection (see Box 14.5 for more detail)

- CS or perineal wound infection
- Symptoms of urinary tract infection
- Delay in involution, heavy lochia, malodourous vaginal discharge
- Productive cough
- Mastitis
- Signs of fetal compromise

BOX.14.4: Assessment of skin changes in women with darker skin

To determine pallor or cyanosis in women with darker skin, the mucous membranes should be examined. This may appear white or greyish when there is not enough circulating oxygen.[18] Does the woman feel she looks unwell if she looks in the mirror? Does her partner think she looks unwell? In the context of poor skin perfusion, brown skin may look yellow-brown and dark skin may look ash grey. Another suggestion is to look at the woman's palms – do they appear pale? It can be useful to compare with a relative who has the same skin tone.[19] A bluish tinge to the skin and mucous membrane of a woman with a lighter skin tone would indicate cyanosis. It should also be noted that oxygen saturation monitoring has been shown to be unreliable in darker skin tones.[20,21] Measuring venous or arterial blood gas offers a more objective measurement of oxygen perfusion and well-being.

Determining an area of inflammation may also be challenging with darker skin tones. The midwife can compare an affected and nonaffected area and see if there is any difference in warmth, skin colour changes and texture.[22]

the pulse is taken, what does her skin feel like – cold, hot, clammy, sweaty? Does she look pale or flushed? Is there any rash?

Some of these features may be more difficult to determine in women with darker skin tones. See Box 14.4 for further detail.

An increased temperature is associated with infection, but in sepsis, due to the abnormal immune response and compensatory changes, a normal temperature or hypothermia can be found. When assessing the temperature, the midwife should enquire if the woman has taken any antipyretic medication such as Paracetamol. Compensatory mechanisms will mean the woman's blood pressure will not drop until sepsis has progressed to septic shock. Frequent monitoring of BP is indicated, using an automated device for consistency.

Neurological impairment, such as confusion, may be an early clinical sign that is noted by caregivers and family. Urine output is a useful indicator of circulation.

A sample of urine should be sent for microscopy, culture and sensitivity (MC&S).

The observations should be plotted on a MEOWS (modified early obstetric warning system) chart to enable triggers for ill health to be identified easily and for monitoring trends. These charts should not replace but rather supplement effective clinical assessment. The Sepsis Trust,[23] in conjunction with NICE,[24] has produced useful checklists with red and amber alerts and algorithms for actions (see further reading and resources).

Diagnosis

There is concern that some women may be escalated on the sepsis management pathway who may

---

BOX 14.5: Head-to-toe Assessment to identify features of infections that may lead to sepsis in pregnant and postpartum women[17]

Increased temperature, heart rate, pain, muscle aching and general feelings of malaise and fatigue are features of infection, but depending on the site and causative organism, other more specific features may be noted. Constant severe abdominal or perineal pain and tenderness that is disproportionate to that which would normally be expected and which is not relieved by usual analgesic medication should be a warning sign. Diarrhoea, in addition to unexplained pain, is characteristic of sepsis. An abnormal fetal heart rate pattern or intrauterine fetal death may indicate maternal disease.

Neurological: *Meningitis*: characteristic rash, photophobia, neck stiffness and headache. Confusion is an early feature of sepsis.

Breasts: *Infective mastitis or breast abscess*: cracked nipples, reddened wedge-shaped discolouration indicating a blocked duct, pain and pus.

Respiratory: *Respiratory infection, pneumonia*: cough, sputum, abnormal breath sounds and increased respiratory rate. Acidosis results in increased respiratory rate.

Uterus: *Chorioamnionitis*: malodorous cloudy amniotic fluid, fetal and maternal tachycardia. *Endometritis*: delayed involution of the uterus, malodorous and/or heavy lochia and abdominal pain.

Wounds: Normal wound healing involves inflammatory processes of redness, swelling, pain and warmth, but where there is increasing redness, swelling, pain, exudate and delayed healing accompanied by systemic features of infection, an infection of the wound is likely.

Abdomen: *Pelvic abscess, appendicitis* and *cholycystitis*: Unusual level and pattern of pain.

Skin: Warm (high temperature), unusual rashes, jaundice and inflammation around IV cannula sites. Pale, cold, clammy skin indicative of compensatory shock indicating significant ill health (see Box 14.4 regarding assessment of darker skin tones). Areas where the skin or mucosa has been broken, such as intravenous cannulae sites, CS or perineal wounds, drains or arterial line sites, should be examined and swabs taken of any discharge.

Urinary tract: Malodourous, cloudy urine. Leucocytes and protein may be found on dipstick of midstream or catheter specimen of urine. Radiating flank pain may be indicative of *pyelonephritis*. Symptoms of urinary infection, such as frequency, urgency and pain on passing urine, may not be present in pregnancy. Quantity of urine output needs to be assessed.

Bowels: Diarrhoea noted as a feature of sepsis.

Legs: *Thrombophlebitis*: pain and swelling.

---

not have an infection. Maternal pyrexia in labour is associated with epidural analgesia, prolonged labour and room temperature. Tachycardia can arise due to dehydration, the physical effort of labour or another medical condition. However, the need to prevent the complications of chorioamnionitis, namely fetal demise, justifies the need to commence antibiotics promptly when there is a suspicion of infection.[5] With concern regarding antibiotic stewardship, better methods of diagnosing infection and determining antibiotic sensitivity are needed. There are some new technologies in development that will facilitate fast identification of organisms and antibiotic sensitivity, including the use of polymerase chain reaction (PCR) to identify gene sequences of organism from blood samples.[5] See Box 14.6 for a list of useful investigations for sepsis that may be ordered.

CARE

The '*Surviving Sepsis Campaign*' is an international effort to improve recognition and management of sepsis.[25] Clinicians should refer to the full guidance. In addition, the RCOG has developed guidelines on the management of sepsis specific for pregnancy and the puerperium.[14,15] These documents and details of how to access them are listed under *Further Reading* at the end of the chapter. Multidisciplinary management with senior clinical leadership will be needed to direct care. The team, in addition to senior maternity

BOX 14.6: Investigations for sepsis[5,15,24]

- Blood culture
- Serum lactate
- FBC and C-reactive protein (CRP)
- Renal and liver function tests
- Coagulation screen
- Samples and swabs taken as indicated by clinical suspicion of the focus of infection. For example, MSU, CSU, vaginal swab, wound swab, throat swab, breast milk
- Imaging – chest x-ray, pelvic USS, CT scan

BOX 14.7: Sepsis Six[26]

Give oxygen to keep saturations above 94%

Take blood cultures

Give IV antibiotics

Give IV Fluids and monitor response

Measure lactate levels

Measure urine output

unit staff, may include an intensive care specialist, general surgeon, microbiologist and the critical care outreach team. Admission to the intensive care unit (ICU) will be indicated by the woman's condition. A venous lactate of >2 mmol/l requires escalation to critical care input, with lactate >4 mmol/l indicating serious deterioration and risk of death.

As a memory aid, the management of sepsis is summarised as the Sepsis Six[26] Investigations will underpin diagnosis and guide treatment (see Box 14.7). Prompt treatment with an adequate dose of appropriate IV antibiotics is essential. The aim is that antibiotics should start within one hour of suspecting sepsis and after samples have been obtained for cultures. While awaiting medical aid, the midwife should give oxygen if available to maintain oxygen saturations above 94%, gain IV access and be ready to give IV fluids as soon as prescribed. This will be a frightening experience for the woman and her family, and the midwife will need to provide information, support and clear guidance. Ongoing assessment by the midwife will include frequent observations of vital signs, including oxygen saturations, neurological assessment, careful records of administration of fluids to prevent fluid overload, assessment of fetal wellbeing and general assessment of the woman's response to treatment.

COVID-19

BOX 14.8: Definition

In March 2020, the World Health Organisation (WHO) declared a global pandemic caused by a coronavirus known as SARS-CoV-2, more commonly known as Covid-19. Since the origins of the virus in humans, a number of variants have arisen and have been named using letters of the Greek alphabet: Alpha, Beta, Delta, Omicron. Variants have differed in the level of transmissibility, common symptoms and incidence of severe illness. Predominantly a respiratory infection, Covid-19 is characterised by a range of symptoms but commonly features fever, a cough, dyspnoea and muscle aching. It has affected people differently. Many with Covid-19 are asymptomatic, others have significant respiratory symptoms but recover, some are left with long-term morbidity and many people have died.

INTRODUCTION

Pregnant women appear no more or less likely to contract Covid-19, and for those who do, the majority (more than 60%) have no symptoms. However, in comparison with non-pregnant women, pregnant women are at increased risk of severe illness.[27] Figures from the WHO Living Systematic Review indicate that around 9% of pregnant women with Covid-19 develop severe infection, 4% require admission to ITU and 2% require invasive ventilation.[27] In the UK, it has been reported that 24 pregnant or postpartum women died of complications of Covid- 19 between March 2020 and March 2021.[28,29]

Features of Covid-19 and recommendations for care are evolving as research aims to identify best practices. As such, practitioners should refer to the most up–to–date national guidelines published by reputable bodies such as the Royal College of Obstetrics and Gynecology (see further reading resources).

PATHOPHYSIOLOGY

Covid-19 is a capsulated single-strand RNA virus that can be readily transmitted via respiratory droplets or secretions, and for most pregnant women, the immune system will effectively deal with the virus. However, pregnant women, particularly in the third trimester of pregnancy, are more at risk of complications. This is due to a combination of the relative immune suppression in pregnancy, increased oxygen requirements and the splinting of the diaphragm by the growing fetus, which restricts lung expansion and hampers the effective clearing of secretions.[30,31] Additionally, in the third trimester, changes in the inflammatory responses of the immune system in preparation for birth make the pregnant women more likely to have a more significant pro- inflammatory response involving an increased production of cytokines to viral pathogens.[32] Cytokines are important in cell signalling and are used to stimulate and control inflammation. There are many types of cytokines, of which interleukin-6 (IL-6) is an example. An excessive production of IL-6 appears to trigger what is known as a 'cytokine storm' and has been noted in patients with severe Covid-19 infection. This 'cytokine storm' causes severe lung inflammation and leads to acute respiratory distress syndrome (ARDS).[32]

Placental lesions have been identified in cases of stillbirth in women with confirmed Covid-19, and these changes, termed 'placentitis', appear to contribute to an increased incidence of small for gestational age babies and stillbirth.[27,33,34] There appears to be no increase in the rate of fetal loss prior to 20 weeks.[35]

Box 14.9 lists the characteristics that may make a pregnant woman more at risk of complications of Covid-19.

Prevention

VACCINATION

Vaccination against Covid-19 is strongly recommended and should be offered to all pregnant women. Analysis of six European countries showed

---

> **BOX 14.9: Risk factors for hospitalisation with Covid-19 in pregnancy[6,29,36,37]**
>
> - Unvaccinated
> - Black, Asian and minority ethnic background
> - BMI >25 kg/m^2
> - Pre-existing medical conditions, including diabetes, asthma and hypertension
> - Age >35years
> - Living in increased socioeconomic deprivation
> - Working in healthcare or an occupation that involves dealing directly with the public

---

that almost all pregnant women admitted to ICU were unvaccinated.[37] Research data from the UK and USA has demonstrated no adverse effects from vaccination. There is currently a preference to vaccinate with Pfizer-BioNTech and Moderna as there is a greater amount of data on the effectiveness and safety of these vaccines.[38,39]

Women will benefit from a discussion with a healthcare professional about the benefits of vaccination and be given the opportunity to discuss any concerns. Vaccines can be given at any stage of pregnancy and are suitable during breastfeeding.[36]

CLINICAL FEATURES

Pregnant women are less likely to develop symptoms compared to women who are not pregnant, although there are characteristics that put them at increased risk (see Box 14.9). If they have symptoms, they are likely to be mild and frequently include cough, fever, sore throat, shortness of breath, myalgia and loss of sense of taste.[13,27]

Where there is a concern about a woman's Covid-19 symptoms and/or there are features of deteriorating respiratory function or concerns about fetal well-being (see Box 14.10), an admission to hospital for assessment and care should be arranged. It is important to remember that pregnant women will compensate effectively but then are liable to rapid deterioration. Complications and the need for admission to hospital are mostly seen in women in the third trimester.

BOX 14.10: Features of deteriorating maternal illness from Covid-19 infection

- Significant feelings of breathlessness
- Increased use of accessory muscles
- Increased respiratory rate >20 breaths/min
- A heart rate over 110 beats per minute
- Not maintaining oxygen saturation levels above 94%
- Concern for fetal well-being
- Any general feeling of anxiety and concern expressed by the women

BOX 14.11: Members of MDT involved in the care of women admitted with Covid-19

- Consultant obstetrician
- Consultant anaesthetist
- Intensive care consultant
- Midwifery coordinator
- Consultant neonatologist (liaison with neonatal intensive care staff)
- Obstetric physician and/or respiratory physician
- Infection control specialist
- Critical Care outreach team

BOX 14.12: Assessment of respiratory function by the midwife

In addition to the usual set of vital signs, the midwife should observe the following features:

- Stridor, cough, wheeze
- Verbal response (Is the woman able to complete a sentence in one breath?)
- Central or peripheral cyanosis
- Decreased capillary refill
- Signs of respiratory distress such as sitting upright and leaning forward, use of accessory muscles when breathing
- Production of sputum – blood-stained/green sputum
- Change in the rate, depth and symmetry of breathing
- Level of consciousness and degree of orientation

The characteristics of Covid-19 infections in pregnancy have changed with the different variants. For example, when the Delta variant was more common, there was an increase in the need for women to be admitted to intensive care.[40] The management of Covid-19 in pregnancy should be followed as closely as possible outside of pregnancy but does require a multidisciplinary approach to ensure joint decision-making between consultants with obstetric and intensive care experience.[29]

CARE FOLLOWING ADMISSION TO HOSPITAL

Box 14.11 lists the potential members of the MDT with responsibility for the care of the mother and fetus/newborn. An urgent MDT meeting should be arranged following the admission of a woman with confirmed or suspected Covid-19. A consideration of the most appropriate location of care (e.g., intensive care unit, isolation room, delivery suite) will be made and adjusted according to developments in the woman's condition. If the woman is cared for away from the maternity unit, an obstetric consultant and a midwife should review the woman at least daily. Good lines of communication will allow timely decisions for delivery should the woman's condition deteriorate.[13]

Women admitted with Covid-19 are likely to require respiratory support to maintain oxygenation, and continuous assessment of their oxygen saturations will be a useful guide. In addition, frequent vital sign assessments – heart rate, respiratory rate and BP (minimum of hourly) – should be recorded on a MEOWS chart and/or a critical care observation sheet. It is important to review trends as well as absolute figures. Assessments by the midwife should include an assessment of respiratory function (see Box 14.12) and all regular antenatal assessments of maternal and fetal well-being. It is important to be alert to the challenges of assessing hypoxic features in women with darker skin tones (see Box 14.4).[18] The midwife should pay special attention to the woman's psychological well-being as this will be a challenging, frightening and isolating experience for her and her family.

Oxygen therapy should be adjusted to maintain oxygen saturations between 94 and 98%. Initially, a nasal cannula might be used. Signs of decompensation, such as an increase in oxygen requirements, a respiratory rate >25/min, reduction in urine output or drowsiness, even if oxygen saturations are normal, will indicate the need for urgent escalation of care to senior members of the MDT experienced in Covid-19 in pregnancy. The critical care outreach team should be alerted.

Further methods of delivery of oxygen to maintain sufficient oxygenation may be needed and include a face mask, venturi mask, non-rebreather mask, non-invasive positive airway pressure (such as continuous positive airway pressure: (CPAP), intubation and ventilation and, in severe cases and only available in specialist centres, extracorporeal membrane oxygenation (ECMO).[41]

Investigations in the context of Covid-19 include the assessment of the extent of complications of Covid-19 itself but are also required to review potential co-existing disorders, including thromboembolism, HELLP syndrome, acute fatty liver disease of pregnancy, acute kidney injury and myocardial infarction.[36,42]

Box 14.13 lists a range of useful investigations in the context of Covid-19 infection. Tests for coagulation are required due to the risk of disseminated intravascular coagulation (DIC), as Covid-19 may cause levels of platelets to drop. (See Chapter 12, Box 12.11 for further details on DIC). If the platelets drop, advice from the haematologist should be sought and any aspirin prophylaxis should be stopped. White cells are normally low in Covid-19 and, if raised, indicate bacterial infection as cause of symptoms and/or deterioration. Both ferritin and C-reactive protein (CRP) are usually raised in Covid-19. Radiological studies should not be withheld, when indicated, over concerns for the fetus.[41]

The incidence of venous thromboembolism is significantly increased in pregnant women with Covid-19.[43] Women admitted to hospital will require a risk assessment for thromboembolism using the RCOG guidelines for risk assessment,[44] (see Chapter 6: Thromboembolism in Pregnancy), with Covid-19 considered an additional transient risk factor. There is a need to balance the level of anticoagulation to take into account labour and birth and to consider that with severe illness, there is also a haemorrhagic risk, so an individualised approach is recommended.

Midwives caring for women with Covid-19 should keep good records of fluid balance using hourly input/output charts, with caution applied to the amounts of intravenous fluids infused.

See Box 14.14 for medication which may be used in the care of women with Covid-19.[36,41]

Labour care

For women with symptoms of Covid-19 at the time of birth, there may be an increased risk of fetal compromise, so birth in an obstetric unit and continuous fetal monitoring is recommended.[36] Those women with severe symptoms require MDT input to determine optimal timing and route for birth. The preterm birth rate (primarily iatrogenic) in women with symptomatic Covid-19 appears to be two to three times higher than the background rate.[27]

The administration of antenatal steroids for lung maturity and magnesium sulphate (MgSo4) for neuroprotection in anticipation of preterm birth should be planned.[36] Liaison with the neonatal team will be essential regarding the birth and care of a preterm infant. Efforts should be made to make the experience of birth fulfilling and positive despite the constraints of the mother's ill health.

BOX 14.13: Laboratory and other investigations for Covid-19[36]

- *Bloods*: FBC, U and E's, LFT, CRP, LDH, coagulation studies, ferritin, troponin, arterial blood gas
- *Chest*: x- ray, computerised tomography (CT)
- *Tests for additional complications and/or alternative diagnosis of respiratory compromise* (cardiac disorder, pulmonary embolism, influenza): ECG, Echocardiogram, ventilation/perfusion (VQ) scan, pulmonary angiography (CTPA)
- *Consider sepsis*: blood cultures and lactate
- Fetal assessment

BOX 14:14 Medication which may be used in the care of women with Covid-19[36,41]

Low molecular weight heparin: to prevent thromboembolism

Corticosteroids

Maternal benefit: Oral prednisolone or IV hydrocortisone

Fetal lung maturity: given according to hospital policy, but any maternal steroid dose may need to be omitted on the days when this is given.

Steroids will affect glucose metabolism, so blood sugar levels must be checked regularly and may need appropriate treatment.

Interlukin-6 (IL-6) receptor antagonists (Tocilizumab): use requires a decision by the MDT in cases where the woman is hypoxic and has systemic inflammation. Safety when breastfeeding needs to be confirmed, but as there are commonly only low levels in breastmilk, it is usually considered suitable.

Neutralising monoclonal antibodies: These attach to virus protein, stopping replication and marking it for disposal.

Due to concerns for fetal and maternal well-being, caesarean section has been more common in women with symptomatic Covid-19.

Women with asymptomatic Covid-19 infection do not require any additional requirements for labour and birth, although measures for personal protective equipment and infection control measures should be adhered to. Every effort should be made to provide personalised midwifery care despite the barriers of face coverings. Water birth is not contraindicated for women who do not have any symptoms of Covid-19.

Postnatal care

Women with Covid-19 should remain with their babies, and separation of mother and baby should be avoided where possible. Infection with Covid-19 is not a contraindication to breastfeeding.

Efforts to reduce transmission to the baby will include handwashing and avoiding coughing and sneezing into the baby's face. The mother could consider wearing a face mask when in close contact.

When the woman is not well enough to breastfeed, she should be helped to express her milk by hand or breast pump, which can be given to the baby. The benefits of breastfeeding outweigh any potential risks of transmission of the virus through breastmilk.

Women should continue on low molecular weight heparin for at least ten days after birth.

INFLUENZA (FLU)

BOX 14.15: Definition

Influenza is a highly infectious, acute respiratory infection caused by influenza viruses. Outbreaks of influenza occur each year in the winter months, although more serious pandemic flu occurs periodically. Morbidity and mortality from influenza vary according to the viral strain, but with all influenza, pregnant women and their newborn offspring are more vulnerable to serious complications.

INTRODUCTION

In the United Kingdom during the period 2009–2012, 36 pregnant women died from 'flu', 32 of which were believed to be from the H1N1 strain commonly known as swine flu.[45] Although swine flu was a relatively mild illness for most people, it was alarming to note the increased susceptibility for pregnant women, who were found to be significantly more likely to die from influenza.[46,47] Co-existing illnesses or conditions contributed to the risk; however, problems also arose in previously healthy women.[47,48] It is considered that delays in recognition, diagnosis and treatment contributed to many of those who died.[49]

Lessons learnt from the swine flu pandemic led to a focus on the impact of seasonal flu, which also contributes to an increased risk of a pregnant woman being admitted to intensive care,[50] and maternal deaths from influenza have been reported in each confidential enquiry review over the last ten years.[4] Midwives need to be alert to the complications of influenza and require skills in the assessment of respiratory disorders to facilitate effective escalation of care. Prevention of influenza with vaccination of pregnant women and the use of antiviral medications within 48 hours of symptoms, are noted as effective ways to reduce deaths.[45,46]

PATHOPHYSIOLOGY

Transmission of the influenza virus occurs via droplets, aerosols or direct contact with respiratory secretions from an infected person, and the usual incubation period is one to three days.[47] For most, influenza is a relatively mild illness, but for some, it may cause considerable morbidity and death. Those at higher risk for complications include those with underlying medical conditions and pregnancy.[51] This risk seems more pronounced in the third trimester.[50]

Although pregnant women are not more likely than non-pregnant women to contract a respiratory infection, when they do, it is more likely to lead to serious complications, including pneumonia, pulmonary oedema and adult respiratory distress syndrome. This is due to a number of anatomical, physiological and immune changes of pregnancy, such as:[52,53,54]

- Increased cardiac output
- Decreased lung capacity
- Splinting of the diaphragm by the enlarging uterus
- Greater oxygen (O_2) requirement
- An increased tendency for fluid to move into the lung interstitial compartment

A primary viral or secondary bacterial pneumonia can complicate the recovery from influenza. Reviews of pregnant women admitted to hospital with H1N1 flu indicated a rapid progression of illness requiring admission to the intensive care unit (ICU) and ventilation. Complications, in addition to pneumonia, included sepsis, disseminated intravascular coagulation, encephalopathy, thromboembolism and psychological trauma.[51]

During the influenza pandemic, the babies of mothers with serious complications of H1N1 flu were much more likely to be delivered prematurely, although very few of them tested positive for H1N1 flu.[55] It is generally thought that the seasonal flu virus does not affect the fetus. However, severe or sustained pyrexia during pregnancy has been associated with an increased risk for birth defects, including neural tube defects,[56] and for this reason, the midwife should advise measures to ensure women do not develop a high temperature.

Prevention

Influenza vaccination is the best way to prevent the spread of influenza. It is recommended to reduce the possibility of complications of flu in the mother with the added benefit of providing immunity to the neonate.[57,58,59] The recommendation of a healthcare provider has been identified as a key factor in improving the uptake of vaccination by pregnant women.[60] Midwives can facilitate women's decision-making with regard to flu vaccination by informing women of their higher risk of complications from flu, that the vaccines have been licensed as safe for use in pregnancy and that side effects are minimal. This has been endorsed by the MBRACCE report,[45] which stated that the deaths of more than half of the women who died from flu could have been prevented if they had been vaccinated.

CLINICAL FEATURES

Influenza may be confused with the common cold, but it is a more serious illness and is caused by a different virus. Cold symptoms come on gradually and include having a stuffy or runny nose and a sore throat. Flu symptoms (see Box 14.16) come on more suddenly and severely. Midwives and other healthcare providers need to educate women about the symptoms of influenza and advise them to seek medical advice promptly so that antiviral treatment (if indicated) can be started as early as possible. Ideally, this would be within 48 hours of the onset of symptoms.[61]

The diagnosis of influenza will be made based on symptoms (Box 14.6), diagnostic tests and exclusion of other complications associated with symptoms of breathlessness. Contact with someone with the flu may increase suspicion but is not conclusive. In common with other severe respiratory illness, the woman may have a raised heart rate, raised respiratory rate and may have low oxygen saturations. One of the challenges of assessment of respiratory illness in pregnancy is distinguishing between the physiological breathlessness experienced by up to 75% of pregnant women and breathlessness of a more serious cause (see Chapter 5, Table 5.1)

Normal breathlessness comes on gradually over a number of weeks and is not associated with other adverse signs or symptoms. The woman may notice it when she is talking, and it can get worse with exercise. Significant breathlessness as a symptom can be a feature of a range of serious illnesses, including other respiratory conditions (Covid-19, pulmonary embolism), cardiac disease, sepsis or a metabolic disturbance such as diabetic ketoacidosis so a number of investigations should be made to confirm a diagnosis (see Box 14.17).

BOX 14.16: Common symptoms of influenza[47]

- Chills
- Sudden onset of fever (temperature of 38°C or above)
- Dry cough and sore throat
- Generalised muscle aches and pains
- Severe headache
- Weakness or fatigue
- Gastrointestinal symptoms (nausea, vomiting, diarrhoea and abdominal pain) were a feature of swine flu in children and adults requiring admission to hospital

BOX 14.17: Investigations for respiratory illness/influenza[13]

- Viral swabs
- FBC
- Blood cultures
- Blood and sputum samples and bacteriological investigations should be collected: bacterial pneumonia may complicate viral flu and will need to be treated with antibiotics.
- CRP: usually raised in cases of influenza which is not common with other viral infections
- Capillary blood sugar
- Venous blood gas (including lactate)
- Chest x-ray
- ECG
- Oxygen saturation

CARE

If a pregnant woman is concerned that she has developed the flu, she should access healthcare to confirm the diagnosis and exclude other causes of ill health. In cases where a woman does become critically unwell with influenza, the involvement of a wider multidisciplinary team is vital and will include a consultant level obstetrician, respiratory physician, obstetric anaesthetist, haematologist, the intensive care team and the infection prevention and control team. The midwife should remain involved, providing an important link for ongoing psychological support for the woman and her family alongside physical care. Box 14.18 lists a summary of considerations for care when a woman is admitted with influenza.

Labour care

A joint, regular review of the woman's condition with the respiratory and obstetric team will be needed to determine the timing and mode of birth.

If a woman is in labour, she would be best cared for in the Delivery Unit with input from the Respiratory team and the Obstetric Anaesthetic team. Close monitoring of maternal and fetal well-being will be essential. Following birth, she may need to be transferred to the clinical area that would be best to provide expert care for her, such as the ICU or a respiratory ward.

Postnatal care

All women with influenza need to be isolated. However, national guidance recommends keeping mother and baby together where possible. Where the baby is premature or has other risk factors, this may not be advised and the neonatal team will have to weigh up the risks involved against the disadvantages of separation.

Women with flu should aim to continue to breastfeed even if they are unwell (if they can). It is not known whether influenza viruses can be passed from mother to baby through breastmilk. However, breastfeeding is recommended as it provides a wealth of anti-infective benefits.[65] If the mother is too ill to feed, feeding the baby with expressed milk should be considered. Women will need to be careful not to cough or

BOX 14.18: Summary of considerations for care when a woman is admitted with influenza[49,51,62,63,64]

Admission should be made to a single room with respiratory isolation. A multidisciplinary decision needs to be made regarding the best place to care for women admitted with influenza. Intensive care unit admission will be indicated if there are signs of respiratory distress, pneumonia, persistent tachycardia (>100 beats per minute) or altered level of consciousness. When the woman is cared for away from the maternity unit, close liaison with obstetric staff needs to be maintained.

- Appropriate infection control measures should be implemented: Infection Prevention and Control Team should be notified, appropriate hand washing should be undertaken, women should be cared for in isolation, women should wear a surgical mask and staff should wear a surgical mask, plastic apron, gloves and eye protection (if there is a risk of eye splash).
- Multidisciplinary assessment is necessary for the exclusion of other pathology or obstetric complications, including pre-eclampsia, chorioamnionitis, urinary tract infection and pulmonary embolism.
- Pulse oximetry and arterial blood gas should be closely monitored, along with routine vital signs. Maternal pyrexia should be controlled to prevent complications, including fetal abnormality and preterm delivery. An early warning tool (MEOWS chart) should be used to facilitate the identification of women whose condition is deteriorating.
- Antiviral medication is recommended.
- Ensure hydration, but careful fluid monitoring and assessment of fluid balance are important.
- A multidisciplinary decision should be made regarding the timing and mode of the birth. Preterm delivery may be indicated to improve the ventilation of a very ill woman.
- Corticosteroids to promote fetal lung maturity may be used with caution. Specialist guidance should be sought.
- Awareness should be maintained of potential complications, including disseminated intravascular coagulation (DIC), cognitive impairment, venous thromboembolism and psychological morbidity.
- Women should be offered appropriate psychological support.

sneeze into their baby's face. It may be useful for mothers with symptoms to wear a face mask when feeding. Vigilant hand washing will also be required.

FOLLOW-UP/LONG-TERM ISSUES

Women who have been unwell/admitted to ICU will require support and follow-up to assess both their physical and psychological recovery.

In the event of another pandemic, midwives will need to access web-based information provided by organisations such as the Royal College of Midwives and the Royal College of Obstetrics and Gynaecology, as happened in the swine flu pandemic and similar to evolving advice with Covid-19.

SUMMARY OF MIDWIFERY RESPONSIBILITIES

- Provide information and administration of flu and Covid-19 vaccination.
- Seek to prevent sepsis and serious respiratory illness through handwashing, effective aseptic techniques, avoiding unnecessary intervention and appropriate infection control measures as indicated.
- Ensure women know how and when to contact the hospital if they have concerns for themselves or their baby.
- Maintain up-to-date knowledge of any evolving changes in recommendations for the care of women with sepsis, Covid-19 and influenza.

- Measure vital signs and record on the MEOWS chart for any woman who appears unwell and/ or has risk factors for developing sepsis or a respiratory illness.
- Monitor usual signs of maternal and fetal well-being.
- Consider other indications of deteriorating health in addition to vital signs and perform a thorough head-to-toe assessment. Consider the challenge of assessing skin features in women with darker skin tones and seek alternative objective measurements to ensure features of ill health are not missed.
- Ensure timely and effective referral to senior obstetrician and anaesthetist of a woman you identify or suspect is becoming unwell.
- Ensure infections are identified and treated effectively to prevent progression to sepsis.
- Administer and assess the effect of prescribed medication, which may include antiviral medication, antibiotics and medication to bring down a maternal temperature.
- Ensure effective use of personal protective equipment as appropriate to protect yourselves and others. Observe strict isolation and infection control measures when indicated.
- Keep accurate documentation of the ongoing assessment of the woman and ensure effective communication between members of the MDT regarding the woman's condition and decisions for her care. This would include a record of vital signs (MEOWS) and accurate records of fluid balance.
- Carry out a risk assessment for thromboprophylaxis for women who are admitted. Remember, Covid-19 is a transient risk factor for VTE. When required, administer and/or teach the woman how to administer regular low molecular weight heparin as indicated.
- Provide assistance with the establishment and maintenance of breastfeeding.
- Support the establishment of close relationships with the mother and baby despite any ongoing challenges to the mother's health.
- Provide psychological support and information for the woman and her family.

FURTHER READING AND RESOURCES

Royal College of Obstetricians and Gynaecologists (RCOG). Green – top guideline no. 64a: bacterial sepsis in pregnancy. 1st ed. London: RCOG. 2012a.

Royal College of Obstetricians and Gynaecologists (RCOG). Green – top guideline no. 64b: bacterial sepsis following pregnancy. 1st ed. London: RCOG; 2012b.

Surviving Sepsis Campaign guidelines provide up-to-date guidance on management and educational resources for diagnosis, management and treatment of sepsis. Available from: www.survivingsepsis.org/Guidelines/Pages/default.aspx </res list>

Nutbeam T, Daniels R, On Behalf of the UK Sepsis Trust, UK Sepsis Trust. Community midwifery sepsis screening and action tool. [Accessed 10 July 2023]. Available from: sepsistrust.org/professional-resources/clinical/

Sepsis Trust Maternal sepsis: causes, symptoms, and support. [Accessed 8 July 2023]. Available from: https://sepsistrust.org/get-support/maternal-sepsis/
Information for women on the features of sepsis and access for support

Royal College of Obstetrics and Gynaecology. Coronavirus (COVID-19) infection and pregnancy: information for healthcare professionals version 16. Dec 2022. [Accessed 21 May 2023]. Available from: https://app.magicapp.org/#/guideline/LqgJ3E
These guidelines have been developed to provide up-to-date information for healthcare professionals. This is reviewed and updated regularly. It is advised to view the most recent version online.

Royal College of Obstetrics and Gynaecology. Coronavirus (COVID-19), infection and pregnancy FAQs advice for women. 2023. [Accessed 21 May 2023]. Available from: www.rcog.org.uk/guidance/coronavirus-covid-19-pregnancy-and-women-s-health/coronavirus-covid-19-infection-in-pregnancy/coronavirus-covid-19-infection-and-pregnancy-faqs/Provides information for women about Covid-19 and includes questions on vaccination, what the woman should do if she develops symptoms, and how Covid-19 might affect her and her baby.

REFERENCES

1. Singer M, Deutschman C, Seymour CW, Shankar-Hari M, Annane D, Bauer M, et al. The third international consensus definitions for sepsis and septic shock (sepsis-3) JAMA. 2016;315(8):801–810. Available from: <doi:10.1001/jama.2016.0287>
2. Gyawali B, Ramakrishna K, Dhamoon AS. Sepsis: the evolution in definition, pathophysiology, and management. SAGE Open Med. 2019 Mar 21;7:2050312119835043. Available from: <doi:10.1177/2050312119835043>. PMID: 30915218; PMCID: PMC6429642.
3. Churchill D, Rodger A, Clift J, Tuffnell D, On Behalf of the MBRRACE-UK Sepsis Chapter Writing Group. Think sepsis. In: Knight M, Kenyon S, Brocklehurst P, Neilson J, Shakespeare J, Kurinczuk J, On Behalf of MBRRACE-UK, editors. Saving lives, improving mothers' care – lessons learned to inform future maternity care from the UK and Ireland confidential enquiries into maternal deaths and morbidity 209–12. Oxford: National Perinatal Epidemiology Unit, University of Oxford; 2014. p. 27–44.
4. Knight M, Bunch K, Patel R, Shakespeare J, Kotnis R, Kenyon S, et al., editors. Saving lives, improving mothers' care core report. Lessons learned to inform maternity care from the UK and Ireland confidential enquiries into maternal deaths and morbidity 2018–20. Oxford: National Perinatal Epidemiology Unit, University of Oxford; 2022.
5. Greer O, Shah NM, Johnson MR. 'Maternal sepsis update: current management and controversies', The Obstetrician & Gynaecologist. 2020;22(1):45–55. Available from: <doi:10.1111/tog.12623>
6. Vousden N, Bunch K, Morris E, et al. The incidence, characteristics and outcomes of pregnant women hospitalized with symptomatic and asymptomatic SARS-CoV-2 infection in the UK from March to September 2020: a national cohort study using the UK Obstetric Surveillance System (UKOSS). PLoS One 2021;16(5):e0251123. (In eng). Available from: <doi:10.1371/journal.pone.0251123>
7. Knowles SJ, O'Sullivan NP, Meenan AM, Hanniffy R, Robson M. Maternal sepsis incidence, aetiology and outcome for mother and fetus: a prospective study. BJOG: An International Journal of Obstetrics and Gynaecology. 2015;122(5):663–671. Available from: <doi:10.1111/1471-0528.12892>
8. Centre for Maternal and Child Enquiries (CMACE). Saving mothers' lives: reviewing maternal deaths to make motherhood safer: 2006–2008. The eighth report of the confidential enquiries into maternal deaths in the United Kingdom. BJOG: An International Journal of Obstetrics and Gynaecology. 2011;118(Suppl. 1):1–203.
9. Acosta CD, Knight M. Sepsis and maternal mortality. Current Opinion in Obstetrics and Gynecology. 2013;25(2):109–116.
10. Acosta C, Kurinczuk J, Lucas D, Tuffnell D, Sellers S, Knight M, UK Obstetric Surveillance System. Severe sepsis in the UK, 2011–2012: a national case-control study. PLoS Medicine. 2014;11(7):e1001672. Available from: <doi:10.1371/journal.pmed.101672>
11. Shields A., de Assis V, Halscott T. Top 10 Pearls for the Recognition, Evaluation, and Management of Maternal Sepsis. Obstetrics & Gynecology. 2021;138(2):289–304. Available from: <doi:10.1097/AOG.0000000000004471>
12. Filetici N, et al. Maternal sepsis. Best Practice & Research Clinical Anaesthesiology. 2022;36(1):165–177. Available from: <doi:10.1016/j.bpa.2022.03.003>
13. Burns R, Dent K. Managing medical and obstetric emergencies and trauma. 4th ed. Wiley. 2022. [Accessed 20 May 2023]. Available from: www.perlego.com/book/3538052/managing-medical-and-obstetric-emergencies-and-trauma-a-practical-approach-pdf
14. Royal College of Obstetricians and Gynaecologists (RCOG). Green – top

guideline no. 64a: bacterial Sepsis in Pregnancy. 1st ed. London: RCOG. 2012a.

15. Royal College of Obstetricians and Gynaecologists (RCOG). Green – top Guideline No.64b: Bacterial Sepsis following Pregnancy. 1st ed. London: RCOG. 2012b.

16. Bothamley J, Boyle M, Costa L, Fisher-van Werkhoven R, Ward L. From ABCDE to BUMP. 2023. Available from: RCMorg.UK/Midwives

17. Boyle M, Bothamley J. Critical care assessment by midwives. Boca Raton: Taylor and Francis; 2018.

18. Raynor M, et al. Decolonising midwifery education part one: how colour aware are you when assessing women with darker skin tones in midwifery practice? Practising Midwife. 2021;24(6):36–43. Available from: <doi:10.55975/gvhn3309>

19. Mukwende M, Tamony P, Turner M. Mind the gap: a handbook of clinical signs in Black and Brown skin. St George's, University of London; 2020. Online resource. Available from: <doi:10.24376/rd.sgul.12769988.v1>

20. Gottlieb ER, Ziegler J, Morley K, Rush B, Celi LA. Assessment of racial and ethnic differences in oxygen supplementation among patients in the intensive care unit. JAMA Intern Med. 2022;182(8):849–858. Available from: <doi:10.1001/jamainternmed.2022.2587>

21. Jamali H, Castillo LT, Morgan CC, Coult J, Muhammad JL, Osobamiro OO, Parsons EC, Adamson R. Racial Disparity in Oxygen Saturation Measurements by Pulse Oximetry: evidence and implications. Ann Am Thorac Soc. 2022 Dec;19(12):1951–1964. Available from: <doi:10.1513/AnnalsATS.202203-270CME>. PMID: 36166259.

22. Pusey-Reid, Eleonor DNP, MEd, RN; Quinn, Lisa PhD, AGACNP-BC, OCN; Samost, Mary E. DNP, RN, CENP; Reidy, Patricia A. DNP, FNP-BC, FNAP, FAAN. Skin Assessment in Patients with Dark Skin Tone. AJN, American Journal of Nursing 123(3): p 36–43, March 2023. | Available from: <doi:10.1097/01.NAJ.0000921800.61980>

23. Nutbeam T, Daniels R on Behalf of the UK Sepsis Trust, UK Sepsis Trust. Community midwifery sepsis screening and action tool. [Accessed 10 July 2023]. Available from: sepsistrust.org/professional-resources/clinical/

24. National Institute for Health and Care Excellence (2016) Sepsis: recognition, diagnosis and early management NICE guideline [NG51]. [Accessed 20 May 2023]. Available from: www.nice.org.uk/guidance/ng51

25. Evans L, Rhodes A, Alhazzani W, Antonelli M, Coopersmith CM, French C, et al. Surviving sepsis campaign. International Guidelines for Management of Sepsis and Septic Shock 2021. Critical Care Medicine. 2021;49(11):p e1063-e1143, November 2021 Available from: <doi:10.1097/CCM.0000000000005337>

26. Daniels R, Nutbeam T, On Behalf of the Sepsis Trust. The Sepsis manual. 6th ed. 2022. [Accessed 4 August 2023]. Available from: https://sepsistrust.org/wp-content/uploads/2022/06/Sepsis-Manual-Sixth-Edition.pdf

27. Allotey J, Stallings E, Bonet M, Yap M, Chatterjee S, Kew T, et al. Clinical manifestations, risk factors, and maternal and perinatal outcomes of coronavirus disease 2019 in pregnancy: living systematic review and meta-analysis. BMJ (Clinical Research ed.). 2020;370:m3320.

28. Knight M, Bunch K, Vousden N, Morris E , Simpson N, Gale C et al. Characteristics and outcomes of pregnant women admitted to hospital with confirmed SARS-CoV-2 infection in UK: national population based cohort study BMJ 2020;369:m2107 doi:10.1136/bmj.m2107

29. Knight M, Bunch K, Cairns A, Cantwell R, Cox P, Kenyon S, et al. Saving Lives, improving mothers' care rapid report 2021: learning from SARS-CoV-2-related and associated maternal deaths in the UK June 2020-March 2021. Oxford: National Perinatal Epidemiology Unit, University of Oxford; 2021.

30. Green J. et al. Part 1: COVID-19 and knowledge for midwifery practice – impact and care of pregnant women part 1. British Journal of Midwifery. 2021;29(4):224–231.

Available from: <doi:10.12968/bjom.2021.29.4.224>

31. Chu J, Johnston TA, Geoghegan J, on Behalf of the Royal College of Obstetricians andGynaecologists. Maternal collapse in pregnancy and the puerperium. BJOG. 2020;127:e14–e52.

32. Obuchowska A, Standyło A, Obuchowska K, Kimber-Trojnar Ż, Leszczyńska-Gorzelak B. Cytokine Storms in the Course of COVID-19 and haemophagocytic lympho-histiocytosis in pregnant and postpartum women. Biomolecules. 2021;11(8):1202. Available from: <doi:10.3390/biom11081202>

33. Dubucs C, Groussolles M, Ousselin J, Sartor A, Van Acker N, Vayssière C, et al. Severe placental lesions due to maternal SARSCoV-2 infection associated to intra-uterine fetal death. Human Pathology. 2022;121:46–55.

34. Schwartz DA, Mulkey SB, Roberts DJ. SARS-CoV-2 placentitis, stillbirth, and maternal COVID-19 vaccination: clinical-pathologic correlations. Am J Obstet Gynecol. 2022;228(3):261–269.

35. Jacoby VL, Murtha A, Afshar Y, Gaw SL, Asiodu I, Tolosa J, et al. Risk of pregnancy loss before 20 weeks' gestation in study participants with COVID-19. Am J Obstet Gynecol. 2021;225(4):456–457.

36. Royal College of Obstetrics and Gynaecology. Coronavirus (COVID-19) infection and pregnancy: information for health-care professionals version 16. Dec 2022. [Accessed 21 May 2023]. Available from: https://app.magicapp.org/#/guideline/LqgJ3E

37. Engjom H, van den Akker T, Aabakke A, Ayras O, Bloemenkamp K, Donati S, et al. Severe COVID-19 in pregnancy is almost exclusively limited to unvaccinated women – time for policies to change. The Lancet Regional Health. Europe. 2022;13:100313.

38. Schrag SJ, Verani JR, Dixon BE, Page JM, Butterfield KA, Gaglani M, et al. Estimation of COVID-19 mRNA vaccine effective-ness against medically attended COVID-19 in pregnancy during periods of delta and omicron variant predominance in the United States. JAMA Network Open. 2022;5(9):e2233273.

39. Department of Health and Social Care. Joint committee on vaccination and immunisation: advice on priority groups for COVID-19 vaccination. London: Department of Health and Social Care; 2020 Dec 30.

40. Vousden N, Ramakrishnan R, Bunch K, Quigley M, Kurinczuk J, Knight M. Severity of maternal infection and perinatal out-comes during periods in which Wildtype, Alpha and Delta SARS-CoV-2 variants were dominant: data from the UK obstetric sur-veillance system national cohort. BMJ Med. 2022;1(1).

41. Nana M, Hodson K, Lucas N, Camporota L, Knight M, Nelson-Piercy C et al. Diagnosis and management of covid-19 in pregnancy. BMJ. 2022;377:e069739. Available from: <doi:10.1136/bmj-2021-069739>

42. Ahmed I, Eltaweel N, Antoun L, Rehal A. Severe pre-eclampsia complicated by acute fatty liver disease of pregnancy, HELLP syndrome and acute kidney injury fol-lowing SARS-CoV-2 infection. BMJ Case Reports. 2020;13(8):1–3. Available from: <doi:10.1136/bcr-2020-237521>

43. Metz TD, Clifton RG, Hughes BL, Sandoval G, Saade GR, Grobman WA, et al. Disease severity and perinatal outcomes of preg-nant patients with coronavirus disease 2019 (COVID-19). Obstetrics and Gynecology. 2021;137(4):571–580.

44. Royal College of Obstetricians and Gynaecologists. Thromboembolic disease in pregnancy and the puerperium: acute management. Green-top guideline 37b. London: Royal College of Obstetricians and Gynaecologists; 2015.

45. Knight M, Kenyon S, Brocklehurst P, Neilson J, Shakespeare J, Kurinczuk J, On behalf of MBRRACE-UK, editors. Saving lives, improving mothers' care – lessons learned to inform future maternity care from the UK and Ireland confidential enquiries into maternal deaths and morbidity 2009–2012. Oxford: National Perinatal Epidemiology Unit, University of Oxford; 2014. p. 57–63.

46. Meijer WJ, van Noortwijk AG, Bruinse HW, Wensing AM. Influenza virus infection in

pregnancy: a review Acta Obstet Gynecol Scand. 2015;94:797–819.

47. UK Health Security Agency. Influenza: the green book, chapter 19. 2022. [Accessed 22 May 2023]. Available from: www.gov.uk/government/publications/influenza-the-green-book-chapter-19

48. Mosby LG, Rasmussen SA, Jamieson DJ. 2009 pandemic influenza A (H1N1) in pregnancy: a systematic review of the literature. Am J Obstet Gynecol. 2011;205(1):10–18.

49. Paterson-Brown S, Howell C., editors. Sepsis. In: The MOET course manual: managing obstetric emergencies and trauma. 3rd ed. Cambridge: Cambridge University Press; 2014.

50. Darling AJ, Federspiel JJ, Wein LE, Swamy GK, Dotters-Katz SK. Morbidity of late-season influenza during pregnancy. American Journal of Obstetrics & Gynecology MFM. 2022;4(1):100487. Available from: <doi:10.1016/j.ajogmf.2021.100487>

51. Lim BH, Mahmood TA. Pandemic H1N1 2009 (swine flu) and pregnancy. Obstetrics Gynaecology and Reproductive Medicine. 2010;20(4):101–106.

52. Tan EK, Tan EL. Alterations in physiology and anatomy during pregnancy. Best Practice & Research Clinical Obstetrics and Gynaecology. 2013;27:791–802.

53. Blackburn ST. Maternal, fetal, & neonatal physiology: a clinical perspective. 5th ed. Philadelphia: Saunders; 2017.

54. Nelson-Piercy C. Handbook of obstetric medicine. Milton: Taylor & Francis Group; 2020.

55. Mendez-Figueroa H, Raker C, Anderson BL. Neonatal characteristics and outcomes of pregnancies complicated by influenza infection during the 2009 pandemic. Am J Obstet Gynecol. 2011;204(6 Suppl. 1):S58–S63.

56. Moretti ME, Bar-Oz B, Fried S, Koren G. Maternal hyperthermia and the risk for neural tube defects in offspring: systematic review and meta-analysis. Epidemiology. 2005;16(2):216–219.

57. Benowitz I, Esposito DB, Gracey KD, Shapiro ED, Vázquez M. Influenza vaccine given to pregnant women reduces hospitalization due to influenza in their infants. Clinical Infectious Diseases. 2010;51(12):1355–1361.

58. Steinhoff MC, MacDonald N, Pfeifer D, Muglia LJ. Influenza vaccine in pregnancy: policy and research strategies. Lancet. 2014;383(9929):1611–1612.

59. Tamma P, Ault K, del Rio C, Steinhoff MC, Halsey NA, Omer SB, et al. Safety of influenza vaccination during pregnancy. Am J Obstet Gynecol. 2009;201(6):547–552.

60. Steelfisher GK, Blendon RJ, Bekheit MM, Mitchell EW, Williams J, Lubell K, et al. Novel pandemic A (H1N1) influenza vaccination among pregnant women: motivators and barriers. Am J Obstet Gynecol. 2011;204(6):S116–S123.

61. Ramussen SA, Kissin DM, Yeung LF, MacFarlane K, Chu SY, Turcios-Ruiz RM. Preparing for influenza after 2009 H1N1: special considerations for pregnant women and newborns. Am J Obstet Gynecol. 2011;204(6):S13–S20.

62. Bothamley J Boyle M. Infections affecting pregnancy and childbirth. London: Radcliffe.

63. Centers for Disease Control and Prevention, National Center for Immunization and Respiratory Diseases (NCIRD). Recommendations for obstetric health care providers related to use of antiviral medications in the treatment and prevention of influenza. 2022. [Accessed 23 May 2023]. Available from: www.cdc.gov/flu/professionals/antivirals/avrec_ob.htm

64. Muthuri SG, Venkatesan S, Myles PR, Leonardi-Bee J, Al Khuwaitir TS, Al Mamun A. Effectiveness of neuraminidase inhibitors in reducing mortality in patients admitted to hospital with influenza A H1N1pdm09 virus infection: a meta-analysis of individual participant data. Lancet Respir Med. 2014 May;2(5):395–404.

65. Tanaka T, Nakajima K, Murashima A, Garcia-Bournissen F, Koren G, Ito S. Safety of neuraminidase inhibitors against novel influenza A (H1N1) in pregnant and breastfeeding women. Canadian Medical Association Journal. 2009;181:55–58.

15

Other causes of potential maternal collapse

ANDREA ARAS-PAYNE

Presenting symptoms   222
Individual conditions   224

References   230

This chapter considers the less common causes of maternal collapse which need emergency or urgent attention. It should be noted that all of these conditions fall outside the midwives' remit and, therefore, their role is to provide a high standard of supportive care after summoning emergency assistance or organising urgent referral.[1] The outcome in several of these serious and life-threatening situations relies on prompt and effective resuscitation (see Chapter 3), many of these conditions are reversible with timely and appropriate treatment and effective team working and communication.[2,3,4]

For most of these conditions, prompt medical or surgical intervention is the only treatment. However, an overview of the potential causes of the woman's symptoms will help the midwife decide how best to provide support, especially in isolated situations, until assistance arrives. It is also possible that, with prior understanding of these conditions, this can lead to earlier suspicion and referral of symptoms which might otherwise have progressed to an emergency situation. Updated knowledge is an important part of professional development.[5]

The overview given in this chapter is intended to be just a brief summary. It is hoped it will provide a starting point; further access to other resources for more in-depth information will be required.

Further information may also be necessary in preparation for discussing and supporting women who have experienced any of these conditions.

The main presenting symptoms of maternal collapse are identified in the first part of this chapter, with the conditions that may be the potential cause listed alphabetically in what follows. Many conditions manifest with various symptoms, depending on the degree of severity or just the individual aetiology, and, therefore, may appear in more than one list. Some of these conditions are discussed in previous chapters. All require urgent care and referral.

A diagnosis of amniotic fluid embolism (see Chapter 13) should be strongly considered in cases of sudden unexplained maternal cardiorespiratory collapse.[6]

PRESENTING SYMPTOMS

Loss of consciousness

The Glasgow Coma scale has been developed to provide a standardised approach when assessing level of consciousness and severity of dysfunction (see www.glasgowcomascale.org for further information). Assessment using this scale allows for a quantitative assessment of responsiveness that can be conveyed alongside other clinical findings.[7]

DOI: 10.4324/9781003382195-15

COMMON CAUSES OF LOSS OF CONSCIOUSNESS

- Acute (formerly adult) respiratory distress syndrome (ARDS) (see page 224).
- Amniotic fluid embolism (see Chapter 13).
- Anaphylaxis (see page 225).
- Aneurysm: ruptured.
- Asthma (see page 226).
- Cerebrovascular accident or stroke (see page 227).
- Diabetic ketoacidosis (see page 227).
- Drug intoxication.
- Epidural: high block (see page 228).
- Eclampsia (see Chapter 7).
- Gastric aspiration (see ARDS).
- Haematoma: paravaginal or paragenital.
- Hyperventilation.
- Hypoglycaemia (see page 229).
- Hypotension.
- Local anaesthetic toxicity.
- Magnesium toxicity (see Chapter 7).
- Myocardial infarction (see Chapter 5).
- Peripartum cardiomyopathy (see Chapter 5).
- Pulmonary embolism (see Chapter 6).
- Thyroid crisis (see page 230).
- Uterine rupture (see Chapter 11)

Chest pain

(Please also refer to Chapter 5: **Cardiac conditions)**

Because heartburn is so common a complaint in pregnancy, chest pain may not be treated with the urgency it may need in some rare cases. However, life-threatening causes usually present with severe pain, unrelieved by common medicine, and are associated with other symptoms (for example, dyspnoea, nausea, vomiting and altered consciousness).[8]

Common causes of chest pain

- Aortic dissection (see Chapter 5).
- Myocardial infarction (see Chapter 5).
- Pericarditis.
- Peripartum cardiomyopathy (see Chapter 5).
- Pleurisy.
- Pneumonia.
- Pneumothorax.
- Pre-eclampsia: fulminating (see Chapter 7).
- Pulmonary embolism (see Chapter 6).
- Sickle-cell crisis (see page 229).

Confusion

Confusion may manifest not only as inappropriate speech but also as aggression or withdrawal of communication. The midwife must make a decision as to whether the cause could be a pathophysiological condition before deciding on the most appropriate action. However, it is worth noting that confusion can often be an early sign of hypoxia.

Common causes of confusion

- ARDS (see page 224).
- Asthma (see page 226).
- Cerebrovascular accident (see page 227).
- Drug intoxication or drug withdrawal.
- Hypoglycaemia (see page 229).
- Hypotension.
- Magnesium toxicity (see Chapter 7).
- Permanent mental disability.
- Pre-eclampsia: fulminating (see Chapter 7).
- Psychiatric illness.
- Pulmonary oedema (see page 229).
- Sepsis (see Chapter 14).
- Thyroid crisis (see page 230).

Shock

See Chapter 3 for a full discussion on the signs, symptoms and related pathophysiology of shock.

Common causes of shock

- ARDS (see page 224).
- Amniotic fluid embolism (see Chapter 13).
- Antepartum haemorrhage (see Chapter 4).
- Appendicitis (see page 226).
- Ectopic pregnancy (see page 228).
- Postpartum haemorrhage (see Chapter 12).
- Pulmonary embolism (see Chapter 6).
- Sepsis (see Chapter 14).
- Uterine inversion (see Chapter 11).
- Uterine rupture (see Chapter 11).

Abdominal pain

Abdominal pain is probably the most common presenting symptom seen by midwives, and as women manifest contraction pain in various ways, it is tempting to assume most abdominal pain is labour. However, it is worth maintaining a degree of suspicion and considering carefully where the pain is, if there is anything that makes it worse or better and – most importantly – is it intermittent, with the uterus relaxing in between? It is also relevant whether gastric symptoms (such as diarrhoea) are present.

Common causes of abdominal pain (other than labour and birth)

- Antepartum haemorrhage (see Chapter 4).
- Appendicitis (see page 226).
- Chorioamnionitis.
- Ectopic pregnancy (see page 228).
- Uterine fibroids (see page 229).
- Haematoma: rectus.
- Pyelonephritis.
- Placental abruption (see Chapter 4)
- Renal stones.
- Sepsis (see Chapter 14).
- Sever pre-eclampsia and eclampsia (see Chapter 7).
- Thyroid crisis (see page 230).
- Uterine inversion (see Chapter 11).
- Uterine rupture (see Chapter 11).

Seizures

Although the most common cause of a seizure in pregnancy, labour or following birth is eclampsia, other, more rare, conditions can first present with a seizure.

Common causes of seizures

- Eclampsia (see Chapter 7).
- Amniotic fluid embolism (see Chapter 13).
- Epilepsy (see page 228)
- Sickle-cell crisis (see page 229).

Trauma

It is always possible that a midwife may be the first person on the scene following an accident, a violent incident or other injuries sustained by a pregnant woman. In these circumstances, it is possible to do no more than provide skilled first aid, remembering that the best way to care for the fetus is to resuscitate the woman adequately (*see* Chapter 3). After calling for emergency help, initial assessment and action should include the emergency measures in Box 15.1.

If a woman is still pregnant during any of the situations discussed within this chapter, alongside caring for the woman, the midwife will also need to monitor fetal wellbeing, usually by cardiotocography (CTG).

BOX 15.1: Emergency care

CALL FOR HELP

- Airway: maintain open. Place in the left lateral (recovery) position or perform manual uterine displacement to the left to relieve aortocaval compression if pregnant (see Chapter 3) while protecting the cervical and remainder of the spine.
- Breathing: assist if necessary.
- Circulation: control obvious bleeding if possible and give cardiac massage if necessary.
- Disability: assess the level of consciousness by noting response to voice or pain.
- Environment: keep warm and safe.

Non-reassuring or abnormal features on a CTG may resolve as the maternal condition improves; however, a deteriorating CTG trace may reflect deterioration in the woman's condition, sometimes evident before other maternal signs and symptoms. Plans for delivery may be needed but will depend on maternal stability and fetal gestation and condition; timing will be made on an individual basis. The midwife will be working as part of a multidisciplinary team to help facilitate the best care while responding to the needs and circumstances of each individual woman, with a particular emphasis on effective communication and cultural sensitivity.

INDIVIDUAL CONDITIONS

Acute respiratory distress syndrome (ARDS)

Most cases of ARDS result from one of the following four causes:

- sepsis from pulmonary or non-pulmonary sources,
- major trauma,
- transfusion related and
- aspiration of gastric contents.

For childbearing women, causes associated with pregnancy need to also be considered, including tocolytic-induced pulmonary oedema, pre-eclampsia, acute fatty liver of pregnancy, peripartum cardiomyopathy, asthma, amniotic fluid embolism, placental abruption, haemorrhage, chorioamnionitis and retained products of conception.[9] Although perinatal mortality rates have been quoted as high,[10] for the survivors, the long-term prognosis, even following prolonged ventilation, is good, with lung function recovery back to normal in four to six months in many women. However, there is also the possibility of complications as a result of ventilation and admission to an intensive therapy unit.

Women will show signs of acute respiratory distress such as dyspnea, orthopnea, tachycardia, tachyapnoea and cyanosis. There will be lung crackles and/or wheezing, and bilateral interstitial infiltrates appear on chest x-ray.[6] Diagnosis is by clinical signs, but the primary cause also needs to be diagnosed and treated concurrently.

Treatment is usually in an intensive care unit (ICU), which means good communication between the maternity and critical care teams is essential. Care is aimed at treating the cause and supporting lung function until the lung heals. Optimum oxygenation must be maintained, and acidosis, anaemia and hypothermia prevented. Careful fluid balance is necessary to prevent pulmonary oedema, and ventilation may be necessary in severe cases.[9]

Anaphylaxis

Anaphylaxis is a severe, life-threating, systemic hypersensitivity reaction.[11] Airway and/or breathing and/or circulation problems suddenly and rapidly develop, typically with accompanying skin and mucosal changes. Anaphylaxis is an acute response with multisystem involvement, resulting from the rapid release of inflammatory mediators to a substance to which the woman has become sensitised. Current estimates suggest an incidence of 1.5 per 100,000 maternities in the UK[12] with a mortality rate of 1%.[4] Common triggers for anaphylaxis include food (most commonly nuts), drugs (most commonly antibiotics but also include anaesthetic, NSAIDSs and aspirin) and stings/venom (such as from a wasp or bee). Latex can also cause a reaction, which is an important consideration when working in a healthcare environment where gloves, catheters, masks and other equipment may contain latex. Severe and sometimes fatal reactions to a trigger can begin rapidly; most reactions appear over several minutes; however,

this can depend on the cause. A response to an IV medication administration may be significantly quicker than to orally ingested foods. Exposure to a known allergen (trigger) can support diagnosis, but it is important to be aware that some women may present with no previous history or obvious trigger.[4,13,14] Mast cell tryptase levels can help with the diagnosis with a series of timed samples taken, but this should not delay resuscitation.[4]

Anaphylaxis is likely when all of the following three criteria are met:

- Sudden onset.
- Rapid progression of symptoms (feels unwell, maybe anxious, 'feels sense of impending doom').
- Life-threatening problems (use ABCDE approach to recognise these):
  - **A**irway (throat and tongue swelling, difficulty swallowing, hoarse voice, stridor [high pitched inspiratory noise]).
    – and/or
  - **B**reathing (shortness of breath, wheezing, confusion [caused by hypoxia] tiredness, cyanosis and respiratory arrest).
    – and/or
  - **C**irculation problems (pale, clammy, tachycardia, hypotension, dizziness, collapse, decreased level of consciousness, ECG changes, cardiac arrest often preceded by bradycardia).
  - **D**isability problems should also be assessed (confusion, agitation and loss of consciousness).
  - **E**xposure (skin and/or mucosal changes should also be observed), including erythema (patchy or generalized red rash), urticaria (welts or hives, may look like nettle stings often surrounded by a red flare and usually itchy) and angioedema (swelling of deeper tissues, most commonly eyelids, lips and sometimes in the mouth and throat).

Once an anaphylactic reaction is recognised, urgent help needs to be summoned and assessment and treatment administered based on the ABCDE approach. The immediate treatment is to stop any drugs and infusions and remove any trigger (e.g., latex, sting). IM Epinephrine (adrenaline) 1 mg/ml is the first-line treatment and should be given to all women with life-threatening symptoms. This should be given again after five minutes if the serious symptoms persist. Consider the best position for the woman; sitting up may be easier if she is experiencing breathing difficulties and laying down if feeling faint or losing consciousness (left lateral if she is pregnant). Establish an airway, administer oxygen and monitor oxygen saturations, also monitor vital signs, obtain intravenous (IV) access and administer fluids to maintain blood pressure. Blood gases must be monitored, and a full blood count, electrolyte assessment and clotting studies must be carried out. An electrocardiograph (ECG) and x-ray may be required. Intubation and ventilation for respiratory support may be necessary. CPR will need to be initiated (see Chapter 3) if the woman has a cardiorespiratory arrest following an anaphylactic reaction.

Further drug therapy is an important part of treatment and may include IV epinephrine (**this should be administered only by those trained to do so**), antihistamines, corticosteroids and bronchodilators.

Women may have a latex allergy, so they need to be asked a specific question at booking regarding any previous reactions to other latex products such as condoms, balloons or household rubber gloves. If a latex allergy is identified, great care is needed to avoid using equipment (such as tape, catheters, masks and gloves) which contain latex. Documentation of any allergy must be made clear within the woman's maternity notes and visible signs, such as a coloured wristband, may help to prevent any errors which may cause a severe reaction.[12] If a woman has had a suspected anaphylactic reaction, it needs investigation, usually by a local allergy clinic.[13]

Appendicitis

Appendicitis is the most common surgical complication in pregnancy, occurring in approximately one in 1,500 pregnant women (similar to that of the non-pregnant population).[15] It is thought to be more common in the first and second trimester, but in the third trimester, an infected appendix is more likely to rupture.[16] A difficulty in diagnosis, a delay in treatment and a possible altered immunological response during pregnancy have all been attributed to this higher incidence of perforation.[17] Peritonitis and other adverse complications

(including postoperative infections, sepsis, bowel obstruction and transfusion) are more common in pregnant women with appendicitis.[15]

Signs and symptoms may include acute abdominal pain, nausea, vomiting, alteration in bowel and urinary habits and possibly pyrexia. During pregnancy, the appendix is displaced by the enlarging gravid uterus, so pain may be experienced higher and more laterally. Ultrasound is usually undertaken to help support the diagnosis, but if this is inconclusive, an MRI assessment may be used.[18] Although medical management may be undertaken, due to the serious adverse outcomes for pregnant women with appendicitis conservative management is usually avoided.[17] Surgical treatment is justified with minimal delay due to increased maternal and perinatal morbidity and mortality.[19]

Asthma

Estimates suggest that asthma may affect up to 7% of pregnancies and is the most common chronic medical disorder seen in pregnancy.[20] A history of asthma can predispose women to complications during pregnancy; 11–18% of pregnant women with asthma will require an emergency visit to hospital, particularly those with severe or poorly controlled asthma.[21] Coordinated multidisciplinary care, urgent assessment and referral if they present with acute respiratory compromise must take place.[2]

For women with asthma, pregnancy can be an unpredictable time. One-third of women experience deterioration in their condition, a third experience an improvement while the remaining third report no change at all. During pregnancy, the risks of taking medication may also be of concern to women; exacerbation of symptoms may, therefore, be caused by a reduction or cessation of prescribed treatment.[22] However, if asthma in pregnancy is well controlled throughout, there is little or no increased risk of adverse outcomes.[21]

Signs and symptoms of acute severe asthma may include increased respiration rate > 25/min, tachycardia > 110/min, Peak Expiratory Flow Rate (PEFR) between 33–50%, coughing, wheezing, bronchospasm, the use of accessory muscles for breathing, chest tightness and a noticeable inability to complete a sentence without taking a breath. They may become frightened and progressively anxious.

As the attack worsens in severity, the woman may start to make only a poor respiratory effort, become exhausted, cyanosed, confused and finally bradycardic and comatose. Life-threatening asthma is considered when oxygen saturation is <92%; there is increasing cyanosis, hypotension is present and weak respiratory effort is being made.[20,23]

Treatment of an asthma exacerbation includes the administration of humidified oxygen and ongoing assessment with pulse oximeter (saturation should be maintained at 94–98%); intravenous access will be required and fluid replacement as appropriate. Drug therapy will include nebulised β2 antagonists (e.g., salbutamol) and early administration of corticosteroids. An ECG and chest x-ray may be indicated (particularly if pneumonia or pneumothorax is suspected – the abdomen will require shielding if pregnant). Arterial/venous blood gases and maternal peak flow (PEFR) should be monitored. Intravenous drugs may be considered, including β2 antagonists and IV magnesium sulphate. With a severe asthma attack that is difficult to treat and progressing to respiratory failure, intubation and ventilation are needed.[20,23]

Cerebrovascular accident

Although considered a condition of old age, strokes happen to childbearing women and, in some cases, can be fatal.[2,24] Women are more susceptible to stroke than men, and this is further increased by the physiologic changes in pregnancy, with the third trimester and puerperium seeming to be the most vulnerable period and the highest risk for hypertensive disorders.[25] Although stroke in pregnancy is rare, the rising prevalence of obesity, hypertension, cardiac disease and older maternal age means women continue to be at risk.[26]

A stroke may be either ischaemic or haemorrhagic, and symptoms are similar, although treatments will differ. An ischaemic stroke is caused by severe loss of blood flow to a specific part of the brain with tissue necrosis; causes include embolism and hypotension. Haemorrhagic stroke is triggered by a ruptured blood vessel, causing blood to spread into the brain tissue (either intracerebral or subarachnoid). This may result from hypertension or traumatic injuries.[27]

Symptoms can range in severity from headache, neck stiffness, visual changes and mild muscle weakness to collapse and cardio or respiratory arrest. Various investigations may be needed to determine a diagnosis, including computed tomography (CT scan), magnetic resonance imaging (MRI), lumbar puncture, cerebral angiography and haematological testing.

Treatment of ischaemic stroke includes possible anticoagulation, while treatment of haemorrhagic stroke is usually surgical.[27] On-going treatment needs will depend on the severity of the stroke.

The standard of care for a stroke should not be altered for pregnant women and, as timely treatment is essential for attaining better outcomes, prompt referral and admission to a Hyperacute Stroke Unit should take place.[2,28]

Diabetic Ketoacidosis (DKA)

Diabetic ketoacidosis (DKA) is a medical and obstetric emergency. Although rare, it is a serious, potentially life-threatening complication for both mother and fetus, with increased morbidity and mortality rates,[2,29] therefore, effective management and prevention are key.[30,31,32,33]

DKA normally affects only those with type I diabetes mellitus (T1DM), but it is not unknown in Type II or even gestational diabetes[33] with cases of DKA cited in the latest MBRRACE report.[2]

Clinical features of DKA include nausea and vomiting, polydipsia and/or polyuria, weakness, fatigue, abdominal pain, signs of dehydration (for example, dry mucous membranes), tachycardia, hypotension and changes in behavior or emotional state, disorientation and, finally, coma. Tachypnea may also be present, with the woman's breath often smelling 'fruity' due to acetone excretion via the lungs. During pregnancy, diabetic women are at increased risk of DKA, which can be more severe, rapid in onset and occur at lower blood glucose levels.[30]

Diagnosis is usually by serum and urinary (dipstick) assessment of ketones, arterial pH and raised plasma glucose levels (noting ketoacidosis can be present at lower glucose levels in pregnancy than if it occurred outside of pregnancy).[28] Management includes appropriate resuscitation, treatment of dehydration and lowering of blood glucose. Transfer to a high dependency area is usual. Underlying causes need to be investigated and treated; these may include infection, hyperemesis, non-compliance with insulin and the use of corticosteroids.[28]

Ectopic pregnancy

An ectopic pregnancy occurs when a fertilised egg develops outside of the uterus.[34] Women with an ectopic pregnancy are at risk of collapse following rupture of the fallopian tube, with the recent MBRRACE report showing that despite a high level of knowledge concerning ectopic pregnancies, women are continuing to die in early pregnancy.[2]

Symptoms of ectopic pregnancy can be varied; commonly, they include abdominal or pelvic pain, amenorrhoea or missed menstrual period and vaginal bleeding. Other reported symptoms include shoulder-tip pain, breast tenderness, dizziness, fainting, rectal pressure or pain on defecation, as well as urinary and gastrointestinal symptoms.[35] Due to the fact that the signs and symptoms of ectopic pregnancy can appear similar to other conditions, such as urinary tract infection and gastrointestinal upset, it is recommended health professionals consider offering a pregnancy test and assessment to all women of childbearing age who present with these symptoms.[35,36] For diagnosis, a transvaginal ultrasound scan is recommended and magnetic resonance imaging (MRI) is used as a means of second-line diagnosis if required. Serum beta-human chorionic gonadotrophin is useful when planning the management of an ectopic pregnancy visualised via an ultrasound.[37]

Treatment involves resuscitation to stabilise the woman's condition, including administering IV fluids (with blood transfusion as necessary) and laparoscopic or abdominal surgery. In some cases, it may be appropriate to treat the condition medically.[35,37]

Epidural/spinal: high block

High regional blocks may occur as a result of an unexpected spread of local anaesthetic after a subarachnoid (spinal) injection or after an accidental subarachnoid injection of an epidural dose of local anaesthetic.[38] This may be due to too much medication, an exaggerated response or an inadvertent injection into the wrong space.[3]

Signs and symptoms are dependent on the height of the block but may include tingling ('pins and needles' in fingers and arms), weakness in hands, nausea, difficulty in breathing, speaking and swallowing, hypotension and/or bradycardia.[3] With a total spinal block, loss of consciousness will occur due to the direct action of local anaesthetic on the brain.

Immediate treatment is to turn off the epidural if running as a continuous infusion, call for urgent help and commence resuscitation if necessary. Oxygen should be given and oxygen saturations should be continuously monitored, with respiratory rate, pulse and frequent blood pressure readings underpinning treatment. Anaesthetists will treat hypotension and bradycardia as appropriate.

Epilepsy

Epilepsy is the most common neurological disorder seen in pregnancy; approximately 0.5% of women of childbearing age are affected.[39] Many women have specific 'triggers' for their seizures (such as sleep deprivation, pain, stress, dehydration and non-compliance with medication due to the fear of its potential teratogenic side effects), and care should be taken to avoid these when possible.[40] For women who do experience seizures during pregnancy, this may be related to epilepsy but may also be caused by other conditions, including eclampsia, infection, drug or alcohol misuse, trauma, metabolic disturbances, cerebral vascular accidents and amniotic fluid embolism.[23,41] It is, therefore, important to consider a differential diagnosis.

A seizure can last for a varying amount of time. Compulsive status epilepticus, which represents a medical emergency, is a continuous prolonged seizure lasting for 30 minutes or more or a series of seizures without full recovery of consciousness in between. Besides having serious potential maternal effects, this can result in premature labour, rupture of membranes, abruption or fetal death.[41]

If a midwife observes or suspects, a seizure, a call for urgent help should be made immediately, and then the woman's safety must be maintained (ensuring she does not hit her head, injure herself or fall). The woman should be placed in the recovery position, with priority given to maintaining a patent airway and administering oxygen if available. If at home, transfer into hospital via ambulance needs to be made. The woman is given IV benzodiazepines and anticonvulsant drugs, and ventilation may be required if the seizure is not controlled.[23] Blood specimens are sent as required (to include toxicology, anti-epileptic drug levels, PET and infection screening). Her normal drug regime should be reviewed, and changes to it may be made. If there is any question of eclampsia, then magnesium sulphate will be given (see Chapter 7).

Fibroids

Fibroids are common benign tumours which can be located in the uterus. The effect on pregnancy and birth can depend on certain characteristics, including number, size and location of the fibroids. Complications can include bleeding, pre-term labour, placental abruption, malpresentation and high rates of caesarean section.[42]

Although fibroids are not usually symptomatic in the antenatal period, women may present with acute abdominal pain due to degeneration, torsion or impaction. Diagnosis is usually by ultrasound, and treatment is generally rehydration and analgesia. Routine myomectomy is not recommended.[43]

Fibroids may contribute to postpartum haemorrhage (see Chapter 12).

Hypoglycaemia

In contrast to DKA, hypoglycaemia can cause a rapid loss of consciousness and can be immediately life-threatening (this can occur when a woman has taken insulin but then not eaten or underestimated the amount of energy she expended). Prior to loss of consciousness, the woman may feel confused or lethargic or start behaving in an unusual way. Hypoglycaemia can also present in a non-diabetic woman, and diagnosis is by measurement of the blood glucose level.[44]

Treatment includes resuscitation as necessary and, following assessment of blood glucose, food/oral glucose should be given immediately (if the woman can tolerate it and is conscious). If this is not possible, IM glucagon 1 mg should be given, but IV administration of a glucose infusion may be required in more severe cases. This should be accompanied by oxygen administration and oxygen saturation monitoring. Any insulin-containing solution should be discontinued until further reassessment is made. An investigation of the underlying cause needs to take place.

Pulmonary Oedema

Pulmonary oedema is a potential complication of many conditions, including pre-eclampsia, septicaemia, pulmonary embolism, amniotic fluid embolism and aspiration of gastric contents or it may be caused by fluid overload and/or tocolytic treatment for premature labour.[6,23] Fluid may enter the alveoli of the lungs due to pulmonary capillary damage or may diffuse from the vessels due to a reduction in colloid oncotic pressure. This fluid will not only block effective oxygenation but also damage the alveoli. Haemodynamic changes in pregnancy make women more susceptible to pulmonary oedema, and it is, therefore, important to monitor fluid balance during any obstetric or non-obstetric procedures.[45]

The woman will appear breathless, have a cough and may display agitation. Other signs are tachycardia, tachypnoea, crackles and wheezing on chest auscultation[2] and decreased oxygen saturations. Diagnosis will be made on clinical signs and by x-ray and ECG findings. Treatment has three aims – to maintain oxygen saturations at >94%, to treat the cause and to relieve symptoms.[6] Management and therapy will include assessment of the maternal condition, including identifying the underlying cause. Diuretics, in particular, will be used, blood pressure may need to be lowered, tocolytic therapy stopped and/or infection treated. Respiratory support may be required, especially if amniotic fluid embolism is suspected. Maternal observations and careful fluid balance monitoring are vital, which may include fluid restriction. Prompt multidisciplinary team involvement is necessary, and consideration is given to transferring the care to an area that best supports this.[46] Pulmonary oedema must be effectively treated, or it may progress to ARDS.

Sickle-cell crisis

Women with sickle cell disease have a high rate of both maternal and fetal complications during pregnancy.[47,48] This includes sickle-cell crisis, which is more common in pregnancy because of increased hypercoagulability, occurring most often in the third trimester and postnatal period. A painful crisis in pregnancy may be caused by nausea and vomiting, anaemia, infection, dehydration, hypothermia, physical exertion and/or increased stress.[47]

All women need to have a pain management plan available for the event of a pain crisis and be available to the multidisciplinary team.[47,49] When a woman with sickle cell disease presents with pain, a thorough investigation needs to take place and pain management initiated and closely monitored. Care must be taken to exclude other possible causes such as abruption, pulmonary embolism or fulminating pre-eclampsia (pregnant women with sickle cell disease are at higher risk of pre-eclampsia).[47] Other signs of sickle-cell crisis may include tachypnoea, acute chest pain, cough, shortness of breath, severe anaemia and, for some women, acute neurological impairment.

Management will include the treatment of any pregnancy complications, as well as oxygen therapy, rehydration (with a strict fluid balance), appropriate analgesia and low-molecular weight heparin prescribed during any antenatal admission to hospital. Prophylactic transfusion is not routinely recommended but may need to be considered in certain circumstances. Assessment of blood results, a chest x-ray, ECG and an infection screen may be required, as well as brain imaging for any woman with neurological impairment. All care should be managed within a multidisciplinary team, including a haematologist.[47,49]

Thyroid crisis (storm)

A thyroid storm is an obstetric emergency and may occur in a woman already being treated for thyrotoxicosis (hyperthyroidism) or in a woman where the disease has not yet been diagnosed. It can be caused by a failure to take prescribed antithyroid medication or be precipitated by events including infection, surgery, trauma, venous thromboembolism or diabetic ketoacidosis.[50] A thyroid crisis may be triggered by labour and birth in women with poorly controlled or untreated thyrotoxicosis.[51] Prompt recognition and critical care unit admission are often required, and prompt treatment from a multidisciplinary team can significantly improve maternal and fetal outcomes.[50]

Signs and symptoms include extreme symptoms of hyperthyroidism, such as pyrexia, tachycardia, tachypnoea, chest pains, palpitations, nausea and vomiting, abdominal pain and/or diarrhoea,

agitation, anxiety and/or confusion, psychosis, seizures and coma. If the woman has not given birth, there may be evidence of fetal tachycardia.[51] It is easier to suspect this condition if the woman has a goitre or known history of thyrotoxicosis. Care will involve gaining IV access, monitoring oxygenation, treatment of underlying causes (exclude or treat infection) and administration of specific thyroid therapies as well as treating any cardiac failure. The maternal condition should be stabilised prior to considering delivery.[50]

REFERENCES

1. Nursing and Midwifery Council. Practicing as a midwife in the UK. London: NMC; 2017, updated 2021.
2. Knight M, Bunch K, Patel R, Shakespeare J, Kotnis R, Kenyon S, Kurinczuk JJ, On Behalf of MBRRACE- UK, editors. Saving lives, improving mothers' care – lessons learned to inform future maternity care from the UK and Ireland confidential enquiries into maternal deaths and morbidity 2018–2020. Oxford: National Perinatal Epidemiology Unit, University of Oxford; 2022.
3. Winter C, Crofts J, Draycott T, Muchatuta N, editors. PROMPT, practical obstetric multi-professional training. Course manual. 3rd ed. Cambridge: Cambridge University Press; 2017. Available from: <doi:10.1017/9781108333627>
4. Chu J, Johnston TA, Geoghegan On Behalf of the Royal College of Obstetricians and Gynaecologists. Maternal collapse in pregnancy and the puerperium. Green top guideline no. 56. London: Royal College of Obstetricians and Gynaecologists; Dec 2019. Available from: <doi:10.1111/1471-0528.15995>
5. Nursing and Midwifery Council. The code: professional standards of practice and behavior for nurses, midwives and nursing associates. London: NMC; 2015 updated 2018.
6. Smith M. Respiratory disease in pregnancy. Chapter 34 In: James D, Steer P, Weiner C, Gonik B, Robson S, editors. High risk pregnancy: management options. 5th ed. Cambridge: Cambridge University Press; 2017. p. 944–973.

7. Burns R, Dent K, editors. The unconscious patient: managing medical and obstetric emergencies and trauma: the Moet course manual, 4th ed. Chichester: Wiley Blackwell; 2022. p. 171–178.

8. Engjom H, Clarke B, Girling J, Hillman S, Holden S, Lucas S, et al. On behalf of the MBRRACE-UK cardiac chapter writing group: lessons on cardiovascular care. In: Knight M, Bunch K, Patel R, Shakespeare J, Kotnis R, Kenyon S, Kurinczuk JJ, On Behalf of MBRRACE-UK, editors. Saving lives, improving mothers' care core report – lessons learned to inform maternity care from the UK and Ireland confidential enquiries into maternal deaths and morbidity 2018–20. Oxford: National Perinatal Epidemiology Unit, University of Oxford; 2022. p. 46–63.

9. Pandya S, Krishna S. Acute respiratory distress syndrome in pregnancy. Indian Journal of Critical Care Medicine. 2021;25(3):241–247. Available from: <doi:10.5005/jp-journals-10071-24036>

10. Muthu V, Agarwal R, Dhooria S, Prasad KT, Aggarwal AN, Suri V, Sehgal IS. Epidemiology, lung mechanics and outcomes of ARDS: a comparison between pregnant and non pregnant subjects. Journal of Critical Care. 2019;50:207–212. Available from: <doi:10.1016/j.jcrc.2018.12.006>

11. Johansson SG, Bieber T, Dahl R, Friedmann PS, Lanier BQ, Lockey RF, et al. Revised nomenclature for allergy for global use: report of the nomenclature review committee of the world allergy organization, October 2003. Journal of Allergy Clinical Immunology. 2004;113(5):832–836. Available from: <doi:10.1016/j.jaci.2003.12.591>

12. McCall SJ, Bonnet M-P, Ayras O, Vandenberghe G, Gissler M, Zhang W-H, et al. Anaphalylaxis in pregnancy: a population – based multinational European study. Anaesthesia. 2020;75(11):1469–1475. Available from: <doi:10.1111/anae.15069>

13. National Institute for Health and Care Excellence. Anaphylaxis: assessment and referral after emergency treatment. CG134. London: NICE; 2011 updated 2020.

14. Resuscitation Council (UK). Emergency treatment of anaphylaxis: guidelines for healthcare providers. London: Resuscitation Council (UK); 2021.

15. Abbasi N, Patenaude V, Abenhaim HA. Management and outcomes of acute appendicitis in pregnancy – population-based study of over 7000 cases. BJOG. 2014;121:1509–1514. Available from: <doi:10.1111/1471-0528.12736>

16. Burns R, Dent K, editors. Abdominal emergencies in pregnancy: managing medical and obstetric emergencies and trauma: the Moet course manual. 4th ed. Chichester: Wiley Blackwell; 2022. p. 198–205.

17. Mahomed K, Kumar S. Abdominal pain in pregnancy Chapter 52. In: James D, Steer P, Weiner C, Gonik B, Robson S, editors. High risk pregnancy: management options. 5th ed. Cambridge: Cambridge University Press; 2017. p. 11523–1543.

18. Wiles R, Hankinson B, Benbow E, Sharp A. Making decisions about radiological imaging in pregnancy. British Medical Journal, BMJ. 2022:377 doi:10.1136/bmj-2022-070486

19. Woodhead N, Nkwam O, Caddick V, Morad S, Mylvaganam S. Surgical causes of acute abdominal pain in pregnancy. The Obstetrician and Gynaecologist. 2019;21:27–25. Available from: <doi:10.1111/tog.12536>

20. Nelson Piercy C. Respiratory disease in handbook of obstetric medicine. 6th ed. Chapter 4. London: CRC Press; 2020. p. 64–85.

21. British Thoracic Society/SIGN. British guideline on the management of asthma. London: British Thoracic Society; 2019.

22. Rohn M, Felder L. Asthma in pregnancy. Topics in Obstetrics and Gynecology. 2021 Feb 3;41:1–7.

23. Bothamley J, Boyle M. Medical conditions affecting pregnancy and childbirth. 2nd ed. London: Routledge; 2021.

24. Elgendy I, Gad M, Mahmoud A, Keeley E, Pepine C. Acute stroke during pregnancy and puerperium. Journal of American College of Cardiology. 2020;75(2):180–190. Available from: <doi:10.1016/j.jacc.2019.10.056>

25. Camargo E, Singhal A. Stroke in pregnancy. Current Obstetrics and Gynecology

Reports. 2023;12:45–56. Available from: <doi:10.1007/s13669-023-00351-0>

26. Boyle M, Bothamley J. Critical care assessment by midwives. Oxon: Routledge; 2021.

27. Miller E, Leffert L. Stroke in pregnancy: a focused update. Anesth Analg. 2020 Apr;130(4):1085–1096. Available from: <doi:10.1213/ANE.0000000000004203>

28. Burns R, Dent K, editors. Cardiac, diabetic and neurological emergencies in pregnancy. managing medical and obstetric emergencies and trauma: the Moet course manual. 4th ed. Chichester: Wiley Blackwell; 2022. p. 241–265.

29. O'Connor M, Kurninczuk JJ, Knight M. UKOSS annual report. 4.3.3 diabetic ketoacidosis in pregnancy. Oxford: National Perinatal Epidemiology Unit; 2019.

30. Sharma S, Tembhare A, Inamdar S, Agarwal H. Impact of diabetic ketoacidosis in pregnancy. Journal of South Asian Federation of Obstetrics and Gynaecology. 2020 Mar–Apr;12(2):113–115. Available from: <doi:10.5005/jp-journals-10006-1761>

31. Dhanasekaran M, Mohan S, Erickson D, Shah P, Szymanski L, Adrian V, Egan A. Diabetic ketoacidosis in pregnancy: clinical risk factors, presentation and outcomes. The Journal of Clinical Endocrinology and Metabolism. 2022 Nov 11;107:3137–3143. Available from: <doi:10.1210/clinem/dgac464>

32. Eshkoli T, Barski L, Faingelernt, Jotkowitz A, Finkel-Oron A, Schwarzfuchs D. Diabetic ketoacidosis in pregnancy – case series, pathophysiology and review of the literature. European Journal of Obstetrics and Gynecology and Reproductive Biology. 2022;269:41–46. Available from: <doi:10.1016/j.ejogrb.2021.12.011>

33. Kamalakannan D, Baskar V, Barton DM, Abdu TAM. Diabetic ketoacidosis in pregnancy. Postgraduate Medical Journal. 2023;79:454–457. Available from: <doi:10.1136/pmj.79.934.454>

34. National Institute for Health and Care Excellence. Ectopic pregnancy and miscarriage. NICE quality standard 69. London: NICE; 2014.

35. National Institute for Health and Care Excellence. Ectopic pregnancy and miscarriage: diagnosis and initial management. NICE clinical guideline 126. London: NICE; 2019.

36. Burns R, Dent K, editors. Saving mothers' lives: lessons from the confidential enquiries. managing medical and obstetric emergencies and trauma: the Moet course manual. 4th ed. Chichester: Wiley Blackwell; 2022. p. 5–13.

37. Elson CJ, Salim R, Potdar N, Chetty M, Ross JA, Kirk EJ, On Behalf of the Royal college of Obstetricians and Gynaecologists. Diagnosis and management of ectopic pregnancy: green top guideline no. 21. London: Royal College of Obstetricians and Gynaecologists; 2016. Available from: <doi:10.1111/1471-0528.14189>

38. Burns R, Dent K, editors. Anaesthetic complications in obstetrics. In: Managing medical and obstetric emergencies and trauma: the Moet course manual. 4th ed. Chichester: Wiley Blackwell; 2022. p. 339–354.

39. Nelson-Piercy C. Handbook of obstetric medicine. Chapter 9, neurological problems. London: CRC Press; 2020. p. 168–196.

40. Royal College of Obstetricians and Gynaecologists. Epilepsy in pregnancy: green-top guideline no. 68. London: RCOG; June 2016.

41. Carhuapoma J, Varner M, Levine S. Neurologic complications in pregnancy Chapter 44. In: James D, Steer P, Weiner C, Gonik B, Robson S, editors. High risk pregnancy: management options. 5th ed. Cambridge: Cambridge University Press, 2017. p. 1273–1321.

42. Datir SG, Bhake A. Mangement of uterine fibroids and its complications during pregnancy: a review of the literature. Cureus. 2022;14(11):1–6. Available from: <doi:10.7759/cureus.31080>

43. Mahomed K, Kumar S. Nonmalignant gynecology in pregnancy Chapter 53. In: James D, Steer P, Weiner C, Gonik B, Robson S. editors. High risk pregnancy: management options. 5th ed. Cambridge: Cambridge University Press, 2017. p. 1544–1556.

44. Burns R, Dent K, editors. Diabetic emergencies in managing medical and obstetric emergencies and trauma: the Moet course

manual. 4th ed. Chichester: Wiley Blackwell; 2022. p. 207–211.

45. Kaur H, Kolli M. Acute pulmonary edema in pregnancy – fluid overload or atypical pre-eclampsia. Cereus. 2021;13(11):1–3. Available from: <doi:10.7759/cureus.19305>

46. Burns R, Dent K, editors. Acute cardiac disease in pregnancy in managing medical and obstetric emergencies and trauma: the Moet course manual. 4th ed. Chichester: Wiley Blackwell; 2022. p. 73–84.

47. Oteng-Ntim E, Pavord S, Howard R, Robinson S, Oakley L, Mackillop L, et al. Management of sickle cell disease in pregnancy: a British society for haematology guideline. British Journal of Haematology. 2021 Sep;194(6):980–995. Available from: <doi:10.1111/bjh.17671>

48. Oakley L, Mitchell S, von Rege I, Hadebe R, Howard J, Robinson S, et al. Perinatal outcomes in women with sickle cell disease: a matched cohort study from London, UK. Bristish Journal of Haematology. 2021;196:1069–1075. Available from: <doi:10.1111/bjh.17983>

49. Stratton P. Standardising care of those at great risk: the importance of sickle cell in pregnancy guidelines. British Journal of Haematology. 2021;194:950–953. Available from: <doi:10.1111/bjh.17667>

50. Goodier C. Endocrine emergencies in obstetrics. Clinical Obstetrics and Gyanecology. 2019;62(2):339–346. Available from: <doi:10.1097/GRF.0000000000000433>

51. Jarvis S, Nelson-Piercy C. Thyroid disease in pregnancy. In: James D, Steer P, Weiner C, Gonik B, Robson S, editors. High risk pregnancy: management options. 5th ed. Cambridge: Cambridge University Press; 2017. p. 1192–1217.

16

Birth trauma and post-traumatic stress disorder

REINA FISHER-VAN WERKHOVEN

Introduction   235
Pathophysiology and contributing factors   235
Clinical presentation   237
Long-term issues   241

Summary of midwifery responsibilities   242
Further reading and resources   242
References   243

BOX 16.1: Post-traumatic stress disorder (PTSD)

A trauma and stressor-related disorder following direct or indirect exposure to, or witnessing of, actual or threatened death, serious injury or sexual violence.[1]
Symptoms must include:

- one intrusive symptom: recurrent, involuntary, distressing memories and/or dreams, dissociative reactions such as flashbacks, intense or prolonged psychological distress to triggers, or marked physiological reactions to triggers;
- one avoidance symptom: avoidance of memories, feelings, or thoughts of trauma or avoidance of external reminders of trauma;
- two negative alterations to cognition or mood related to the trauma: dissociate amnesia, negative beliefs of self or the world, persistent negative emotional state, anhedonia (reduced ability to experience pleasure), feelings of detachment or estrangement from others, inability to experience positive emotions;
- two symptoms of marked alterations in arousal and reactivity: irritability or anger outbursts, reckless or self-destructive behaviours, hyper-vigilance, exaggerated startle response, problems with concentration, sleep disturbance.

There may also be persistent dissociative symptoms such as depersonalization (feeling detached from oneself, as if observing from out of body) or derealization (feelings of the unreality of the environment).[2]
Post-traumatic stress disorder (PTSD) may develop following exposure to an extremely threatening or horrific event or series of events. It is characterised by all of the following:

DOI: 10.4324/9781003382195-16

1) re-experiencing the traumatic event or events in the present in the form of vivid intrusive memories, flashbacks or nightmares. Re-experiencing may occur via one or multiple sensory modalities and is typically accompanied by strong or overwhelming emotions, particularly fear or horror, and strong physical sensations;
2) avoidance of thoughts and memories of the event or events, or avoidance of activities, situations or people reminiscent of the event(s); and
3) persistent perceptions of heightened current threat, for example, as indicated by hypervigilance or an enhanced startle reaction to stimuli such as unexpected noises.

The symptoms persist for at least several weeks and cause significant impairment in personal, family, social, educational, occupational or other important areas of functioning.[3]

INTRODUCTION

Birth is generally considered a positive life event;[4] however, recent research shows that 4–6% of women present with (postnatal) post-traumatic stress disorder.[5,6,7] This was found to be significantly higher in women who experienced a high-risk pregnancy or birth.[7] In women whose babies died, rates of PTSD of up to 39% have been found.[8] Post-traumatic stress disorder (PTSD) presents with intrusive flashbacks, avoidance of triggering circumstances, fear, irritability, guilt and shame.[1]

There is also a significant group of women who do not meet the full PTSD criteria but who still experienced the birth as traumatic.[9,10] When the experience of that traumatic birth causes ongoing distress, this is referred to as 'birth trauma.'[10] Women with birth trauma do not meet all the criteria to be diagnosed with PTSD but do display symptoms of traumatic stress similar to those found in PTSD.[11,12] Post-traumatic stress symptoms have been found in 14–17% of postnatal women.[6,13]

Both medical interventions during childbirth and women's subjective feelings of poor-quality care have been identified as contributing factors to Birth Trauma and postnatal PTSD.[6,14] It is estimated that 70% of adults have experienced psychological trauma at some point in their lives,[12] and childbirth is a time where many of these experiences can be relived and revisited, sometimes for the first time ever.[15]

Birth trauma has been found often to be co-morbid with other mental health issues such as depression,[14] anxiety[7] and fear of birth.[16] Sometimes, that has led to PTSD being missed as the underlying issue and the diagnosis of PTSD has been missed or delayed.[5,17]

Although there was an awareness of people experiencing physical and psychological symptoms following trauma during the 19th century, it was during the First World War that these were prevalent and recognised on a large scale. Initially, the cause was thought to be related to the physical effect of being near the exploding shells, and the condition became known as 'shellshock,' but later was recognised and treated as a psychological condition.[18] In 1980, it was first officially recognised and named as PTSD in the Diagnostic and Statistical Manual of Mental Disorders-3 (DSM-3). Based on ongoing research, it was understood that traumatic events other than war, such as natural disasters, airplane or car accidents, and, more commonly, rape and sexual abuse, could cause PTSD.[18] Gradually, the DSM has adjusted its definition and criteria of a traumatic event, which now includes the possibility of including birth as such.[1] There is even an argument that childbirth-related PTSD (CB-PTS) should be considered a recognised subtype of PTSD due to its unique traumatic event, its unique characteristics and phenomenology, its unique family implications and its unique survivors.[4]

These facts are important to consider, particularly in the context of childbirth emergencies. Even when a birth emergency has been managed effectively, resulting in a physically positive outcome, the long-term psychological impact of the event on the woman and her birth partner – and ultimately – the infant, should not be overlooked.

PATHOPHYSIOLOGY AND CONTRIBUTING FACTORS

Many of the emergencies described in this book could potentially cause the woman and her partner to have a traumatic birth experience. Some of these women and their partners[21] will experience PTSS, and a significant number of women are likely to

BOX 16.2: Definitions of conditions associated with PTSD

Complex post-traumatic stress disorder (Complex PTSD) is a disorder that may develop following exposure to an event or series of events of an extremely threatening or horrific nature, most commonly prolonged or repetitive events from which escape is difficult or impossible (e.g., torture, slavery, genocide campaigns, prolonged domestic violence and repeated childhood sexual or physical abuse).

All diagnostic requirements for PTSD are met. In addition, Complex PTSD is characterised by severe and persistent:

1) problems in affect regulation;
2) beliefs about oneself as diminished, defeated or worthless, accompanied by feelings of shame, guilt or failure related to the traumatic event; and
3) difficulties in sustaining relationships and in feeling close to others.

These symptoms cause significant impairment in personal, family, social, educational, occupational or other important areas of functioning.[1]

POST-TRAUMATIC STRESS SYMPTOMS (PTSS):

Women display symptoms of post-traumatic stress such as re-experiencing, avoidance, hyper-arousal and negative alterations in mood and thinking, but all criteria for PTSD are not met.[19]

BIRTH TRAUMA:

Any difficult experience on the journey: from trying to conceive (for example, reproductive trauma) to pregnancy (for example, hyperemesis gravidarum), the birth itself and beyond (for example, breastfeeding trauma) – any experience that left a woman feeling intensely afraid, out of control or helpless. Women may experience PTSS but do not meet the criteria for PTSD.[10,12]

TRAUMATIC BIRTH:

This includes births, whether preterm or full term, which are physically traumatic (for example, assisted deliveries or emergency caesarean sections, severe perineal tears, postpartum haemorrhage) and births that are experienced as traumatic, even when the birth is obstetrically straightforward.[20]

develop PTSD.[7,8] However, that is not the case for all women.

Multifactorial elements have been identified as contributing to the development of birth trauma/PTSD. Complications and obstetric interventions have been found to be contributing factors for the development of Postnatal PTSD.[22,13] However, it has also been identified that not all women who experience birth complications develop PTSD, but that particularly the subjective experience of the birth contributes to the development of PTSD.[14,6,18] 'Trauma is in the eye of the beholder.'[23]

Also, Garthus-Niegel et al.[24] identified that women who subjectively experience the birth as traumatising are more likely to develop PTSD.

This includes experiencing high levels of distress, fear for her own life and/or that of the baby, lack of control and feeling unsupported, and this was again demonstrated by Baptie et al.[25] Elmir et al.[10] describe how women's experiences of feeling a victim, feeling invisible and out of control and being treated inhumanely contributed to the birth being experienced as traumatic. General trauma literature shows evidence that trauma where a person is the cause of the trauma (rather than war or natural disaster) leads to more serious forms of PTSD,[14,18] and this is important to consider when providing maternity care. Simpson and Catling,[26] in a literature review to understand psychologically traumatic birth experiences, identified the impact of poor verbal and non-verbal communication of care providers in meeting the woman's need for a sense of control and dignity and meeting cultural and birth expectations on the development of PTSD[27]. A recent study by Ertan et al.[28] identified that previous exposure to trauma (such as sexual trauma, childhood trauma and abuse), as well as birth-related factors (such as an emergency caesarean section, major surgery or labour pain) and the lack of support (social support in general or lack of support from medical staff) were all risk factors for the development of PTSD following childbirth.

It is important to recognise the growing evidence that racial factors play a role in women experiencing birth trauma,[29] captured under the terminology of 'racial trauma.' These are important considerations for health professionals involved in caring for women and their partners in these circumstances. Black women have reported experiencing gendered racism during childbirth, which leads to potentially traumatic events and poorer birth outcomes.[29,30,31,32] A further group of women that should be considered at high risk for previous trauma are those who have arrived in the country as refugees or asylum seekers and may have been exposed to war, rape, natural disasters, been forced to leave their homes and families, lost family members and have arrived in a country they do not know and where they may not understand and speak the language.[33]

According to Garthus-Niegel et al.,[24] risk factors can be divided into pre-disposing and precipitating factors. Pre-disposing factors are pre-existing factors in a woman's life that make her more vulnerable to developing PTSD, and precipitating factors trigger events for PTSD to develop (see Table 16.1).

Pregnancy and birth can be a time which often includes intimate physical examinations and the involvement of many different male and female maternity care providers, affording many opportunities to trigger previous traumatic experiences where women revisit previous traumatic experiences, sometimes for the very first time (where these experiences have been repressed for many years). These can include previous birth trauma, previous perinatal loss, adverse childhood experiences (such as abuse or neglect, attachment trauma), sexual abuse and assault and intimate partner violence.[32] This is even more significant when a birth emergency occurs and many obstetric interventions happen, often without much time for discussion and explanation to the woman and her birth partner, with the risk of consequent physical as well as psychological trauma.[35]

CLINICAL PRESENTATION

Signs and symptoms

In order to meet the clinical diagnosis of PTSD, women need to meet the criteria as defined in Box 16.1. For examples of intrusive symptoms and avoidance, see Box 16.3.

Table 16.1 Pre-disposing and precipitating factors[24,34]

Pre-disposing factors:	Precipitating factors:

• Psychiatric history
• Previous counselling, depression, anxiety, PTSD
• Socio-economic and socio-demographic factors
• Primiparity
• Current anxiety, depression
• Previous childbirth-related trauma, sexual abuse
• Fear of upcoming childbirth (pre-traumatic distress)
• Low stress coping (low self-esteem and self-efficacy)
• Critical life events
	• Difficult pregnancy, abnormal screening results
	• Instrumental/operative delivery, duration, type and number of interventions
	• Fear of harm to self or baby
	• Perception of poor care
	• Unmet expectations
	• Negative perception of staff-mother interactions:
	  o Poor communication,
	  o Feeling not being listened to
	  o Not taken seriously
	  o false reassurance
	• Feeling dehumanised
	• Loss of control, feeling of powerlessness
	• High levels of pain, inadequate pain relief
	• Perceived low levels of social or partner support

BOX 16.3: Examples of intrusive symptoms and avoidance

INTRUSIVE SYMPTOMS

"I was walking into supermarkets and couldn't cope with the fans or the lights or smell of lavender, watching things like 'Finding Dory' or anything to do with running water. It's the most horrific thing I've ever been through in my life . . . I couldn't bath my kids properly for ages. Having a shower, all the things I'd normally do to relax, massively brought on flashbacks" (Carys, who spent much of her labour in a birthing pool).[18, p.33]

AVOIDANCE

"I've got a perpetual fear of hospitals and I can't watch any programme where anyone gives birth at all. Anything at all, even if it's just a very short thing. One Born Every Minute – that's right out of the window. And even Pampers adverts are quite triggering, not just for the reminder of the pain, but because there's always a lot of care and love, and I didn't feel that at all" (Sam, who had a traumatic birth due to the fact she felt she wasn't cared for as expected and at times felt abandoned by staff during her birth).[18, pp.34,35]

Women will show symptoms of negative alterations in cognition or mood: they may feel depressed and guilty, have low self-confidence and feel that they have failed their baby.[18,10] They will also exhibit symptoms of altered arousal and reactivity: hyper-vigilance for the baby's wellbeing, irritability, anxiousness and anger or aggression, which can affect the relationship with the partner or family.[18,10] While some of these symptoms can be present soon after birth, a formal diagnosis of PTSD can only be made when they have been present for more than one month, and they will generally have a significant impact on social and occupational functioning and cause significant distress. It needs to be established that these signs and symptoms are not caused by alcohol, substances or medication.[18] These signs and symptoms can be delayed and only appear at six months after the events.[7]

Women may also experience feelings of:

Dissociation, including 'depersonalisation': a persistent or recurrent sense of unreality of self or body, or time moving slowly, feeling detached and observing oneself from a distance, or
Derealisation: persistent or recurrent experience of the unreality of surroundings, living in an unreal, dreamlike, distant or distorted world.[2,18]

The factor uniting all the signs and symptoms of PTSD is the fact that the woman feels that the trauma is still happening; the same response of fear and being ready to respond to the real or perceived danger is still present.[18] It is important to understand what physical processes underpin the development of PTSD. The brain recognises danger and responds to this with the fight-or-flight response. The thalamus receives the message of an outside threat and will process this information to interpret the threat. This information is then passed on to the amygdala and the frontal lobes (conscious awareness).[18] The amygdala sends a message to the hypothalamus, and the hypothalamus will initiate a hormonal response to stressful stimuli (the real or perceived danger/threat) via the hypothalamic-pituitary-adrenal (HPA) axis.[36] The response of the amygdala, as an instinctive response, is faster than the processing of the information in the frontal lobes. The ability of the rational brain to override the unconscious response is limited, so the body's response to a threat is most commonly to go into fight-or-flight mode. Once the threat has disappeared, the body returns to normal; however, if the potential threat persists, the stress response (fight-or-flight mode) will also continue.[18] Studies suggest that dysregulation of the hypothalamus and interactions with other brain structures may cause an excessive or prolonged stress response, which can lead to the development of PTSD.[37] This area needs further research.[36]

MRI scans performed on people suffering from PTSD, compared with scans in those who don't, show increased activation of the amygdala when there is a reminder of the trauma ('trigger') and the volume of the hippocampus (the part of the brain involved in controlling stress responses) processing memories and fear conditioning is reduced in people with PTSD.[38] This may indicate that those with PTSD are not processing traumatic memories properly: they are not processed and stored in the long-term memory but remain active in the short-term memory, which possibly explains the sense of being on a constant high alert that women have described.[39]

Preconception care and screening

Screening tools for PTSD are either non-childbirth specific[28] or, if developed for childbirth-related PTSD, they do not meet the DSM-5 criteria (Perinatal PTSD Questionnaire) and have not been fully tested and validated (Traumatic Event Scale).[5] Screening for postpartum PTSD has, therefore, been limited, which probably means that many women with PTSD have not been identified[5] or misdiagnosed with postnatal depression, as comorbidity with postnatal depression is high.[14,17] In 2018, Ayers, Wright and Thornton developed the City Birth Trauma scale based on the current Diagnostic and Statistical Manual of Mental Disorders, Fifth Edition (DSM-5)[1] PTSD criteria and found this to have good reliability and some indication of validity.[5] It consists of a self-reported questionnaire, which includes 31 items, aiming to identify the frequency of PTSD symptoms over the last week; a higher score indicates an increased risk for PTSD. It can be used between six weeks and one year postpartum.[18] Since then, the City Birth Trauma scale has been tested in different languages and cultural settings[28,40] and also for use with fathers and birth partners.[41]

Women with known pre-disposing factors and vulnerabilities, particularly previous traumatic birth or existing mental health issues, would benefit from accessing therapy before their next pregnancy. Contrary to other traumatic situations, women may need to decide whether they are willing to expose themselves to this 'trauma' again, and women are hesitant to become pregnant and give birth again,[42] particularly if the trauma was related to their first pregnancy and birth, and there is often a prolonged interval between pregnancies.[43,44] It would reduce the risk of further PTSD if they could access preconception care before embarking on a new pregnancy. Therapy

and medication could help them to deal with any pre-existing traumas to enable them to feel more confident before getting pregnant again.[18]

Antenatal care

It is important that maternity healthcare professionals are aware of women's previous psychosocial history.[9] The booking appointment is a critical time to identify any pre-disposing factors and vulnerabilities for PTSD.[14,20] Risk factors for PTSD can be assessed in pregnancy, particularly depression, severe fear of childbirth and pre-traumatic stress in view of the forthcoming birth, poor health or complications in pregnancy, a history of PTSD or previous counselling for issues related to pregnancy or birth.[45,14] A detailed history of psycho-social factors, as well as previous births and reviewing notes of previous birth(s), could identify pre-disposing factors for PTSD/birth trauma in the current pregnancy.[9]

NHS England supports the use of a trauma-informed care model in the perinatal period,[32] which emphasises the importance of creating an environment where choice, control and psychological safety are paramount, with the purpose of actively resisting re-traumatisation. This is built on the following principles:

- **Compassion and recognition:** recognising the prevalence of trauma and how this can impact women.
- **Communication and collaboration:** clear communication. Acknowledging different communication needs. Using trauma-sensitive language will empower women to collaborate with healthcare professionals and make informed choices.
- **Consistency and continuity:** continuity of care, coordinated care and correct referral pathways for women with previous trauma.
- **Recognising diversity and facilitating recovery:** recognising that each woman's experience of trauma is unique, which will inform how to support her recovery and care for a consecutive pregnancy and birth; also recognising cultural and gender diversity and how these factors may impact people's lives.

When women disclose a history of a traumatic birth, referral to the Perinatal Mental Health team is essential to support the woman through this new pregnancy.[20] It is important that a detailed birth plan is made with the woman and, where appropriate, her partner to avoid a traumatic birth this time. This can support the woman's sense of control and being listened to.[32] The traumatic birth experience is known to contribute to secondary tokophobia and may lead to a request for an elective caesarean section[26] or a home birth.[18] Discussing the benefits, risks and alternatives should be part of the antenatal conversation and planning.[32] Since unmet birth expectations have been found to contribute to a traumatic birth experience,[26] midwives have an important role in discussing realistic birth expectations with women.[28] Cross et al.[46] found that when women received antenatal information that included normality as well as broader focused information, including information on obstetric complications, this was found to be beneficial in reducing women experiencing the birth as traumatic. Greenfield et al.[47] found that during consecutive pregnancies, women themselves are also ensuring they are informed and aware of their choices, aiming to avoid a repeat of their previous experience and to avoid loss of control during the birth. Women have also found peer support groups to be helpful.[18]

Labour care

Based on the research into causes and risk factors for postnatal PTSD, it is important that women are treated with respect and dignity and are given every opportunity to consent and the option of informed choice.[10,11,28] A supportive birth environment, where the woman is encouraged to have a sense of autonomy, has been found to have a buffering effect against a complicated birth with obstetric intervention.[48] Any previous or current sexual abuse should be clearly recorded and taken into consideration when examinations or any form of touch are needed. Equally, maternity staff should be aware that the language that is sometimes used, such as 'open your legs' or 'cooperate' can trigger the memory of rape or abuse,[18] as well as any situation where women are lying down, with others standing around them, making them feel powerless and helpless.

A positive and supportive birth experience has been demonstrated to mediate and negate the traumatic effects of complications and the need for obstetric interventions.[25] Where a birth plan

has been made, this should be followed as much as possible. As Greenfield et al.[47] state, the midwife needs to regain the trust of a woman who has experienced a previous traumatic birth, and it is, therefore, important that she understands and acknowledges the previous trauma. Using a continuity-of-care model can enhance the building of a trusting relationship in this situation.[42,43,47] The continuous presence of the midwife during birth and being given physical comfort measures has been identified by women as making a positive difference during difficult labour.[42]

Support from close friends and family throughout pregnancy and in the postnatal period has been found to reduce the risk of PTSD developing or enhancing recovery,[43] and is particularly important to consider during the birth.

Mapp and Hudson,[35] in a qualitative study on women's experiences during obstetric emergencies, identified a number of simple but effective strategies that could help reduce the emotional impact and traumatic experience. These included identifying one member of staff to support the woman and birth partner during the emergency, the use of touch (with consent), hand holding, being aware of facial expressions, a reassuring smile, providing brief and simple explanations of the events, informing them that a detailed explanation will be given when the emergency is over and the person leading the emergency to briefly engage with the woman, even if just by saying her name. It is important to validate and acknowledge the woman and partner's concerns, and telling them "not to worry" should be avoided.[35] Adequate pain relief is important, as this has frequently been described as a reason for the birth to be traumatic,[28,42,43] often in relation to a lack of control.[42]

Women should be observed for behaviour that may indicate previous trauma, such as dissociation during labour and birth, which is a strong risk factor for postnatal PTSD,[14,49] extreme fear, lack of trust, extreme emotion/absolute silence, intense need for control, extreme modesty and mistrust of their body.

Postnatal care

Following a traumatic birth, it is essential that women and partners are not left alone, as women have described that it made them anxious to be alone, or they may be experiencing flashbacks or nightmares.[35] It is important that women and their partners have an opportunity to understand what has happened, although it has been recognised that women may suffer from cognitive impairment in the initial postnatal period.[35]

Skin-to-skin and breastfeeding support should be offered, although midwives should be aware that the child can be a trigger to relive the birth trauma,[50] and breastfeeding can be linked to a previous traumatic experience.[10] A negative breastfeeding experience can increase the trauma.[11] However, breastfeeding has also been perceived as a way to overcome the trauma and prove success as a mother.[10] The effects of oxytocin can also help a woman to feel more positive.[51]

Midwives should ensure that women have effective pain relief,[43] and it is important that women have an opportunity to sleep, as there is some research to suggest that insomnia can contribute to PTSD.[24]

Before discharge, women and their partners should have had an opportunity for a conversation with the midwife or obstetrician to discuss the birth and have their immediate questions answered,[34] and this can be followed up during postnatal care in the community.

There should be information for the woman and her partner about further opportunities to discuss the birth at a later stage. Women generally want to talk about the birth; however, it is important that this happens when they feel ready to do so and in an unstructured format. Telling their story, being listened to, being able to ask questions and reading through the notes together with the midwife, thus gaining a better understanding of their birthing experience, may be valuable. Birth Reflection[42] or Birth Afterthoughts services[52] have been found useful for this. Formal structured debriefing with an emphasis on reliving the event is no longer recommended for women experiencing postnatal PTSD[20] as there is insufficient evidence to support its use,[53] and some evidence to suggest that it could increase the trauma.[35] However, 'meaning making,' the process through which people assess and come to understand potentially stressful situations in the context of the birth experience has demonstrated better postpartum adjustment.[54]

A detailed handover of the details of the birth and immediate postnatal period to the community midwife, the GP and the Health Visitor (HV) is essential to allow for a close follow-up by community services. This is important as signs and symptoms of PTSD can still develop at a later stage, and PTSD can only be diagnosed when signs and symptoms have been present for at least one month.[34] The City Birth Trauma Scale could be used around six weeks after birth to assess for the presence of PTSD.[55,18]

Where PTSS has been identified and/or a diagnosis of PTSD has been made, the woman should be referred to high-intensity psychological intervention, such as trauma-focused cognitive behavioural therapy (CBT) or eye-movement desensitisation and reprocessing (EMDR). Women who have received one of these treatments often make a near-complete recovery. The traumatic memory does not disappear but has lost its intrusive character.[18] In addition, medication such as Sertraline (a selective serotonin reuptake inhibitor [SSRI]) or an antipsychotic such as risperidone may be prescribed.[18]

Other treatments, such as Emotional Freedom Technique (EFT) or Rewind Therapy – specific to treat PTSD, known as birth trauma resolution (BTR), may also be available, and some midwives are being trained in this by the RCM.[18,35] Self-help programmes have not been demonstrated to be effective for the treatment of PTSD, and yoga and mindfulness seem to demonstrate limited effectiveness and need to be used with caution.[18]

Peer support groups, including online platforms, while having limited research evidence to demonstrate effective treatment for PTSD, are providing support to women that they experience as beneficial, based on anecdotal evidence.[18]

LONG-TERM ISSUES

Research into women's experience of birth trauma and PTSD has shown that women felt they had failed their babies, particularly when they struggled to establish a bond. Breastfeeding has been found to be helpful in a way of compensating for the birth and giving the baby the best possible start in life.[10] They also expressed that they felt a great sense of loss in relation to their experience of childbirth, motherhood, self and the ideal family.[26] Women have reported feeling severely depressed and having suicidal ideation.[26] Difficulty in bonding with the baby and the negative impact of PTSD on the mother/infant relationship was also demonstrated by Ertan et al.[28] The couple relationship has also been shown to be affected by the woman experiencing PTSD:[28] sexual intimacy was found to be a constant reminder of the birth, combined with the fear of another pregnancy. Some women did not want to be touched at all. Women felt traumatic experiences were not always acknowledged by their partners. Partners can feel rejected and frustrated by the loss of intimacy, and in some instances, this has resulted in relationship breakdown.[10,56]

Research has shown that birth partners (partners, family member or close friends) are also at risk of developing a birth trauma, and up to 8% of partners are reported to have developed PTSD[57] from being present at a traumatic birth.[58,19] The City Birth Trauma Scale has now been adapted for use with birth partners, too.[41] Fathers/birth partners have described emotional aspects such as fear of death for their partners or their child, feeling helpless, feeling isolated and abandoned, increasing anxiety, loss of positive shared experience around the birth, feeling dismissed or not cared for by staff and feeling things happened in a blur and seemed to take forever (distortion of perception).[58] Where women's most common PTSS seems to be re-experiencing the trauma, for partners, this seems to be avoidance,[58,19] which, in itself, may lead to PTSD in partners being underdiagnosed. PTSD in partners can, in turn, impact PTSD in women.[34]

Cook, Ayers and Horsch,[59] in a systematic review looking at maternal PTSD during the perinatal period and child outcomes, found that maternal PTSD is associated with low birth weight and lower breastfeeding rates but the evidence for a link with pre-term birth, fetal growth, head circumference, mother-infant interaction and relationship or child development was contradictory, although they acknowledged that some of the inconclusive outcomes might be related to the methodological limitations of the research. A more recent systematic review[60] indicates that there is a suggested link between childbirth-related PTSD and mother-infant attachment problems and also problems in child behaviour. Thomas and McCann,[18] also reviewing anecdotal evidence and qualitative data based on women's experiences, suggest that women with postnatal PTSD do experience difficulties in bonding with their babies, despite the fact they want to and feel guilty about this. At the moment, there is insufficient evidence to demonstrate a long-term negative impact on the parent-child bond.[18]

Finally, it should be recognised that maternity staff can also experience PTSD from being involved in caring for women who have traumatic births.[34] Equally, midwives will face their own personal traumas and the daily effect of working in a healthcare system that is very challenging.[52] There is growing acknowledgement of the fact that these factors may affect not only how midwives care for women but also the importance of supporting midwives to provide individualised, person-centred care that will help to prevent women from experiencing childbirth-related PTSD.[12,61]

SUMMARY OF MIDWIFERY RESPONSIBILITIES

- Use a trauma-informed care model.
- Screen for risk factors and vulnerabilities for PTSD.
- Referral to PNMH specialist support if these are identified.
- Clear documentation and handover between professionals.
- Continuity of care.
- Support women in setting realistic expectations.
- Clear communication, verbal and non-verbal.
- Informed consent and choice.
- Acknowledge and support the (birth) partner.
- Pain relief.
- Sensitively support breastfeeding and skin-to-skin.
- Listen and answer questions postnatally.
- Ensure the woman receives information about birth reflection services.

FURTHER READING AND RESOURCES

Brodrick A, Wilson E. Listening to women after childbirth. London: Routledge; 2020.
Birth Trauma Association, Available from: https://birthtraumaassociation.org.uk/#
     This is a peer support organisation for parents who have experienced a traumatic birth and also provides training materials on birth trauma for professionals.
Birth Trauma Resolution. Available from: www.birthtraumaresolution.com/
     Information about the Birth Trauma Resolution Training.

Making Birth Better. Available from: www.make
birthbetter.org/

This organisation involves a group of
experts who bring together lived experience
and extensive professional knowledge of birth
trauma and vicarious trauma and provides support for women and professionals.

National Institute for Health and Care Excellence
(NICE). Antenatal and postnatal mental health:
clinical management and service guidance, CG
12. 2014, last updated 2020. Available from:
www.nice.org.uk/guidance/cg192

National Institute for Health and Care Excellence
(NICE). Post-traumatic stress disorder, NG116.
2018. Available from: www.nice.org.uk/
guidance/NG116

Thomas K, McCan S. Postnatal PTSD – a guide for
health professionals. London: Jessica Kingsley
Publishers; 2022.

REFERENCES

1. American Psychiatric Association, DSM-5
   Task Force. Diagnostic and statistical
   manual of mental disorders: DSM-5™ (5th
   ed.). Washington, DC: American Psychiatric
   Publishing, Inc.; 2013. Available from:
   <doi:10.1176/appi.books.9780890425596>
2. Schraeder C, Ross A. A review of PTSD
   and current treatment strategies. Missouri
   Medicine. 2021;118(5):546–551. PMID:
   34924624 PMCID: PMC8672952.
3. WHO. International classification of diseases
   11th revision (ICD-11), version 01/2023. 2019.
   [Accessed 3 September 2023]. Available
   from: https://icd.who.int/browse11/l-m/en
4. Horesh D, Garthus-Niegel S, Horsch, A.
   Childbirth-related PTSD: is it a unique post-
   traumatic disorder? Journal of Reproductive
   and Infant Psychology. 2021;39:221–224.
   Available from: <doi:10.1080/02646838.202
   1.1930739>
5. Ayers S, Wright DB, Thornton A.
   Development of a measure of postpartum
   PTSD: the city birth trauma scale. Frontiers
   in Psychiatry. 2018;9(409). Available from:
   <doi:10.3389/fpsyt.2018.00409>
6. Dekel S, Stuebe C, Dishy G. Childbirth
   induced posttraumatic stress syndrome:
   a systematic review of prevalence and
   risk factors. Frontiers in Psychology.
   2017;8. Available from: <doi:10.3389/
   fpsyg.2017.00560>
7. Dikmen-Yildiz P, Ayers S, Phillips L. The
   prevalence of posttraumatic stress disorder
   in pregnancy and after birth: a systematic
   review and meta-analysis. Journal of
   Affective Disorders. 2018;2017:634–645.
   Available from: <doi:10.1016/j.jad.2016.
   10.009>
8. Christiansen DM. Posttraumatic stress
   disorder in parents following infant death:
   a systematic review. Clinical Psychology
   Review. 2017;51:60–74. Available from:
   <doi:10.1016/j.cpr.2016.10.007>
9. Alcorn KL, O'Donovan A, Patrick JC,
   Creedy D, Devilly GJ. A prospective longitudinal study of the prevalence of post-
   traumatic stress disorder resulting from
   childbirth events. Psychological Medicine.
   2010;40:1849–1859. Available from:
   <doi:10.1017/S0033291709992224>
10. Elmir R, Schmied V, Wilkes L, Jackson
    D. Women's perceptions and experi-
    ences of a traumatic birth: a meta-
    ethnography. Journal of Advanced Nursing,
    2010;66(10):2142–2153. Available from:
    <doi:10.1111/j.1365-2648.2010.05391.x>
11. Ayers S. Delivery as a traumatic event:
    prevalence, risk factors, screening & treat-
    ment. Clinical Obstetrics & Gynecology.
    2004;47(3):552–567. Available from:
    <doi:10.1097/01.grf.0000129919.00756.9c>
12. Make Birth Better. What is birth trauma.
    n.d. [Accessed 3 September 2023].
    Available from: www.makebirthbetter.org/
    what-is-birth-trauma
13. Boorman RJ, Devilly GJ, Gamble J,
    Creedy DK, Fenwick J. Childbirth and
    criteria for traumatic events. Midwifery.
    2014;30(2):255–261. Available from:
    <doi:10.1016/j.midw.2013.03.001>
14. Ayers S, Bond R, Bertullies S, Wijma K. The
    aetiology of post-traumatic stress following
    childbirth: a meta-analysis and theoreti-
    cal framework. Psychological Medicine.
    2016;46:1121–1134. Available from:
    <doi:10.1017/S0033291715002706>
15. Montgomery E, Pope C, Rogers J. The
    re-enactment of childhood sexual abuse
    in maternity care: a qualitative study. BMC
    Pregnancy and Childbirth. 2015;15(1):1–7.

16. Dencker A, Nilsson C, Begley C, Jangsten E, Mollberg M, Patel H, et al. Causes and outcomes in studies of fear of childbirth: a systematic review. Women Birth. 2019 Apr;32(2):99–111. Available from: <doi:10.1016/j.wombi.2018.07.004>. Epub 2018 Aug 14. PMID: 30115515.

17. Coates R, de Visser R, Ayers S. Not identifying with postnatal depression: a qualitative study of womens postnatal symptoms of distress and need for support. Journal of Psychosomatic Obstetrics and Gynecology. 2015;36(3):114–121. Available from: <doi:10.3109/0167482X.2015.1059418>

18. Thomas K, McCan S. Postnatal PTSD – a guide for health professionals. London: Jessica Kingsley Publishers; 2022.

19. Delicate A, Ayers S, McMullen S. 'Healthcare practitioners' assessment and observations of birth trauma in mothers and partners. Journal of Reproductive and Infant Psychology. 2022;40(1):34–46. Available from: <doi:10.1080/02646838.2020.1788210>

20. National Institute for Health and Care Excellence (NICE). Antenatal and postnatal mental health: clinical management and service guidance, CG 12. 2014, last updated 2020. Available from: www.nice.org.uk/guidance/cg192

21. Etheridge J, Slade P. 'Nothing's actually happened to me': the experiences of fathers who found childbirth traumatic. BMC Pregnancy Childbirth. 2017 Mar 7;17(1):80. Available from: <doi:10.1186/s12884-017-1259-y>. PMID: 28270116; PMCID: PMC5341171.

22. Adewuya AO, Ologun YA, Ibigbami OS. Post-traumatic stress disorder after childbirth in Nigerian women: prevalence and risk factors. BJOG. 2006;113(3):284–288. Available from: <doi:10.1111/j.1471-0528.2006.00861.x.45.22>

23. Beck CT. Birth trauma: in the eye of the beholder. Nursing Research. 2004;53(1):28–35. ISSN: 0029-6562, eISSN: 1538-9847.

24. Garthus-Niegel S, Von Soest T, Vollrath M, Eberhard-Gran M. The impact of subjective birth experiences on post-traumatic stress symptoms: a longitudinal study. Arch Womens Ment Health. 2013;16:1–10. Available from: <doi:10.1007/s00737-012-0301-3>

25. Baptie G, Andrade J, Bacon AM, Norman A. Birth trauma: the mediating effects of perceived support. British Journal of Midwifery. 2020;28(10):724–730. Available from: <doi:10.12968/bjom.2020.28.10.724>

26. Simpson M, Catling C. Understanding psychological traumatic birth experiences: a literature review. Women and Birth. 2016;29:203–207. Available from: <doi:10.1016/j.wombi.2015.10.009>

27. Sorenson DSS, Tschetter L. Prevalence of negative birth perception, disaffirmation, perinatal trauma symptoms, and depression among postpartum women. Perspectives in Psychiatric Care. 2010 Jan;46(1):14–25. Available from: <doi:10.1111/j.1744-6163.2009.00234.x>

28. Ertan D, Hingray C, Burlacu E, Sterlé A, El-Hage W. Post-traumatic stress disorder following childbirth. BMC Psychiatry, 2021;21(155):1–9. Available from: <doi:10.1186/s12888-021-03158-6>

29. Markin RD, Coleman MN. Intersections of gendered racial trauma and childbirth trauma: clinical interventions for Black women. Psychotherapy (Chic). 2023 Mar;60(1):27–38. Available from: <doi:10.1037/pst0000403>. Epub 2021 Nov 29. PMID: 34843315.

30. Bunch K, Knight M. Maternal mortality in the UK 2017–19: surveillance and epidemiology. In Knight M, Bunch K, Tuffnell D, Patel R, Shakespeare J, Kotnis R, Kenyon S, Kurinczuk JJ, On Behalf of MBRRACE-UK, editors. Saving lives, improving mothers' care – lessons learned to inform maternity care from the UK and Ireland confidential enquiries into maternal deaths and morbidity 2017–19. Oxford: National Perinatal Epidemiology Unit, University of Oxford; 2021. p. 5–23.

31. Bunch K, Knight M. Maternal mortality in the UK 2018–20: surveillance and epidemiology. In: Knight M, Bunch K, Patel R, Shakespeare J, Kotnis R, Kenyon S, Kurinczuk JJ, On behalf of MBRRACE-UK, editors. Saving lives, improving mothers' care core report – lessons learned to inform maternity care from the UK and Ireland

confidential enquiries into maternal deaths and morbidity 2018–20. Oxford: National Perinatal Epidemiology Unit, University of Oxford; 2022. pp. 2–20.

32. Law et al for NHS England. A good practice guide to support implementation of trauma-informed care in the perinatal period. 2021. Available from: www.england.nhs.uk/publication/a-good-practice-guide-to-support-implementation-of-trauma-informed-care-in-the-perinatal-period/

33. Evans M, Plows J, McCarthy R, McConville B, Haith-Cooper M. What refugee women want from maternity care: a qualitative study. BJOM. 2022;30(9):502–511. Available from: <doi:10.12968/bjom.2022.30.9.502>

34. Aimee P, McKenzie-Mcharg K. The experience of PTSD following childbirth. British Journal of Mental Health Nursing. 2015;4:122–128.

35. Mapp T. Feelings and fears post obstetric emergencies. Br J Midwifery 2005;13(1):36–40. Available from: <doi:10.12968/bjom.2005.13.1.17320>

36. Raise-Abdullahi P, Meamar M, Vafaei AA, Alizadeh M, Dadkhah M, Shafia S, et al. Hypothalamus and post-traumatic stress disorder: a review. Brain Sci. 2023 Jun 29;13(7):1010. Available from: <doi:10.3390/brainsci13071010>. PMID: 37508942; PMCID: PMC10377115.

37. Joëls M, Baram TZ. The neuro-symphony of stress. Nat Rev Neurosci. 2009;10:459–466.

38. Sherin JE, Nemeroff CB. Post-traumatic stress disorder: the neurobiological impact of psychological trauma. Dialogues in Clinical Neuroscience. 2011;13(3):263–278. Available from: <doi:10.31887/DCNS.2011.13.2/jsherin>

39. Duval ER, Javanbakht A, Liberzon I. Neural circuits in anxiety and stress disorders: a focused review. Ther Clin Risk Manag. 2015 Jan 23;11:115–126. Available from: <doi:10.2147/TCRM.S48528>. PMID: 25670901; PMCID: PMC4315464.

40. Stén G, Ayers S, Malmquist A, Nieminen K, Grundström H. Assessment of maternal posttraumatic stress disorder following childbirth: psychometric properties of the Swedish version of city birth trauma scale. Psychological Trauma: Theory, Research, Practice, and Policy. 2023;15(7):1153–1163. Available from: <doi:10.1037/tra0001465>

41. Webb R, et al. Development and validation of a measure of birth-related PTSD for fathers and birth partners: the city birth trauma scale (partner version). 2021. Available from: https://www.frontiersin.org/journals/psychology/articles/10.3389/fpsyg.2021.596779/full

42. Baxter J. An exploration of reasons why some women may leave the birth experience with emotional distress. British Journal of Midwifery. 2020;28(1). Available from: <doi:10.12968/bjom.2020.28.1.2442>

43. Fenwick J, Toohill J, Gamble J, Creedy DK, Buist A, Turkstra E, et al. Effects of a midwife psycho-education intervention to reduce childbirth fear on women's birth outcomes and postpartum psychological wellbeing. BMC Pregnancy Childbirth. 2015 Oct 30;15:284. Available from: <doi:10.1186/s12884-015-0721-y>. PMID: 26518597; PMCID: PMC4628230.

44. Dencker A, Nilsson C, Begley C, Jangsten E, Mollberg M, Patel H, et al. Causes and outcomes in studies of fear of childbirth: a systematic review. Women Birth. 2019 Apr;32(2):99–111. Available from: <doi:10.1016/j.wombi.2018.07.004>. Epub 2018 Aug 14. PMID: 30115515.

45. Söderquist J, Wijma B, Thorbert G, Wijma K. Risk factors in pregnancy for post-traumatic stres and depression after childbirth. BJOG An International Journal of Obstetrics and Gynaecology. 2009;116:672–680. Available from: <doi:10.1111/j.1471-0528.2008.02083.x>

46. Cross H, Krahé C, Spilby H, Slade P. Do antenatal preparation and obstetric complications and procedures interact to affect birth experience and postnatal mental health? BMC Pregnancy and Childbirth. 2023;543:1–14. Available from: <doi:10.1186/s12884-023-05846-5>

47. Greenfield M, Jomeen J, Glover V. 'It can't be like last time' – choices made in early pregnancy by women who have previously experienced a traumatic birth. Front Psychol. 2019 Jan 25;10. Available from: <doi:10.3389/fpsyg.2019.00056>

48. Ford E, Ayers S. Stressful events and support during birth: the effect on anxiety,

mood and perceived control. Journal of Anxiety Disorders. 2009;23(2):260–268. Available from: <doi:10.1016/j.janxdis.2008.07.009>

49. Haagen F, Moerbeek M, Olde E, Van Der Hart O, Kleber RJ. PTSD after childbirth: a predictive ethological model for symptom development. Journal of Affective Disorders. 2015;185:135. Available from: <doi:10.1016/j.jad.2015.06.049>

50. Brodrick A, Williamson E. Birth afterthoughts. London: Routledge; 2020. Available from: <doi:10.4324/9781351118422-4>

51. Bastos M, Furuta M, Small R, McKenzie-McHarg K, Bick D. Debriefing interventions for the prevention of psychological trauma in women following childbirth. Cochrane Database of Systematic Reviews. 2015(4):CD007194. Available from: <doi:10.1002/14651858.CD007194.pub2>

52. Birth Trauma Association. Available from: https://birthtraumaassociation.org.uk/#50

53. Yoon S, Kim YK. The role of the oxytocin system in anxiety disorders. Adv Exp Med Biol. 2020;1191:103–120. Available from: <doi:10.1007/978-981-32-9705-0_7>. PMID: 32002925.

54. Corner G, Rasmussen H, Khaled M, Alyssa R, Hannah B, et al. The birth of a story: childbirth experiences, meaning-making and postpartum adjustment. Journal of Family Psychology. 2023 Aug;37(5): 667–679. Available from: <doi:10.1037/fam0001062>

55. Birth Trauma Resolution. Birth trauma resolution practitioner training programme. n.d. [Accessed 9 September 2023]. Available from: www.birthtraumaresolution.com/

56. Ayers S, Eagle A, Waring H. The effects of childbirth-related post-traumatic stress disorder on women and their relationships: a qualitative study. Psychol Health Med. 2006 Nov;11(4):389–398. Available from: <doi:10.1080/13548500600708409>. PMID: 17129916.

57. Bohren MA, Berger BO, Munthe-Kaas H, Tunçalp Ö. Perceptions and experiences of labour companionship: a qualitative evidence synthesis. Cochrane Database Syst Rev. 2019:CD012449. Available from: <doi:10.1002/14651858.CD012449.pub2>

58. Etheridge J, Slade P. 'Nothing's actually happened to me': the experiences of fathers who found childbirth traumatic. BMC Pregnancy and Childbirth. 2017;17:80. Available from: <doi:10.1186/s12884-017-1259-y>

59. Cook N, Ayers S, Horsch A. Maternal posttraumatic stress disorder during the perinatal period and child outcomes: a systematic review. J Affect Disord. 2018 Jan 1;225:18–31. Available from: <doi:10.1016/j.jad.2017.07.045>. Epub 2017 Jul 27. PMID: 28777972.

60. Van Sieleghem S, Danckaerts M, Rieken R, Okkerse JME, de Jonge E, Bramer WM, Lambregtse-van den Berg MP. Childbirth related PTSD and its association with infant outcome: a systematic review. Early Hum Dev. 2022 Nov;174:105667. Available from: <doi:10.1016/j.earlhumdev.2022.105667>. Epub 2022 Sep 16. PMID: 36152399.

61. RCM. Strengthening perinatal mental health. 2023. Available from: www.rcm.org.uk/media-releases/2023/august/midwives-need-the-time-to-care-says-the-rcm-as-it-calls-for-perinatal-mental-health-support/

17

Postpartum psychosis

REINA FISHER-VAN WERKHOVEN

Introduction	247	Summary of midwifery responsibilities	254
Pathophysiology	248	Further reading and resources	254
Clinical features	249	References	255
Follow-up/long-term issues	254		

BOX 17.1: Definitions

Postpartum psychosis (also known as puerperal psychosis or peripartum psychosis)

- Brief psychotic disorder with postpartum onset: if onset of brief psychotic disorder symptoms is during pregnancy or within 4 weeks after birth.[1]
- Psychosis often with mania and/or depressive symptoms in the immediate postnatal period, which can become very severe extremely quickly.[2]
- Mental or behavioural disorders associated with pregnancy, childbirth or the puerperium, with psychotic symptoms:
  A syndrome associated with pregnancy or the puerperium (commencing within about 6 weeks after delivery) that involves significant mental and behavioural features, including delusions, hallucinations, or other psychotic symptoms. Mood symptoms (depressive and/or manic) are also typically present. If the symptoms meet the diagnostic requirements for a specific mental disorder, that diagnosis should also be assigned.[3]

INTRODUCTION

Postpartum psychosis is classified as a severe mental illness[2] and affects 1–2:1,000 births in the UK and globally.[4,5] In the UK, this equates to more than 1,400 women who experience postpartum psychosis each year.[6]

Postpartum psychosis can be characterised as an episode of mood disorder: mania with or without psychotic features or depression with psychosis which occurs soon after birth.[4] It mostly has a sudden onset and a rapid deterioration[7] and presents itself with a 'kaleidoscopic' clinical picture which includes severe mood swings, hallucinations and delusions, confusion, bewilderment and perplexity, interspersed with brief intervals of lucidity.[8,4,7]

To date, there is no universally accepted definition of postpartum psychosis,[4] and the aetiology of this condition remains poorly understood.[9]

Whilst postpartum psychosis is considered a less common perinatal mental health condition, the implications for the woman, the infant and her family are significant,[10,9] and postpartum psychosis is known to be an important contributing factor to maternal suicide, which is still the second direct cause of maternal death within the period of up to one year after birth in the UK.[11]

However, better identification of potential risk factors antenatal and prompt detection and

DOI: 10.4324/9781003382195-17

interventions postnatally can make a difference in the outcomes for women and families,[12] and following the correct treatment, the prognosis of recovery from an initial episode of postpartum psychosis is overall very good,[4] although the process of recovery can be complex and long-lasting effects of postpartum psychosis have been identified.[13]

PATHOPHYSIOLOGY

The pathophysiology of postpartum psychosis remains poorly understood[9] and can best be explained by considering a complex interaction of biological, psychological and social factors.[4]

It is important to exclude other causes for psychosis, known as 'organic' psychoses, which could include sepsis, severe anaemia, alcohol or substance withdrawal, encephalitis, subdural hematomas and right hemisphere dysfunction.[14,15]

There is growing evidence that supports a strong link between postpartum psychosis and bipolar disorder. Women with a history of bipolar disorder are 37.2% more likely to experience postpartum psychosis, and in addition, women with a first onset psychosis or mania in the postpartum period are *sometimes* consequently diagnosed with bipolar disorder.[16]

More than 40% of women who experience postpartum psychosis do not have a history of severe mental illness, but for the remainder, this is a recurrence of a pre-existing psychiatric illness, often a psychotic or mood disorder.[17,4]

An episode of postpartum psychosis can be considered a situation where a woman with an underlying tendency to develop postpartum psychosis now experiences a specific puerperal trigger. Several triggers have been identified.[7]

There is a strong indication that **genetic factors** play a role in the pathophysiology of postpartum psychosis, as is the case with mood disorders in general.[4] This same genetic susceptibility has been identified from family, twin and adoption studies.[13] Evidence shows that 40–50% of women with postpartum psychosis have a first-degree relative with a mood disorder, including bipolar disorder.[7,13] Women with bipolar disorder have a one in four risk of suffering a psychotic episode following birth.[7]

Women with bipolar disorder who have suffered a previous episode of postpartum psychosis or with a family history of postpartum psychosis have a greater than one in two risk of developing postpartum psychosis.[7] Although there is a strong indication for this genetic link, research is still ongoing to identify specific genes that would be indicative of an increased risk of postpartum psychosis.[4]

Certain **obstetric risk factors** have also been identified, such as primiparity, complications during pregnancy and birth, cesarean section, having a female infant and premature birth.[18] Primiparity has the only consistent findings, however, and it is thought that the biological characteristics, such as hormonal and immunological differences associated with a first pregnancy could contribute to this.[19,4] Women themselves have reported obstetric emergencies as contributing to the development of their postpartum psychosis.[20,21] Ngyen et al.,[22] in a recent systematic review, were unable to demonstrate a consistent link between childbirth complications and postpartum psychosis but suggest that these can be considered as one of several culminating factors resulting in first onset postpartum psychosis.

Immune system dysregulation (with increased macrophage activity and a reduced number of T cells) has been found in women with postpartum psychosis and has been suggested as a trigger for the onset of postpartum psychosis. A similar pattern has been found in the aetiology of psychoses not related to childbirth, specifically bipolar disorder. Other immune disorders, such as rheumatoid arthritis and multiple sclerosis, are also typically exacerbated in the postpartum period.[4]

Sleep deprivation, which is known as a trigger for bipolar disorder, has been considered a possible trigger for the onset of postpartum psychosis and could be linked to long labour and a birth at night as risk factors.[23,4] It was found that ongoing sleep deprivation, such as due to nighttime feeding, affected primiparous women more than multiparous women.[23] The disruption of the circadian rhythm could affect neurotransmitters such as dopamine and serotonin, which are known to play a role in mood disorders.[4]

The fact that pregnant women often have come off mood stabilising **medication,** such as lithium, in the preconception period or early pregnancy because of the risk of toxicity to the fetus increases the risk of developing postpartum psychosis following birth.[7] However, there is still the additional effect of pregnancy itself, as research shows that, compared to non-pregnant women who discontinued mood stabilising medication, the risk of psychosis developing at 40–41 weeks after that was greater for those women who had given birth.[24] More recent evidence suggests that particularly where there has been a recent relapse, taking mood stabilising medication in pregnancy does not seem to reduce the incidence of relapse postpartum.[25]

The sudden change in **hormone levels** following birth, especially oestrogen and progesterone, has been hypothesised to contribute to the development of postpartum psychosis, particularly given the sudden onset of postpartum psychosis.[7,9]

This would probably also involve the interaction with other reproductive hormones and neurotransmitters, such as dopamine. Prolactin inhibitors, such as Bromocriptine (a dopamine D2 receptor antagonist), have been shown to potentially increase the risk of psychosis in the postnatal period and should, therefore, no longer be used for lactation suppression.[26] This could also be linked to the fact that sudden cessation of breastfeeding and the resumption of menstrual periods have been suggested to contribute to the development of postpartum psychosis.[9]

There are some case reports of psychosis during pregnancy, after termination of pregnancy, miscarriage or hydatidiform mole pregnancy. Many of these women suffered postpartum psychosis after a subsequent pregnancy that resulted in a term birth.[14]

The main aetiology of postpartum psychosis has mostly been described as being within the biomedical model, without evidence to support the possibility that life events, personality traits, temperament and other psycho-social factors are involved in the development of postpartum psychosis.[4,7,27,28] A small study by Glover et al.[20] exploring women's own experiences of postpartum psychosis indicated that women themselves described stressful events before and during the pregnancy as the path leading to postpartum psychosis, factors which have also been identified as precursors to non-postpartum psychosis. In addition, the perceived lack of support from family and those close to them seemed to be detrimental to their recovery. Consequently, Glover et al.[20] argue that a more holistic, multidimensional understanding of postpartum psychosis may be needed and needs to be explored in further research.

CLINICAL FEATURES

Risk/pre-disposing factors

While the aetiology of postpartum psychosis is complex, and many women who develop postpartum psychosis have no history of psychiatric illness, some features have been identified as a trigger for postpartum psychosis (see Box 17.2).

Pre-conception care

While in 40% of cases, postpartum psychosis occurs in women without a previous history of psychiatric illness, it is important for the remaining 60% to access preconception care to discuss the risk of postpartum psychosis/relapse and what can be done to mitigate this risk.[9,16]

If women are using antipsychotic or mood-stabilising medication such as Valproate or lithium, this should be reviewed by a perinatal psychiatrist with a view to changing to medication that is safe in pregnancy or stopping completely with intensive support from mental health practitioners. It should be noted, however, that girls and women of childbearing potential should not be taking/prescribed Valproate, as recommended by the Medicines and Healthcare products Regulatory Agency (MHRA) safety advice on the use of Valproate[29] due to the

---

BOX 17.2: Possible risk/ pre-disposing factors[7,22,19,21,9]

- Previous episode of postpartum psychosis
- Women with bipolar disorder or other psychotic illnesses
- First-degree relative with bipolar disorder and/or episode of postpartum psychosis
- Primiparous women
- Change in mood stabilising medication such as lithium
- Sleep deprivation and circadian rhythm disruption
- Abrupt cessation of breastfeeding
- Resumption of menstrual periods
- Comorbidities such as anaemia, infection and pre-eclampsia
- Complications in pregnancy and labour

risks of serious congenital malformations and neuro-developmental disorders.[2]

Wesseloo et al.[16] found that the overall relapse rate for women with bipolar disorder was 37.2%. The relapse rate for women with bipolar disorder was, however, found to be significantly higher without the use of lithium during pregnancy (66% vs 23% compared to women who did use lithium during pregnancy). The relapse rate for women with a previous postpartum psychosis was 31%, but it was noted that the relapses in women with previous postpartum psychosis were more severe in nature. The use of prophylactic lithium in the immediate postpartum period was found to be highly effective in preventing a relapse postpartum and avoided the woman needing to use lithium during pregnancy. Taylor et al.[25] identified that the risk of postpartum relapse is increased if there has been a recent relapse in the two years before or during pregnancy. They were not able to demonstrate that women who used medication in the third trimester and immediate postpartum period were not at greater risk of relapse postpartum, although acknowledged that women may have been undertreated due to the pharmacokinetic changes in pregnancy (e.g., increased clearance of medication) and lack of compliance. It is, therefore, important that a risk-benefit analysis should be done with women on an individual basis to determine the best risk-mitigating strategy.[16,25,2]

Signs and symptoms

The International Classification of Diseases (ICD) version 11[3] definition of postpartum psychosis indicates the multiple signs and symptoms with which the disorder can present. While there is no universal definition of postpartum psychosis, "the term generally refers to a manic, mixed, or major depressive episode with psychotic features, a psychotic disorder not otherwise specified, and a brief psychotic disorder within four weeks postpartum."[23,p 2;30]

The majority of cases of postpartum psychosis occur within the first two weeks after birth, with 50% of cases occurring in the first three days, while 22% of onsets occur on day one.[31,32] Other studies describe an average onset at day eight postpartum; however, prodromal symptoms were seen at an earlier stage.[33] Brockington[34] describes a few cases of onset immediately before or during labour.

Postpartum psychosis is typically characterised by a sudden onset and a rapid deterioration.[7]

Clinical features that can be observed in women experiencing postpartum psychosis include mood symptoms: these can be signs of elation, hyperactivity, talking incessantly but incoherently and mania, but also apathy and – severe – depression. There can be a variety of psychotic phenomena, including hallucinations and delusions (see Box 17.3), and a general disturbance of consciousness, presented as confusion, bewilderment or perplexity, and judgment and decision-making capacity are impaired.[7,12,8] The clinical picture can be very changeable and fluctuating – described as 'kaleidoscopic' – and can be interspersed with moments of lucidity.[8]

Kamperman et al.,[36] in their study of 130 women admitted to a Mother and Baby Unit (MBU) for postpartum psychosis, found that irritability was the most common symptom (73%), closely followed by abnormal thought content (72%) and anxiety (71%).

Delusions have been described as 'persecutory,' where women believe that people may harm them or their baby, or 'grandiose,' where women feel that they or their baby are chosen or possess special gifts,[12] which could lead to risk-taking behaviour.

Lewis, Blake and Seneviratne[15] describe the Delusional Misidentification Syndrome (DSM), sometimes seen in postpartum psychosis delusions: this could include the perception that a familiar person or object has been replaced by a duplicate or impostor (Capgras syndrome) or strangers are believed to be familiar persons in disguise (Fregoli syndrome). This often includes those emotionally close, such as the partner or infant. DSM often results in hostility towards the person who has

---

BOX 17.3: Examples of psychotic phenomena[12,35]

Hallucinations: perceptual abnormalities – a person perceives to see, hear, smell, taste or feel something that does not exist in reality

Delusions: firmly held ideas that are not based on reason or evidence and not in keeping with the woman's usual cultural and religious concepts

been the object of misidentification and could, therefore, disrupt the bonding between the woman and the child, which, in turn, could result in the risk of neglect, violence or infanticide. Friedman et al.,[37] reviewing a case series of 39 women, a third of which committed infanticide, found that the majority of these women were experiencing hallucinations, hearing voices commanding them to kill their children and/or had delusions, which included beliefs that the child was possessed by the devil or that something terrible would happen to the child and that the killing was seen as an altruistic act. Infanticide can be part of an extended suicide. Infanticide was found to be five-fold higher in women who had psychosis with depression rather than psychosis alone (without depression).[32,9]

Suicide attempts and suicidal ideation, the process of contemplating or wishing to commit suicide, are common in women who experience postpartum psychosis, specifically among those with depression.[9] Brockington[32] found that suicide is not common in the acute stage of postpartum psychosis but is more likely to occur during the final quarter of the first year postpartum. This is significant in the context that suicide is still the main cause of maternal death during the first year postpartum.[10] The recent Enquiries into Maternal Deaths (MBRRACE reports) have shown that maternal suicides, including from mental health causes, are lowest in the first six weeks postpartum and most common between six weeks and nine months.[38,11] These reports also show that violent deaths are common in women who commit suicide, with hanging the most common mode of death (52%), followed by overdose (16%) and fall from height (16%).[11] Violent mode of death indicates that these women had a clear intent to commit suicide,[38] and it is, therefore, important that midwives and other health care providers ask women about suicidal ideation, including harming or killing their children.[36] When women express any suicidal thoughts, these should be taken seriously, and appropriate follow-up by mental health services should be initiated.[38]

In the Diagnostic and Statistical Manual of Mental Disorders 5 (DSM-5),[1] postpartum psychosis is not recognised as a distinct disorder but is classified under general mania or psychotic depression, but with the postpartum onset specifier. As is evident from the different definitions used to describe postpartum psychosis,[1,2,3]

criteria for a diagnosis of postpartum psychosis lack clarity regarding the number of symptoms required to be diagnosed with postpartum psychosis, and neither is the duration of the symptoms clearly specified. Because of this lack of clarity, it is suggested that the actual number of women experiencing postpartum psychosis may be underreported.[9]

Antenatal screening and specific care

Screening for risk factors is an important aspect of the booking appointment; however, it is important to note that 40% of women who develop postpartum psychosis do not have known risk factors.[4] At the booking appointment, the midwife should ask depression identification questions and questions to identify anxiety according to the NICE guideline[2] (see Box 17.4).

The woman should be asked about any past or present severe mental illness (SMI) or treatment by specialist mental health services (including in-patient care) as part of the medical history at booking.[2] This is important because, due to the cyclic nature of bipolar disorder and the generally good recovery from postpartum psychosis, women at risk are often well at the time of booking.[7] This should also include a family history of severe mental illness, as it is known that having a first-degree female relative with bipolar disorder and/or postpartum psychosis is a significant risk factor for the development of postpartum psychosis.[7,9] It is important that these questions are asked

---

BOX 17.4: Questions to identify depression/anxiety[2, p.32]

- "During the past month, have you often been bothered by feeling down, depressed or hopeless?
- "During the past month, have you often been bothered by having little interest or pleasure in doing things?
- "Over the last 2 weeks, how often have you been bothered by feeling nervous, anxious or on edge?
- "Over the last 2 weeks, how often have you been bothered by not being able to stop or control worrying?"

in a sensitive manner, as it is known that women are reluctant to disclose mental health illness due to a fear of stigmatisation and the fear of children being taken into care.[39] It is also important that these questions, as well as a general assessment of the woman's well-being, are repeated throughout pregnancy and in the postnatal period.[2]

The use of an interpreter has been found to be essential in getting clearer responses to these questions when the woman does not speak English.[38]

It has been identified that effective communication between healthcare professionals, including GP and mental health practitioners and maternity services, where there is a previous history or family history of severe mental illness, has contributed to much better outcomes.[39,38]

Where a current or previous SMI has been identified, the woman should be referred to a secondary mental health service. The involvement of specialist perinatal mental health (PMH) services would be preferred.[2]

In the case of current SMI, such as bipolar disorder, medication should be reviewed by a perinatal psychiatrist and, where possible, changed to ones that are safe in pregnancy or stopped with intensive support from mental health professionals.[2] If the woman needs to continue with lithium because no other effective medication could be identified, it is important that this is monitored carefully. This should include checking plasma levels every four weeks and weekly from 36 weeks and adjusting the dose if required to ensure the levels stay within the woman's therapeutic range. The woman should be made aware that there is a risk of fetal heart malformations if lithium is taken in the first trimester (although the size of the risk is uncertain) and that high lithium levels in breastmilk could pose a risk of toxicity for the baby.[2]

The specialist perinatal mental health team, together with the woman and, if possible, her partner and family, should develop a detailed care plan. This should set out the care for the antenatal, intra-partum and postpartum periods. The plan needs to include details of medication, appointments with PMH services and names and contact details of key professionals. This should be available in the notes so that all professionals involved can have access to it, and a copy should be given to the woman herself.[2] It is essential that this plan is carefully followed throughout pregnancy, labour and the postnatal period.

Continuity of care, coordinated by the Specialist Perinatal Mental Health midwife and provided by vulnerable women team midwives and mental health specialists, is known to contribute to better outcomes.[40,41]

Women can be asked to complete a mood diary to monitor changes in mood and sleep, and information from the partner or a family member may be used alongside this to identify any changes that may indicate psychosis.[9] Some studies suggest that there may be prepartum indications of postpartum psychosis: this could present itself in the form of euphoria, reduced sleep requirements or inability to sleep and feeling active or energetic and over-talkative; these are symptoms that will then worsen postpartum.[34]

Care during labour

During labour, it is important to provide one-to-one midwifery care. Research suggests that women's experiences with poor maternity care, such as delays being attended to in labour, midwives not being aware of their mental health history and a stressful hospital environment, contributed to the development of postpartum psychosis.[21] It is important to avoid exhaustion and sleep deprivation as much as possible. Women have reported the importance of having their partner stay with them in hospital when they felt they needed support.[21]

If women have continued with lithium during pregnancy, a hospital birth is advised due to the risk of neonatal lithium toxicity and the need for regular lithium level monitoring during labour.[42] Lithium should be stopped during labour; lithium levels should be monitored during labour and a careful fluid balance should be maintained to avoid dehydration and, thereby, lithium toxicity.[2]

It is important for the midwife and partner to monitor for early indications of postpartum psychosis, as there have been incidences where these became apparent during labour.[34]

Postnatal care

Avoidance of possible triggers for postpartum psychosis needs to continue in the postnatal period. Sleep deprivation should be avoided by ensuring a quiet room and support with feeding and changing the baby during the night. The partner can be instructed and supported to take an active role in the baby's care[39] to facilitate this.

Continued observation of early signs and symptoms of postpartum psychosis needs to be maintained following the birth. Any indication of agitation, incessant talkativeness, confusion, elation or depression needs to be escalated to the specialist perinatal mental health team for immediate assessment. Assessment should take place within four hours of referral,[2] and clear pathways for referral should be in place for both hospital and community settings. The safety of the woman and infant is paramount,[12] and women requiring in-patient psychiatric care should be admitted to a Mother and Baby Unit.[39,2,14]

It is important that midwives are aware of the possibility of a rapidly changing clinical picture.[7] Women have reported that staff at the maternity unit were not aware of their pre-existing mental health diagnosis and the possibility of a rapidly deteriorating condition.[21]

From reviewing maternal morbidity and mortality due to postpartum psychosis, clear red and amber flags have been identified in the 2015 and 2016 MBRRACE-UK Reports[38,43] to improve timely recognition of the risk factors for, and signs and symptoms of, postpartum psychosis and to ensure appropriate referral takes place (see Boxes 17.5 and 17.6).

Following birth, lithium will need to be continued at the pre-pregnancy dose.[14] Women need to

---

BOX 17.5: MBRRACE-UK red flags for severe maternal illness[38, p. 22]

"The following are 'red flag' signs for severe maternal illness and require urgent senior psychiatric assessment:

- "Recent significant change in mental state or emergence of new symptoms,
- "New thoughts or acts of violent self-harm,
- "New and persistent expressions of incompetency as a mother or estrangement from the infant.

"Admission to a mother and baby unit should always be considered where a woman has any of the following:

- "rapidly changing mental state,
- "suicidal ideation (particularly of a violent nature),
- "pervasive guilt or hopelessness,
- "significant estrangement from the infant,
- "new or persistent beliefs of inadequacy as a mother,
- "evidence of psychosis."

BOX 17.6: MBRRACE-UK amber flags to prompt heightened awareness of change in mental state[43, p. 42]

- "Women with any past history of psychotic disorder, even where not diagnosed as postpartum psychosis or bipolar disorder, should be regarded as at elevated risk in future postpartum periods and should be referred to mental health services in pregnancy to receive an individualised assessment of risk and development of a postpartum plan.
- "Women with a family history of postpartum major mental illness should be closely monitored by maternity and primary care services in late pregnancy and the early postpartum

period. Where they themselves are currently unwell in pregnancy or have had previous postpartum mood destabilisation, they should be referred to mental health services as soon as possible in pregnancy to receive an individualised assessment of risk and development of a management plan

"The personal and familial pattern of occurrence and re-occurrence of postpartum mood disorder should inform risk minimisation strategies."

be aware that the dose of lithium may be high in breastmilk, with the potential risk of toxicity for the baby, and a conversation should be had with women on the risks and benefits of breastfeeding while taking lithium.[44] Although most commonly, breastfeeding is discouraged, there have been case reports of women successfully breastfeeding while taking lithium with careful monitoring of neonatal lithium levels.[44] The infant of a woman having taken any psychotropic medication will need to be reviewed by the neonatologist and observed for signs of withdrawal or toxicity.[44] Infants of women who have taken lithium during pregnancy will need a lithium level assessed soon after birth.[41]

Prior to discharge from midwifery care, clear communication with the GP, Health Visitor and specialist perinatal mental health service need to ensure that a comprehensive care plan is in place. Safeguarding concerns need to be addressed, although it is rare that babies are removed from maternal care due to mental health illness. This will only occur where, even with support, the woman and her family are unable to provide the care that the infant needs or to protect the infant from harm.[39]

FOLLOW-UP/LONG-TERM ISSUES

Early recognition and appropriate treatment are known to contribute to a good prognosis for the recovery of postpartum psychosis,[13,21] although long-term disability has been described.

Treatment commonly includes a combination of psychotherapy and medication, such as lithium, benzodiazepines and antipsychotics, although the complex presentation of postpartum psychosis can make it difficult to find the right treatment.[9]

It is known that women with postpartum psychosis respond well to Electroconvulsive therapy, and only a few transient side effects for the women and no adverse effects on breastfed infants have been described.[14]

Qualitative studies into women's experiences of postpartum psychosis and recovery from postpartum psychosis have demonstrated that postpartum psychosis has a significant impact on women and their partners and that the recovery is a complex process.[13,20,45,21] Women described a sense of loss and disruption to many aspects of their lives, guilt, shame, fear of stigma, a sense of fear and hopelessness, difficulty in bonding with the baby and mixed emotions regarding their relationship with family.[13,45] Women also reported concerns about their partners not receiving support.[21] Holford et al.,[10] in a study exploring the impact of postpartum psychosis on partners, described that they also experience loss and trauma and can feel guilt or self-blame while facing the impact on the couple's relationship and the challenge of having to take on multiple roles in this situation.

Access to peer support groups has been found helpful by both women and their partners in the long-term recovery process of postpartum psychosis.[13]

SUMMARY OF MIDWIFERY RESPONSIBILITIES

- Screen for anxiety, depression and serious mental health illness at booking and throughout pregnancy.
- Referral to specialist PMH team.
- Awareness of women's mental health history when providing care.
- Avoidance of postpartum psychosis triggers during labour and the postpartum period.
- Monitor for signs and symptoms of postpartum psychosis.
- Urgent escalation to specialist PMH team in case of Red Flags for Severe Mental Illness.
- Follow guidance on the use of lithium.
- Undertake neonatal observation following the use of lithium or other psychotropic medication.
- Support the partner and family.
- Clear communication with GP, Health Visitor and Mental Health specialist to ensure continuity of care.

FURTHER READING AND RESOURCES

Action on Postpartum Psychosis (APP). Available from: www.apostpartum psychosis-network. org/about-us/
    A charity for women and families affected by postpartum psychosis; also provides training for professionals.
Maternal Mental Health Alliance (MMHA). Available from: https://maternalmentalhealthalliance.org/
    A UK-wide charity providing support to parents and guidance to professionals to ensure

women and families receive the best possible perinatal mental health care.

National Institute for Health and Care Excellence (NICE). Antenatal and postnatal mental health: clinical management and service guidance, CG 12. 2014. Available from: www.nice.org.uk/guidance/cg192

Royal College of Midwives (RCM). Caring for women with mental health problems. 2015. Available from: www.rcm.org.uk/publications/

Royal College of Psychiatrists information on Postpartum Psychosis for women and their families. available from: www.rcpsych.ac.uk/mental-health/mental-illnesses-and-mental-health-problems/postpartum-psychosis

REFERENCES

1. American Psychiatric Association (APA). Diagnostic and statistical manual of mental disorders. Revised 5th ed. (DSM-V-Text Revision 2022). Arlington VA: APA Publishing; 2013.

2. National Institute for Health and Care Excellence (NICE). Antenatal and postnatal mental health: clinical management and service guidance, CG 12. 2014, last updated 2020. [Accessed 7 August 2023]. Available from: www.nice.org.uk/guidance/cg192

3. World Health Organization (WHO). International classification of diseases, eleventh revision-version 01/2023 (ICD-11). 2019. Available from: www.icd.who.int/browse11

4. Perry A, Gordon-Smith K, Jones L, Jones I. Phenomenology, epidemiology and aetiology of postpartum psychosis: a review. Brain Sciences. 2021;11(47). Available from: <doi:10.3390/brainsci11010047>

5. VanderKruik R, Barreix M, Chou D, Allen T, Sau L, Cohen LS, On behalf of the Maternal Morbidity Working Group. The global prevalence of postpartum psychosis: a systematic review. BMC Psychiatry. 2017;17(272). Available from: <doi:10.1186/s12888-017-1427-7>

6. Action on Postpartum Psychosis. What we do. n.d. [Accessed 25 August 2023]. Available from: www.app-network.org/about-us/what-we-do/

7. Di Florio A, Smith S, Jones I. Postpartum psychosis. The Obstetrician & Gynaecologist. 2013:145–150. Available from: <doi:10.1111/tog.12041>

8. Klompenhouwer JL, van Hulst AM, Tulen JH, Jacobs ML, Jacobs BC, Segers F. The clinical features of postpartum psychosis. European Psychiatry. 1995;10:355–367. Available from: <doi:10.1016/0924-9338(96)80337-3>

9. Sharma V, Mazmanian D, Palagini L, Bramante A. Postpartum psychosis: revisting the phenomenology, nosology and treatment. Journal of Affective Disorders Reports. 2022;10. Available from: <doi:10.1016/j.adr.2022.100378>

10. Holford N, Channon S, Heron J, Jones I. The impact of postpartum psychosis on partners. BMC Pregnancy and Childbirth. 2018;18(414). Available from: <doi:10.1186/s12884-018-2055-z>

11. Cairns A, Kenyon S, Pathel R, Bunch K, Knight M, On Behalf of the MBRRACE-UK Mental Health Chapter-Writing Group. Improving mental health care and care for women with multiple adversity. In: Knight M, Bunch K, Patel R, Shakespeare J, Kotnis R, Kenyon S, Kurinczuk JJ, On Behalf of MBRRACE-UK, editors. Saving Lives, Improving Mothers' Care Core Report – Lessons learned to inform maternity care from the UK and Ireland Confidential Enquiries into Maternal Deaths and Morbidity 2018–20. Oxford: National Perinatal Epidemiology Unit, University of Oxford; 2022. p. 34–44.

12. Berrisford G, Lambert A, Heron J. Understanding postpartum psychosis. Community Practitioner. 2015:23. PMID:26364332.

13. McGrath L, Peters S, Wieck A, Wittkowski A. The process of recovery in women who experienced psychosis following childbirth. BioMed Central Psychiatry. 2013;13(341). Available from: <doi:10.1186/1471-244X-13-341>

14. Henshaw C, Cox J, Barton J. Modern management of perinatal psychiatric disorders. 2nd ed. Cambridge: Cambridge University Press; 2017.

15. Lewis G, Blake L, Seneviratne G. Delusional misidentification syndromes in postpartum psychosis: a systematic review.

Psychopathology. 2023;56:285–294. Available from: <doi:10.1159/000526129>

16. Wesseloo R, Kamperman AM, Munk-Olsen T, Pop VJM, Kushner SA, Bergink V. Risk of postpartum relapse in bipolar disorder and postpartum psychosis: a systematic review and meta-analysis. American Journal of Psychiatry. 2016;173(2):117–127. Available from: <doi:10.1176/appi.ajp.2015.15010124>

17. Langan Martin J, McLean G, Cantwell R, Smith DJ. Admission to psychiatric hospital in the early and late postpartum periods: Scottish national linkage study. BMJ Open. 2016;6. Available from: <doi:10.1136/bmjopen-2015008758>

18. Di Florio A, Jones L, Forty L, Gordon-Smith K, Robertson Blackmore E, Heron J, et al. Mood disorders and parity – a clue to the aetiology of the postpartum trigger. Journal of Affective Disorders. 2014;152–154: 334–339. Available from: <doi:10.1016/j.jad.2013.09.034>

19. Robertson Blackmore E, Jones I, Doshi M, Haque S, Holder R, Brockington I, Craddock N. Obstetric variables associated with bipolar affective puerperal psychosis. British Journal of Psychiatry. 2006;188:32–36. Available from: <doi:10.1192/bjp.188.1.32>

20. Glover L, Jomeen J, Urquhart T, Martin CR. Puerperal psychosis – a qualitative study of women's experiences. Journal of Reproductive and Infant Psychology. 2014;32(3):254–269. Available from: <doi:10.1080/02646838.2014.883597>

21. Roxburgh E, Morant N, Dolman C, Johnson S, Tayler BL. Experiences of mental health care among women treated for postpartum psychosis in England: a qualitative study. Community Mental Health Journal. 2023;59:243–252. Available from: <doi:10.1007/s10597-022-01002-z>

22. Nguyen K, Mukona LT, Nalbandyan L, Yar N, St. Fler G, Mukona L, et al. Peripartum complications as risk factors for postpartum psychosis: a systemic review. Cureus. 2022;14(9):1–7. Available from: <doi:10.7759/cureus.29224>

23. Sharma V, Smith A, Khan M. The relationship between duration of labour, time of delivery, and puerperal psychosis. Journal of Affective Disorders. 2004;83:215–220.

Available from: <doi:10.1016/j.jad.2004.04.014>

24. Viguera AC, Nonacs R, Cohen LS, Tondo L, Murray A, Baldessarini RJ. Risk of recurrence of bipolar disorder in pregnant and nonpregnant women after discontinuing lithium maintenance. Am J Psychiatry. 2000;157:179–184. Available from: <doi:10.1176/appi.ajp.157.2.179>

25. Taylor CL, Stewart RJ, Howard LM. Relapse in the first three months postpartum in women with history of serious mental illness. Schizophrenia Research. 2019;204: 46–54. Available from: <doi:10.1016/j.schres.2018.07.037>

26. Snellen M, Power J, Blankley G, Galbally M. Pharmacological lactation suppression with D 2 receptor agonists and risk of postpartum psychosis: a systematic review. R Aust NZ J Obstet Gynaecol. 2016:1–5. Available from: <doi:10.1111/ajo.12479>

27. Perry A, Gordon-Smith K, Di Florio A, Forty L, Craddock N, Jones, L, et al. Adverse childhood events and postpartum psychosis in bipolar disorder. Journal of Affective Disorders. 2016;205:69–72. Available from: <doi:10.1016/j.jad.2016.06.061>

28. Perry A, Gordon-Smith K, Webb I, Fone E, Di Florio A, Craddock N, et al. Postpartum psychosis in bipolar disorder: no evidence of association with personality traits, cognitive style or affective temperaments. BMC Psychiatry. 2019;19(395):1–10. Available from: <doi:10.1186/s12888-019-2392-0>

29. Medicines & Healthcare products Regulatory Agency (MHRA). Information on the risks of valproate use in girls (of any age) and women of childbearing potential (Epilim, Depakote, Convulex, Episenta, Epival, Kentlim, Orlept, Sodium Valproate, Syonell, Valpal, Belvo & Dyzantil). 2021. Available from: www.gov.uk/guidance/valproate-use-by-women-and-girls

30. Bergink V, Bouvy PF, Vervoort JRS, Koorengevel KM, Steegers EAP, Kushner SA. Prevention of postpartum psychosis and mania in women at high risk. American Journal of Psychiatry. 2012;169:609–615. Available from: <doi:10.1176/appi.ajp.2012.11071047>

31. Heron J, McGuinness, M, Robertson Blackmore E, Craddock N, Jones I. No 'latent

period' in the onset of bipolar affective puerperal psychosis. Archives of Women's Mental Health. 2007;10:79–81. Available from: <doi:10.1007/s00737-007-0174-z>

32. Brockington I. Suicide and filicide in post-partum psychosis. Archives of Women's Mental Health. 2017a;20:63–69. Available from: <doi:10.1007/s00737-016-0675-8>

33. Bergink V, Lambregtse-van den Berg MP, Koorengevel KM, Kupka R, Kushner SA. First onset psychosis occurring in the post-partum period: a prospective cohort study. Journal of Clinical Psychiatry. 2011;72:1531–1537. Available from: <doi:10.4088/JCP.10m06648>

34. Brockington I. Some unusual forms of early onset postpartum psychosis. Archives of Women's Mental Health. 2017b;20:71–76. Available from: <doi:10.1007/s00737-016-0676-7>

35. Klimowicz A, Best E. Severe perinatal mental health difficulties. In: Gellhorn S, editor. Postnatal depression and maternal mental health. Hove: Pavilion Publishing and Media Ltd.; 2016.

36. Kamperman A, Veldman-Hoek M, Wesseloo R, Robertson-Blackmore E, Bergink V. Phenotypical characteristics of postpartum psychosis: a clinical cohort study. Bipolar Disorders. 2017;19(6):450–457. Available from: <doi:10.1111/bdi.12523>

37. Friedman SH, McCue Horwitz S, Resnick PJ. Child murder by mothers: a critical analysis of the current state of knowledge and a research agenda. Am J Psychiatry. 2005;162(9):1578–1587. Available from: <doi:10.1176/appi.ajp.162.9.1578>

38. Cantwell R, Knight M, Oates M, Shakespeare J, On Behalf of the MBRRACE-UK Mental Health Chapter Writing Group. Lessons on maternal mental health. In: Knight M, Tuffnell D, Kenyon S, Shakespeare J, Gray R, Kurinczuk JJ, On Behalf of MBRRACE-UK, editors. Saving lives, improving mothers' care – surveillance of maternal deaths in the UK 2011–13 and lessons learned to inform maternity care from the UK and Ireland confidential enquiries into maternal deaths and morbidity 2009–13. Oxford: National Perinatal Epidemiology Unit, University of Oxford; 2015. p. 22–41.

39. Hogg S. Prevention in mind: all babies count: spotlight on perinatal mental health. 2013. Available from: learning.nspcc.org.uk/services-children-families/pregnancy-in-mind

40. Maternal Mental Health Alliance (MMHA), National Society of the Prevention of Cruelty to Children (NSPCC), Royal College of Midwives (RCM). Specialist mental health midwives – what they do and why they matter? 2015. Available from: maternalmentalhealthalliance.org/projects/specialist-maternal-mental-health-midwives/

41. Royal College of Midwives (RCM). Caring for women with mental health problems. 2015. Available from: www.rcm.org.uk/publications/

42. UK Teratology Information Service (UKTIS). Use of Lithium in pregnancy. 2022. [Accessed 5 August 2023]. Available from: www.uktis.org/monographs/use-of-lithium-in-pregnancy/#:~:text=National%20Institute%20for%20Health%20and,and%20then%20weekly%20until%20delivery

43. Cantwell R, Gray R, Knight M, On Behalf of the MBRRACE-UK Psychosis Chapter-Writing Group. Caring for women with psychosis. In: Knight M, Nair M, Tuffnell D, Shakespeare J, Kenyon S, Kurinczuk JJ, On Behalf of MBRRACE-UK, editors. Saving lives, improving mothers' care – lessons learned to inform maternity care from the UK and Ireland confidential enquiries into maternal deaths and morbidity 2013–15. Oxford: National Perinatal Epidemiology Unit, University of Oxford; 2017. p. 37–49.

44. McAllister-Williams RH, Baldwin DS, Cantwell R, Easter A, Gilvarry E, Glover V, et al. British association for psychopharmacology consensus guidance on the use of psychotropic medication preconception, in pregnancy and postpartum 2017. J Psychopharmacol. 2017:1–34. Available from: <doi:10.1177/0269881117699361>

45. Forde R, Peters S, Wittkowski A. Recovery of postpartum psychosis: a systematic review and metasynthesis of women's and families' experiences. Arch Women's Ment Health. 2020:1–16. Available from: <doi:10.1007s00737-020-01025-z>

Index

Note: Page numbers in *italic* indicate a figure on the corresponding page; page numbers in **bold** indicate a table.

ABCDE approach 38, 225
abdominal pain 223–224
abdominal palpation 57, 125–127, 170
abnormal placentation 168
ABUO *see* antepartum bleeding of unknown origin
accountability 3, 21–*22*
ACR *see* albumin:creatinine ratio (ACR)
action on pre-eclampsia (apec) 104
acute coronary syndrome 83
acute fatty liver of pregnancy (AFLP): antenatal care 118; care in labour 119; clinical features of 118–119; complications 119; definition 117; diagnosis of 118; follow-up/long-term issues 119; midwifery responsibilities 119–120; overview 117; pathophysiology of 117–118; postnatal care 119; preconception care 117; risk factors 117; signs and symptoms of 118; Swansea criteria for diagnosis 118; *see also* eclampsia; HELLP syndrome; pre-eclampsia; severe pre-eclampsia
acute kidney injury 70
acute respiratory distress syndrome (ARDS) 224–225
AD *see* aortic dissection (AD)
advanced life support in obstetrics 38–40; defibrillation 36, 38;

drugs 40, **40**; fluid replacement 40; *see also* maternal resuscitation
AEDs *see* automated external defibrillators
AES *see* anti-embolic stockings
AFE *see* amniotic fluid embolism (AFE)
AFLP *see* acute fatty liver of pregnancy
albumin:creatinine ratio (ACR) 108
amniotic fluid embolism (AFE): care for 198–199; clinical features of 196–198; deaths from 195; definition 194, 197; drugs 199; follow-up/long-term issues 200; midwifery responsibilities 200; overview 194–195; pathophysiology of 195–196; potential investigations 199; risk factors 196; signs and symptoms of 196–198; treatment aims 198; tumultuous labour 196
amniotomy 130
anaemia 70, 183–184
anaphylactoid syndrome of pregnancy *see* amniotic fluid embolism (AFE)
anaphylaxis 225–226
antenatal thromboprophylaxis with LMWH 93, 94
antepartum bleeding of unknown origin (ABUO) 57
antepartum haemorrhage (APH): blood tests 69; care in hospital

setting 67–68; care prior to hospital admission 67; causes of **57**; definitions 56, **67**; fetal/baby outcomes 70; follow-up/long-term issues 70; immediate care of 68–69; maternal outcomes 69–70; midwifery responsibilities 71; older maternal age 60; overview 57; recurrence 70; risk and predisposing factors for 57, **58**; team members for managing 68; unclassified bleeding 57; *see also* placental abruption; placenta praevia; Primary postpartum haemorrhage (Primary PPH)
anticoagulation treatment: education, advice and support 98–99; follow-up/long-term issues 99; labour care 97; low molecular weight heparin 96, 97; midwifery responsibilities 99; postnatal care 98; unfractionated (standard) heparin 97; warfarin 97; *see also* thromboembolism
anti-embolic stockings (AES) 92–93
aortal compression *35*
aortic dissection (AD) 84
APEC *see* action on pre-eclampsia (APEC)
APH *see* antepartum haemorrhage (APH)
appendicitis 226

ARDS *see* acute respiratory distress syndrome (ARDS)
asthma 226–227
automated external defibrillators (AEDs) 39–40

Bandl's ring 170; *see also* Uterine rupture
basic life support 36–39; advanced life support 38–40; hand position for maternal chest compression *38*; resuscitation algorithm *37*; sequence of events 36–39; *see also* maternal resuscitation
bimanual compression 188, 189, *189*
birth trauma 235, 236; *see also* post-traumatic stress disorder (PTSD)
Black Maternity Experience Survey 26
blood gas levels **36**
blood pH levels 35
blood pressure 34–35, 103, 107–108, 119
bohr effect 44
Bolam test 24, 25
Bracht manoeuvre *132*
breech: abdominal examination 127; alternative and complementary therapies 128–129; antenatal diagnosis 127; care during labour 130–131; care for 127–133; to cephalic presentation 127–128; classification of *125*; clinical features of 126–127; complications 133; ECV 125, 127–128; emergency extraction 132; historical context 125–126; incidence of 125; Løvset's manoeuvre 131; manoeuvres for arms 131–132; manoeuvres for head 132; MSV 132; overview 125; pathophysiology of 126; posture and positioning 129; risk factors 126; undiagnosed 129–130; vaginal breech delivery 130, 133; vaginal examination 129, 130; *see also* malpresentation

Breech Trial 126
brow presentation 136–137; *see also* malpresentation

caesarean section: breech presentation 125; classical (longitudinal) incision 167; emergency 41–42; and uterine rupture 166–167; and venous thromboembolism 92
carboprost 188
cardiac arrest, maternal 33; drugs **40**; modifications 41–43; numbers of 42; survival rates 36, 42; *see also* maternal resuscitation
cardiac compressions, newborn 50–51
cardiac disease: actions with suspected conditions 80; blood tests 81; changes to cardiovascular systems in labour and postnatal period 77–78; changes to cardiovascular systems in pregnancy 77; clinical features of 78–80; conditions complicating pregnancy 83–84; initial care 80; labour 80; long-term issues 83–84; midwifery responsibilities 81, 84; overview 76–77; pathophysiology of 77–78; postnatal care 82–83; preconception care 80; risk factors 78; signs and symptoms of 78, **79**; sinus rhythm, normal *82*
cardiac failure 83
cardiac valve compromise 84
Care Quality Commission (CQC) 20
case law 19
CCT *see* controlled cord traction (CCT)
cell salvage 188–189
cerebral venous thrombosis (cvt) 87, 94
cerebrovascular accident 227
chest compressions *38*, 39
chest pain 79, 223
childbed fever *see* puerperal sepsis

chronic inversion 172
classical (longitudinal) incision 167
Clinical Negligence Scheme for Trusts (CNST) 22
CNST *see* Clinical Negligence Scheme for Trusts (CNST)
Code, The *see* NMC Code
Compassion in Practice 9
complete rupture 165, 166
compound presentation 135–136
compression stockings 92–93
compulsive status epilepticus 228
concealed haemorrhage 59
consent, informed 23–26
controlled cord traction (CCT) 173
cord, clamping and cutting 45–46
cord presentation 143
cord prolapse: care for 145; clinical features of 144–145; definition 143; diagnosis of 144–145; filling the bladder after 145; incidence of 143; management 145–147, *146*, *147*, **148**; midwifery responsibilities 149; mode of birth 147–148; outcome/follow-up 148; overview 143–144; pathophysiology of 144; professional considerations 149; risk factors **144**
couvelaire uterus 59
COVID-19 43; care for 211–213; clinical features of 210–211; definition 209; deteriorating maternal illness 211; drugs 213; incidence of 209; investigations for 212; labour care 212–213; MDT involvement 211; overview 209–210; pathophysiology of 210; postnatal care 213; prevention 210; respiratory function 211; risk factors 210; vaccination 210
CQC *see* Care Quality Commission (CQC)
culture, positive 6–7
CVT *see* cerebral venous thrombosis (CVT)
cytokines 210

Data Protection Act 9
deep vein thrombosis (DVT): anticoagulation treatment

96–97; definition 87; diagnosis of 94–95; follow-up/long-term issues 99; medical and midwifery measures 92; midwifery responsibilities 99; treatment of 95

defibrillation 36, 38

Delusional Misidentification Syndrome (DSM) 250

delusions 250

derealisation 238

diabetic ketoacidosis (DKA) 227

Diagnostic and Statistical Manual of Mental Disorders (DSM) 235, 239, 251

DIC see Disseminated intravascular coagulation (DIC)

disseminated intravascular coagulation (DIC) 69, 191, 212

dissociation 238

DKA see diabetic ketoacidosis (DKA)

drugs: for amniotic fluid embolism 199; for cardiac arrest **40**; for COVID-19 213; for newborn resuscitation 51, **52**; and postpartum psychosis risk 248–249; for primary postpartum haemorrhage 184, 187, 188

DSM see Delusional Misidentification Syndrome (DSM); Diagnostic and Statistical Manual of Mental Disorders (DSM)

Duty of care 3, 22–23

DVT see Deep vein thrombosis (DVT)

eclampsia: care for women with magnesium sulphate infusion 114; definition 113; immediate care 113, 114; ongoing care 113–115; overview 113; pathophysiology of 113; see also acute fatty liver of pregnancy (AFLP); HELLP syndrome; Pre-eclampsia; Severe pre-eclampsia

ectopic pregnancy 228

ECV see external cephalic version (ECV)

EFT see Emotional Freedom Technique (EFT)

emergency care 26–27

Emotional Freedom Technique (EFT) 241

E-P-A see European Pathway Association (E-P-A)

epilepsy 228–229

equality act 20

European Pathway Association (E-P-A) 8

external cephalic version (ECV) 125; contraindications 127; description of 128; risks associated with 128

face presentation 137–138; see also malpresentation

FBC see Full blood count (FBC)

fetal adaptations in utero **45**

fetal hypoxia 70

fetal physiology 44–45

fetus, rights of 28

fibroids 229

flu see influenza (flu)

fluid replacement 40

four H's 34

four T's 34, 182

framing effect 27

fulminating pre-eclampsia 103

GAS see Group A betahaemolytic streptococcus

gas device, pressurised 46

GCS see graduated compression stockings (GCS)

graduated compression stockings (GCS) 93

Group A betahaemolytic streptococcus 205

hallucinations 250

Hannah Trial 126

HCPC see Health and Care Professions Council (HCPC)

Health and Care Professions Council (HCPC) 5

healthcare organisations: accountability and duty of care 3; Being Open Framework 9; care bundles 8; care pathways 8; communication 8–9; Compassion in Practice 9; Data Protection Act 9; human factors contributing to risk **4**; leadership 6; local interprofessional training 7; multiprofessional communication 8; National Reporting and Learning System (NRLS) 4; Nursing and Midwifery Order 2001 5; positive culture creation 6–7; professional issues and safe practice 1; professional standards of practice **2**; record keeping 9–11; risk assessment and management 3–5; social media 11; teamwork and multiprofessional training 7

HELLP syndrome: antenatal care 115–116; care for 116; clinical features of 115–117; complications 116–117; definition 115; diagnosis of 115; overview 115; pathophysiology of 115; signs and symptoms of 116; see also acute fatty liver of pregnancy (AFLP); eclampsia; pre-eclampsia

heparin 96, 97, 98

hepatic hematoma 117

high regional blocks 228

Human Rights Act 19–20, 28; application to midwifery **20–21**

hydralazine 110

hydrostatic method 175

hypercoagulability 88

hypertension 103, 104, 107, 119

hypoglycaemia 229

hypotension 34

hysterectomy 69, 190

ICM see International Confederation of Midwives (ICM)

immune system dysregulation 248

incomplete uterine rupture 165, 166, 170

induction of labour 19

infections: influenza (flu); sepsis: APH outcome 70; definition 204;

midwifery responsibilities 216–217; see also COVID-19

influenza (flu): breathlessness 214–215; care for 215; clinical features of 214–215; considerations for 216; deaths from 213; definition 213; diagnosis of 214; follow-up/long-term issues 216; investigations for 215; labour care 215; midwifery responsibilities 216–217; overview 213–214; pathophysiology of 214; postnatal care 215–216; prevention 214; symptoms 215; vaccination 214; see also infections

informed consent 23–26; during labour 27; Montgomery v Lanarkshire Health Board 24–26, 25; NMC Code 24; principles of 25

intermittent pneumatic compression devices 93

internal bimanual compression 189

internal iliac artery ligation 190

International Confederation of Midwives (ICM) 3

interprofessional training 7

interventional radiology 189

intrapartum haemorrhage (IPH) see primary postpartum haemorrhage (primary PPH)

intrauterine tamponade 189

ischaemic stroke 227

ischemic heart disease 83

Johnson's manoeuvre 174

Kehr's sign 169

Labetalol 110

leadership 6

legal issues in emergency care: accountability 21–22; capacity 27–28; definitions 17; duty of care 22–23; Human Rights Act 19–21; informed consent 23–26; intrapartum and emergency care 26–27; law, defining 18–19; law, types of 19; maternity statistics 23; overview 18;

protected title and function of midwife 18; rights of the fetus 28

lithium 248, 250, 252, 253–254

liver function tests 109

LMWH see low molecular weight heparin (LMWH)

loss of consciousness 222–223

Løvset's manoeuvre 131, 131

low-lying placenta 56, 62–63; care for 66; diagnosis of 65; pathophysiology of 63–65; signs and symptoms of 65

low molecular weight heparin (LMWH) 96; education, advice and support 98–99; midwifery responsibilities 98

macrosomia 154

magnesium sulphate 111, 114

malpresentation 124; breech presentation see breech;brow presentation 136–137; complications 139; compound presentation 135–136; definition 124; face presentation 137–138; midwifery responsibilities 139; transverse or oblique lie 133–135

MAP see mean arterial pressure (MAP)

Maternal cardiac arrest 34; see also cardiac disease

Maternal collapse: abdominal pain 223–224; anaphylaxis 225–226; appendicitis 226; ARDS 224–225; asthma 226–227; causes of 34; cerebrovascular accident 227; chest pain 223; confusion 223; definition 34; DKA 227; ectopic pregnancy 228; emergency care 224; epilepsy 228–229; fibroids 229; high regional blocks 228; hypoglycaemia 229; individual conditions 224–230; loss of consciousness 222–223; overview 222; presenting symptoms 222–224; pulmonary oedema 229; recognition of 36; seizures 224; shock 223; sickle cell crisis 229–230; thyroid crisis 230; trauma 224

maternal deaths: causes of 34; number of 33

maternal resuscitation: 4 H's and 4 T's 34; aortal and inferior vena caval compression 35; basic life support 36–39; COVID-19 and 43; equipment 34; maternal cardiac arrest 34; midwifery responsibilities 42–44; modifications 41–43; normal blood pH levels 35, 36; overview 33–34; physiological changes affecting 34–36; uterine displacement 41–43; see also advanced life support in obstetrics; basic life support

Mauriceau-Cronk manoeuvre 132

Mauriceau-Smellie-Veit (MSV) 132

McRoberts position 156

mean arterial pressure (MAP) 108

Mental Health Capacity Act 2005 27–28, 28

methyldopa 110

MI see myocardial infarction (MI)

Midwifery and human rights: a practitioners guide 20–21

midwifery responsibilities: in acute fatty liver of pregnancy 119–120; in amniotic fluid embolism 200; anticoagulation treatment 99; in APH 71; in cardiac disease 81, 84; in cord prolapse 149; in deep vein thrombosis 99; for infections 216–217; low molecular weight heparin (LMWH) 98; in malpresentation 139; in maternal resuscitation 42–44; in newborn resuscitation 44, 52–53; for postpartum psychosis 254; in pre-eclampsia 111, 112; in primary postpartum haemorrhage 191; in PTSD 242; in pulmonary embolism 96; in sepsis 206–207; in shoulder dystocia 160; in thromboembolism 99; in uterine inversion 176; in uterine rupture 171; in venous thromboembolism 99

midwives: accountability and duty of care 3; overview 1; protected

title and function of 18; *see also* healthcare organisations; nurses
misoprostol 188
mixed haemorrhage *59*
Modified Mauriceau-Smellie-Veit (MSV) 132; *see also* Breech
Montgomery v Lanarkshire Health Board 24–26, *25*
moxibustion 128–129
MSV *see* Modified Mauriceau-Smellie-Veit (MSV)
multiprofessional communication 8
multi-professional training 5
myocardial infarction (MI) 83

National Health Service Litigation Authority (NHSLA) 4
National Health Service (NHS) Constitution 1
National Patient Safety Association (NPSA) 4
National Reporting and Learning System (NRLS) 4
negligence 22
newborn life support *49*
newborn resuscitation: bag/valve mask 46; Bohr effect 44; care following resuscitation 52; 'C' grip for holding the mask 46, *48*; clamping and cutting cord 45–46; definition 434; drugs 51, **52**; equipment 46, *47*; failure to respond 52; fetal adaptations in utero *45*; fetal physiology 44–45; finger positions for neonate chest compressions *51*; head position for optimum airway opening *50*; meconium 51–52; midwifery responsibilities 44, 52–53; newborn life support *49*; overview 43; oxygen 46; oxygen saturation levels 48; risk-predisposing factors 44; single-handed jaw thrust 46; thermoregulation 45; two-person jaw thrust *50*; *in utero* to *ex utero* transition support 46–51
'Newborn Resuscitation and Support of Transition of Infants at Birth Guidelines' 43

NHSLA *see* National Health Service Litigation Authority (NHSLA)
NHS Resolution 4, 22, *23*
Nifedipine (Adalat') 110
NMC *see* Nursing Midwifery Council (NMC)
NMC Code: accountability and duty of care 3, 21; human rights 19; informed consent **24**; record keeping 9; resuscitation 33; summary **2**
NPSA *see* National Health Service Litigation Authority (NHSLA)
NRLA *see* National Reporting and Learning System (NRLS)
Nursing and Midwifery Order 2001 5
Nursing Midwifery Council (NMC) 1, 18

OASIS *see* Obstetric Anal Sphincter Injury (OASIS)
oblique lie 133–135
obstetric anal sphincter injury (OASIS) 157
obstetric haemorrhage 56; *see also* antepartum haemorrhage (APH); primary postpartum haemorrhage (Primary PPH)
occult cord prolapse 143
Organisation with a Memory, A (report) 3–4
overt cord prolapse 143
oxytocin 184

PAS *see* placenta accreta spectrum (PAS)
Patient Safety Alerts 4
Patient Safety Incident Management System 4
Pawlik's grip 127
PCR *see* polymerase chain reaction (PCR); protein:creatinine ratio (PCR)
PE *see* pulmonary embolism (PE)
PEA *see* pulseless electrical activity (PEA)
peri-mortem caesarean section 41–42
peripartum cardiomyopathy (PPCM) 82, 83

peripartum psychosis *see* postpartum psychosis
PET screening 108
physiological changes in pregnancy affecting resuscitation 34–36
PlGF *see* Placental Growth Factor (PlGF)
Placenta accreta spectrum (PAS) 64, 186
Placenta increta 64
Placental abruption: acute inflammatory pathway 60; acute processes 60; aetiology and risk factors 59–60; care for 62, 66; chorioamnionitis 60; chronis processes 60; clinical features of 59–62; definition 56; direct trauma to abdomen 60; overview 59; pathophysiology of 59; placental implantation 60; risk and predisposing factors for **58**; symptoms 60–62, **61**; vascular changes 60; *see also* antepartum haemorrhage (APH)
Placental Growth Factor (PlGF) 105
placental hypertrophy 65
placenta, manual removal of 185, *186*
placenta percreta 64, 168
placenta praevia: care for 66; classification of **63**, *63*; definition 56; diagnosis of 65; overview 62–63; pathophysiology of 63–65; risk and predisposing factors for **58**; signs and symptoms of 65; *see also* antepartum haemorrhage (APH)
placentitis 210
PMA *see* Professional Midwifery Advocate (PMA)
polymerase chain reaction (PCR) 208
positive culture 6–7
postnatal depression 70
postpartum haemorrhage *see* primary postpartum haemorrhage (primary PPH) 69
postpartum hypopituitary (Sheehan's) syndrome 70

postpartum psychosis: antenatal screening and care 251–252; care during labour 252–254; clinical features of 249–254; definition 250, 257; examples of 250; follow-up/long-term issues 254; midwifery responsibilities 254; overview 247–248; pathophysiology of 248–249; preconception care 249–250; questions to identify 251; red flags 253; risk factors 249; signs and symptoms of 250

post-thrombotic syndrome (PTS) 99

post-traumatic stress disorder (PTSD) 70, 234, 241–242; antenatal care 239–240; clinical features of 237–241; conditions associated with 236; definition 234–235; DSM criteria for 235, 239; labour care 240; midwifery responsibilities 242; overview 235; pathophysiology of 235–237; postnatal care 240–241; preconception care and screening 239; risk factors 237; signs and symptoms of 237–239, 238

PPCM see peripartum cardiomyopathy (PPCM)

Practical Obstetric Multi-professional Training (PROMPT) see Simulation and Firedrill Evaluation (SaFE)

Pre-eclampsia 92 antenatal care 107–111; antenatal screening 106; blood pressure 107–108; blood tests 108; care in labour 112; clinical features of 106–112; complications 112; definition 103; fetal assessment 111; fluid balance 109; full blood count 109; liver function tests 109; MAP 108; medication 110–111; midwifery responsibilities 111, 112; multidisciplinary team 109–110; overview 104; pathophysiology of 104–105; PET screening 108; postnatal care 112; preconception care 106; prediction 106; prevention 106; proteinuria 103, 104, 108; rates of 104; renal function tests 109; risk factors 105; self-assessment 107; signs and symptoms of 106; see also acute fatty liver of pregnancy (AFLP); eclampsia; HELLP syndrome; severe pre-eclampsia

pressurised gas device 46

primary postpartum haemorrhage (primary PPH): antenatal and labour care 183–185; care for 183–191; causes of 182; clinical features of 183; deaths from 181; definition 181; DIC 191; first line drugs 187; four T's 182; management 185–190; manual removal of placenta 185, 186; midwifery responsibilities 191; overview 181–182; pathophysiology of 182; postnatal care 190–191; record keeping 11; risk factors 182–183; risks following 190; rubbing up contraction 187; second line drugs 188; symptoms 184

primary PPH see primary postpartum haemorrhage (Primary PPH)

pro-coagulant factors 88

prodromal phase 113

professionalism 1, 2

Professional Midwifery Advocate (PMA) 5

proformas 10

PROMPT see Practical Obstetric Multi-professional Training (PROMPT)

protein:creatinine ratio (PCR) 103, 108

proteinuria 103, 104, 108

PTS see post-thrombotic syndrome (PTS)

PTSD see post-traumatic stress disorder (PTSD)

puerperal psychosis see postpartum psychosis

puerperal sepsis 205

pulmonary embolism (PE): anticoagulation treatment 96–97; definition 87; diagnosis of 95, 96; midwifery responsibilities 96; signs and symptoms of 95; treatment of 95–96

pulmonary oedema 229

pulseless electrical activity (PEA) 40

racial inequalities 26

racial trauma 237

record keeping 9–11; critical points 11; functions of 10

renal function tests 109

Resuscitation Council (UK) 34; equipment for newborn resuscitation 47; newborn life support 49; obstetric cardiac arrest 42; resuscitation algorithm 37; Resuscitation Council Guidelines 43

revealed haemorrhage 59

rewind therapy 241

rights of the fetus 28

risk assessment and management 3–5; human factors 4

risk management 3–5

SaFE see Simulation and Firedrill Evaluation (SaFE)

Safer Births Initiative 5

SCAD see Spontaneous coronary artery dissection (SCAD)

seizures 224, 228

sepsis: assessment 208; care for 208–209; clinical features of 206–208; definition 204; diagnosis of 207–208; GAS 205; investigations for 209; midwifery responsibilities 206–207; overview 204–205; pathophysiology of 205–206; risk factors 206; sepsis six 8, 209; signs and symptoms of 207; skin changes in darker skin 207; see also infections

septic shock 204

severe pre-eclampsia 103

shock 173, 223

shortness of breath 79
shoulder dystocia: clinical features of 154–160; complications 158, 159; definition 152; delivery of posterior arm 157, 158; incidence of 152; internal manoeuvres 157–158; labour care 155–158; McRoberts position 156; midwifery responsibilities 160; moving disacromial diameter 157–158; multidisciplinary team 155; overview 152, 153; pathophysiology of 153; postnatal care 158–160; preconception/antenatal care 154–155; record keeping 11; risk factors 153–154; signs of 155; suprapubic pressure 156–157, 158
sickle cell disease 229–230
sims position 147
Simulation and Firedrill Evaluation (SaFE) 7, 10
sinus rhythm, normal 82
social media 11
spontaneous coronary artery dissection (SCAD) 83
standards of practice 1, 2
standards of proficiency 3
statute law 19
stroke 227
subacute uterine inversion 172
suicide 251
supine hypotension 34
suprapubic pressure 156–157, 158
Surviving Sepsis Campaign 208
Swansea criteria for diagnosis of AFLP 118
syntocinon 168
syntometrine 184

T1DM see Type I diabetes mellitus (T1DM)
TCM see Traditional Chinese medicine (TCM)
Teamwork 7
TEDS see thromboembolic deterrent stockings (TEDS)
thermoregulation 45
thrombin 182
thrombocytopenia 110, 115

thromboembolic deterrent stockings (teds) 92–93
thromboembolism 70; deep vein thrombosis (DVT); pulmonary embolism (PE); venous thromboembolism (VTE); antenatal care 93–94; antenatal thromboprophylaxis with LMWH 93, 94; caesarean section 92; compression stockings 92–93; definition 87; intermittent pneumatic compression devices 93; labour care 97; medical and midwifery measures 92; midwifery responsibilities 99; overview 87; pathophysiology of 88; postnatal care 97–98; preconception care 88; pre-eclampsia 92; prophylactic measures 92; risk assessment 89, 90–91; risk factors 89–92; signs and symptoms of 94; thrombophilia conditions 89; see also anticoagulation treatment
thrombophilia 89
thyroid storm 230
tonic-clonic phase 113
tranexamic acid 188
transverse lie 133–135
traumatic birth 236; see also post-traumatic stress disorder (PTSD)
tumultuous labour 196
two-person jaw thrust 50
type I diabetes mellitus (T1DM) 227

UH see unfractionated (standard) heparin (UH)
umbilical cord prolapse see cord prolapse
umbilical venous catheter (UVC) 51
unfractionated (standard) heparin (UH) 97
uterine atony 182
uterine complications see uterine inversion; uterine rupture
uterine dehiscence 170
uterine displacement 41–43
uterine inversion: care for 174–175; clinical features of 173–174;

definition 171; diagnosis of 173–174; follow-up/long-term issues 175–176; hydrostatic method 175; immediate actions 174; incidence of 171–172; Johnson's manoeuvre 174; manual repositioning 174; midwifery responsibilities 176; overview 171–172; pathophysiology of 172; replacement of uterus 174–175; risk factors 172–173; severity of 172; signs and symptoms of 173; timing 172
uterine rupture 56; actions with suspected condition 170; care for 170; clinical features of 169–170; complete 165; complete/incomplete 166; definition 165; follow-up/long-term issues 170–171; incidence of 165–166; incomplete 165, 170; midwifery responsibilities 171; overview 165–166; pathophysiology of 166; prediction 170; risk factors 166–168; signs and symptoms of 169
uteroplacental apoplexy 59
UVC see umbilical venous catheter (UVC)

vaccinations: COVID-19 210; flu 214
vaginal birth after caesarean (VBAC) 166
vasa praevia 56, 57
vascular damage 88
VBAC see vaginal birth after caesarean (VBAC)
vena caval compression 35
venous stasis 88
venous thromboembolism (VTE): and COVID-19 212; definition 87; follow-up/long-term issues 99; labour care 97; midwifery responsibilities 99; postnatal care 97–98; risk factors 89–92; triad of factors 88
VTE see venous thromboembolism (VTE)

warfarin 97

Printed in the United States
by Baker & Taylor Publisher Services